A
History
of
Medicine

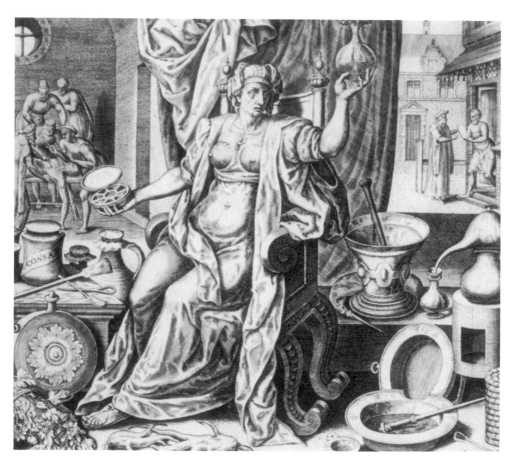

Panacea

A
History
of
Medicine

Lois N. Magner
Department of History
Purdue University
West Lafayette, Indiana

Marcel Dekker, Inc.   New York • Basel • Hong Kong

Library of Congress Cataloging-in-Publication Data

Magner, Lois N.
    A history of medicine / Lois N. Magner.
        p.   cm.
    Includes bibliographical references and index.
    ISBN 0-8247-8673-4 (alk. paper)
    1. Medicine -- History.   I. Title.
    [DNLM: 1. History of Medicine. WZ 40 M196h]
R131.M179   1992
610' .9--dc20
DNLM/DLC
for Library of Congress   92-4425
                                                            CIP

This book is printed on acid-free paper.

MARCEL DEKKER, INC.
270 Madison Avenue, New York, New York 10016

Current printing (last digit):
10 9 8 7 6 5 4 3

PRINTED IN THE UNITED STATES OF AMERICA

To Ki-Han and Oliver

FOREWORD

Lois Magner's *A History of Medicine* is a welcome addition to the literature of medical history. There has long been a need for a good English-language textbook of the history of medicine. Existing works that cover the subject are out of print and/or inadequate for the purposes of undergraduate instruction. For example, Garrison's *History of Medicine* is dated (having last been revised in 1928) and more of an encyclopedic reference work than a textbook. Ackerknecht's *Short History of Medicine,* although a well-written and perceptive book, is too brief to provide more than superficial coverage of its subject, especially in the period after 1800.

That Dr. Magner's text will find a ready audience is suggested by a recent report of the Education Committee of the American Association for the History of Medicine. Of 152 history of medicine courses identified in a survey of undergraduate instruction in American and Canadian universities, some 65% were either "Western surveys" or courses devoted to "Western topics." Professor Magner's book could well serve as an appropriate main text or supplementary reading for these and other medical history courses.

A History of Medicine is carefully researched and eminently readable. Dr. Magner has managed to condense thousands of years of medical history into a cohesive and interesting account, making excellent use of "case studies" (e.g., of a disease such as syphilis) to represent broader issues and trends. Although focusing largely on Western medicine, Dr. Magner devotes significant attention to developments in the Near and Far East. Her sense of humor, reflected throughout the work, is refreshingly unusual in a textbook. I recommend this book with enthusiasm to anyone interested in a general introduction to the history of medicine.

John Parascandola, Ph.D.
Chief
History of Medicine Division
National Library of Medicine
Bethesda, Maryland

PREFACE

Many changes have taken place in the history of medicine since 1940 when Henry E. Sigerist called for a new direction in the field, a move away from the study of the great physicians and their texts towards a new concept of medical history as social and cultural history. New theories and methods evolved as scholars raised new questions about patients, healers, institutions, economics, race, gender, etc. Some arguments about the nature of the field remain, but there certainly is general agreement that medical history is not simply an account of the path from past darkness to modern scientific enlightenment. Given the vitality, diversity, and growing tendency to specialization characteristic of the field today, finding a way to present all of these aspects of the history of medicine in a one-volume introductory text has probably become an impossible mission. Yet most teachers will acknowledge the need for books aimed at a general audience to introduce beginners to the field, including some aspects of recent developments in the biomedical sciences. Thus, a selective approach based on a consideration of the needs and interests of readers who are first approaching the field seems appropriate.

After teaching undergraduate courses in the history of medicine and the life sciences for about 20 years, I have come to the conclusion that there is no one great lesson that should be imposed upon an undergraduate course. Students seek out courses in the history of medicine for many different reasons and take very different lessons from their experience. Some even come to agree with me that the history of medicine is so intrinsically fascinating that like beauty it has its own excuse for being. Over the years, I have used a variety of texts, articles, and abstracts, but finding a text that is useful to students has been a continuous problem. Generally, I have tried to assign one general history of medicine and one or more specialized texts which have included biographies and studies of particular diseases. The major problem in adopting this pattern is that questions and issues that are of great interest to professional historians of medicine, and the subject of excellent recent scholarship, often fail to meet the needs of undergraduate students who are looking at the subject for the first time. Based on my experience, I have written a text for use in a one-semester survey course, which I hope will also be of interest to many general readers, and to teachers who are trying to add historical materials to their science courses or science to their history courses.

Of course, no one book, and no one-semester course can adequately cover a field as vast as the history of medicine. Rather than trying to include allusions to everything and everyone, I have selected particular examples of theories, diseases, professions, healers, and scientists, and attempted to allow them to illuminate particular themes. It is, of course, very difficult to determine what should be included and what should be omitted in a general survey. My goal is to make my book, and my course, comprehensible to students with little or no background in the history of medicine. Being comprehensible seems to be more important at this level than being comprehensive. The themes that I have included are generally those that I think are essential for raising fundamental questions about health, disease, and history.

The central problem of any survey of the history of medicine may well be the question of balance. Achieving a degree of balance among themes and topics that will be satisfactory to historians in various specialties is essentially impossible. My preference is for themes of general interest rather than those which are of purely internal interest to specialists in the history of medicine. My general approach in teaching has been, if at all possible, to emphasize concepts in inverse proportion to student familiarity with a given topic. That is, students are well aware of modern medicine, bacteriology, Europe, America, cancer, heart disease. They have heard of acupuncture, but do not know that this is only one small item in a very ancient and complex medical tradition. They have heard promotions for "Ayurvedic remedies," but are unfamiliar with Indian history and culture. Cutting out topics, especially when following the advice of experts rather than personal preference, has been particularly painful. In some cases, like the history of nursing, the challenge of cholera, and medical education, there are excellent and accessible studies which can be used to supplement a general text. However, the suggestion that all "non-Western" materials be removed was one I found unacceptable.

The history of medicine comes closer, I think, than any other discipline to approaching a universal and global framework. Medical concepts and practices can provide a most sensitive probe of the intimate network of interactions in a society, as well as traces of the introduction, diffusion, and transformation of novel or foreign ideas and techniques. Medical problems concern the most fundamental and revealing aspects of any society—health and disease, wealth and poverty, birth, aging, disability, suffering, and death. All people, in every period of history, have encountered the problems of disease, distress, and traumatic injury and have developed means of dealing with the problems faced by patients and practitioners. Thus, the variety of responses provides a valuable focus for examining different cultures. For example, bleeding has been a well-respected tradition in Western medicine but was not adopted by Chinese physicians. Human dissection has been a dominant theme in Western medicine, and is often thought to be a key prerequisite for advances in surgery. However, Indian medicine developed a strong surgical tradition without an emphasis on human dissection. Thus, I think that it is important to include Chinese and Indian medicine as a counterweight to Western assumptions. The idea that a book, course, or curriculum can achieve "balance" by eliminating the history and culture of more than half the world's peoples is, I think, very dangerous.

It should also be noted that I have used a framework that historians of medicine tend to find incongruous with current historiographical trends. That is, the book is arranged in a roughly chronological, but largely thematic manner. Historians of medicine may well object to discussing Hansen's disease and its status and treatment in the 1990s in a chapter that primarily deals with the Middle Ages. This is an excellent example of how the perspective of historians of medicine differs from that of the nonspecialist. I have found that once the question of the medical, social, and psychological meaning of "leprosy" is introduced, it is essential to deal with the question of modern victims of Hansen's disease, why the disease still exists, what it means to call people with AIDS "lepers," and so forth. Whether my audience is an undergraduate class, the Caduceus Club, the Optimists, the Sophomore Science Students, or the American Association of Retired People, the questions that people want answered when any fairly exotic disease is mentioned are: Does it still exist? and How is it treated? Therefore, I think that if historians of medicine wish to serve a broader audience we should acknowledge and answer such questions.

Many students come to a course in the history of medicine with the preconceived notion that the medical practices of the past were, to put it mildly, not very specific or efficacious, in the sense that we would judge by a modern clinical trial. Of course, a major objective of a survey of the history of medicine is to show students that the concept of the clinical trial has nothing to do with most of the history of medicine. Students must deal with the very difficult task of looking at medical theory and practice within a context that is very different from their own. They must also cope with the fact that many people question the value of modern medicine and many others accept the most remarkable forms of superstition as valid. Asking students to think critically about past and present seems a worthwhile thing to do, even if we sometimes stop and deliberately ask a question that is totally anachronistic in order to do so. The most important aspect of teaching the history of medicine is to allow students to discover for themselves a feeling of kinship with patients and practitioners past and present, a sense of humility with respect to disease and nature, and a critical approach to our present medical problems.

Perhaps the survey of the teaching of the history of medicine in colleges and universities in the United States and Canada, conducted by the Education Committee of the American Association for the History of Medicine in 1990, provides some support for the approach I have used in my courses and my text (Eyler et al., 1990).

Many of the courses in the history of medicine currently offered are general surveys covering a broad sweep of Western history. The editors of the report were rather surprised that course offerings did not mirror recent trends in historical scholarship. They were not surprised to find that the emphasis on European and American subjects in surveys and specialized courses came at the expense of almost total neglect of non-Western medical history. The survey also discovered that students expressed an interest in history of medicine courses, but faculty members who would like to develop such courses felt that finding teaching materials and texts would be a problem. Recent recommendations for the reform of the undergraduate liberal arts curriculum also suggest that broadly based courses in the history of medicine could play a valuable role in helping students understand the development of science and technology, cultural traditions, and human values (Association of American Colleges, 1990). Professional schools, including medical colleges, are also calling for reform of the undergraduate curriculum in order to encourage more sensitivity to human values and the social context of the health care professions (Association of American Medical Colleges, 1984).

Perhaps, in the midst of the great debate about what the new history of medicine represents and what it can contribute to undergraduate education, we should stop and reflect on how strange it is to be writing about the history of medicine in 1991 when one can read newspaper articles about remarkable new diagnostic and therapeutic technologies, the soaring costs of medical care in the United States, the resurgence of syphilis and tuberculosis, epidemic cholera in Latin America and Africa, and the threat of epidemic diseases, including typhoid fever in Iraq as the aftermath of war. In 1976, when the United States was celebrating its bicentennial, it was widely believed that the infectious diseases had been conquered, except for the nuisance of the common cold. Diseases like tuberculosis, cholera, smallpox, and even poliomyelitis were of little concern to the people of the wealthy industrialized nations. Indeed, most college students in the 1990s have no vaccination scars to remind them of an era in which smallpox remained endemic in much of the world. Only the threat of AIDS, a viral disease with no preventive vaccine and no known cure, has served to temper our optimism and arrogance concerning the conquest of disease.

Of course, we expect the history of medicine to throw light on these changing patterns of health and disease, as well as questions of medical practice, professionalization, institutions, education, medical costs, innovation, and resistance to change. In essence, the history of medicine can be seen as the study of the encounter between patient and practitioner, but this must inevitably be broadened to include all the relationships in society that intersect at the point where the sick person meets the healer. We often assume that interest in the care and cure of the sick are inseparable components of the historical role of the physician. As Dr. Francis Peabody reminded his colleagues in 1927, "The secret of the care of the patient is in caring for the patient." Yet a close examination of the work of eminent physicians throughout the course of Western history reveals a pattern of what might be called "uncoupling" between attention to the patient and a focus on scientific matters not directly linked to the care of the patient. At the extremes we can visualize physicians who considered close observation of the patient the central precept of medicine and viewed science as peripheral, and experimental scientists who believed that disease and therapy could be reduced to problems to be solved by the methods of physics, chemistry, and mathematics. Medical research since the end of the nineteenth century has flourished by following what might be called the "gospel of specific etiology"— that is, the concept that if we understand the causative agent of a disease, or the specific molecular events of the pathological process, we can totally understand and control the disease. This view fails to take into account the complex social, ethical, economic, and geopolitical aspects of disease in a world drawn closer together by modern communications and transportation, while simultaneously being torn apart by vast and growing differences between wealth and poverty.

Public debates about medicine today no longer seem concerned with fundamental aspects of the art and science of medicine; instead, the questions most insistently examined have to do with health care costs, availability, access, and equity. Comparisons among the medical systems of many different nations in the 1980s suggest that despite differences in form, philosophy, organization, and goals, all experience stresses caused by rising costs and expectations and pressure on limited resources. Government officials, policy analysts, and health care professionals have increasingly focused their energies and attention on the management of cost containment measures. Rarely is an attempt made to question the entire enterprise in terms of the issues raised by demographers, historians, and epidemiologists as to the relative value of modern medicine and more broadly based environmental reforms in lowering death rates from disease and extending life expectancy. Even the call for more emphasis on prevention has not touched on fundamental issues. Complicating the evaluation of the impact of any particular parameter is the shift in disease patterns from one in which the major killers were infectious diseases to one in which chronic and degenerative diseases predominate, and the demographic shift from an era of high infant mortality to one with increased life expectancy at birth and an aging population.

After years of celebrating the obvious achievements of biomedical science, as exemplified by such contributions as vaccines, anesthesia, insulin, organ transplantation, and the hope that infectious epidemic diseases would follow smallpox into oblivion, deep and disturbing questions are being raised about the discrepancy between the astronomical costs of modern medicine and the actual role that medicine has played in terms of patterns of morbidity and mortality. Expectations for medical miracles appear to be hugely exaggerated. Many drugs and diagnostic and therapeutic interventions have failed to live up to expectations and some, such as thalidomide and diethylstilbestrol (DES) have proved to be disastrous. Careful analysis of the role of medicine and that of social and environmental factors in determining the health of the people has led to the conclusion that medical technology is not a panacea for either epidemic and acute disease, or endemic and chronic disease. This is a lesson that is very difficult to accept and assimilate in an era that worships progress.

A general survey of the history of medicine reinforces the fundamental principle that medicine alone has never been the answer to the ills of the individual or the ills of society, but human beings have never stopped looking to the healing arts to provide cure, consolation, relief, and rehabilitation. Perhaps an introductory survey can serve as a first step in rethinking the evolution of medicine, and a point of entry into a diverse and fascinating literature.

ACKNOWLEDGMENTS

I would like to express my deep appreciation to John Parascandola and Ann Carmichael for their invaluable advice and criticism concerning a draft of the entire text. For their suggestions concerning particular parts of the manuscript, I would like to thank John Contreni, Leonard Gordon, and Karen Reeds. For their suggestions and criticism of previous drafts of this work, I would like to thank the anonymous readers. Of course, all remaining errors of omission and commission remain my own. I am particularly indebted to the staff of the Department of History for their patience, help, and support. Without the cooperation and assistance of the staff of the Inter-Library Loan Division of the HSSE Library, it would have been impossible to complete this project. I would also like to acknowledge the History of Medicine Division, National Library of Medicine, for providing the illustrations used in this book and the World Health Organization for the photograph of the last case of smallpox in the Indian subcontinent. I would particularly like to thank Lucy Keister and John Parascandola of the History of Medicine Division, National Library of Medicine, for their valuable help and advice in selecting the illustrations.

Lois N. Magner
Department of History
Purdue University

SUGGESTED READINGS

In order to keep the size of this book within reasonable limits, only brief lists of suggested readings have been attached to each chapter. The emphasis has been on recent books which should be readily available and can be used to obtain information about previous books, articles, and primary sources. Readers should also be aware of the following selected sources.

Association of American Medical Colleges (1984). *Physicians for the Twenty-First Century*, Washington, D.C.: Association of American Medical Colleges.

Association of American Colleges (1990). *Liberal Learning and the History Major*. Washington, D.C.: American Historical Association.

Bibliography of the History of Medicine. (1965–). Bethesda, MD: National Institutes of Health, National Library of Medicine.

Corsi, Pietro and Weindling, Paul, eds. (1983). *Information Sources in the History of Science and Medicine*. London: Butterworth Scientific.

Current Work in the History of Medicine. An International Bibliography. (Quarterly index of periodical articles on the history of medicine and allied sciences). London: The Wellcome Institute for the History of Medicine.

Erlen, Jonathan (1984). *The History of the Health Care Sciences and Health Care, 1700–1980. A Selective Annotated Bibliography*. New York: Garland.

Eyler, John M., Gevitz, Norman, and Tuchman, Arleen M. (1991). *History of Medicine in the Undergraduate Curriculum: Report of a Survey of Colleges and Universities in the United States and Canada During 1990*. American Association for the History of Medicine.

Gillispie, Charles Coulston, ed. (1970–1980). *Dictionary of Scientific Biography*. 16 vols. New York: Scribner's.

Greene, Rebecca, ed. (1988). *History of Medicine. Trends in History* Volume 4, Numbers 2/3. New York: The Institute for Research in History and The Haworth Press.

Index Catalog of the Surgeon General's Office. 58 volumes, 1880–1955. (Continues as *Bibliography of the History of Medicine, 1965–* , National Library of Medicine).

Leavitt, Judith Walzer (1990). Medicine in Context: A Review Essay of the History of Medicine. *American Historical Review* 95: 1471–1484.

Morton, Leslie T. and Norman, Jeremy M. (1991). *Morton's Medical Bibliography: An Annotated Checklist of Texts Illustrating the History of Medicine (Garrison and Morton)*. 5th edition. Brookfield, VT: Gower Publishing Company Ltd.

Neu, John, ed. (1980). *Isis Cumulative Bibliography 1966–1975. A Bibliography of the History of Science Formed from Isis Critical Bibliographies 91–100. Indexing Literature Published from 1965 to 1974*. London: Mansell.

Whitrow, Magda, ed. (1971–1976). *Isis Cumulative Bibliography: A Bibliography of the History of Science Formed from Isis Critical Bibliographies 1–90, 1913–1965*. 3 volumes London: Mansell.

CONTENTS

A
History
of
Medicine

1
PALEOPATHOLOGY AND PALEOMEDICINE

O ne of our most appealing and persistent myths is that of the Golden Age, a time before the discovery of good and evil, when death and disease were unknown. But scientific evidence—meager, fragmentary, and tantalizing though it often is—proves that disease is older than the human race. Thus, understanding the pattern of disease and injury that afflicted our earliest ancestors requires the perspective of the paleopathologist. Sir Marc Armand Ruffer (1859–1917), one of the founders of paleopathology, defined it as the science of the diseases that can be demonstrated in human and animal remains of ancient times. In order to explore the problem of disease in this remote time period, we will need to survey some aspects of human evolution, both biological and cultural.

Evidence from the study of fossils, stratigraphy, and molecular biology suggests that separation of the human line from that of the apes took place in Africa some 5 million years ago. It took several million years before large-brained, tool-making modern human beings evolved. *Homo sapiens sapiens*, the oldest human beings of morphologically modern character, appeared approximately 50,000 years ago.

The Paleolithic Era, or Old Stone Age, when the most important steps in cultural evolution occurred, coincides with the geological epoch known as the Pleistocene, or Great Ice Age, which ended about 10,000 years ago with the last retreat of the glaciers. Early humans were hunter-gatherers, that is, opportunistic omnivores, who learned to make tools, build shelters, carry and share food, and create uniquely human social structures. Although Paleolithic technology is characterized by the manufacture

1

of crude tools made of bone and chipped stones and the absence of pottery and metal objects, the people of this era produced the dramatic cave paintings at Lascaux, France, and Altamira, Spain. Presumably, they also produced useful inventions that were fully biodegradable and left no traces in the fossil record. Indeed, during the 1960s feminist scientists challenged prevailing assumptions about the importance of hunting as a source of food among hunter-gatherers; the vegetables and small animals gathered by women probably constituted the more reliable component of the Paleolithic diet. Moreover, because women were often burdened by carrying infants, they probably invented disposable digging sticks and biodegradable bags or baskets in which to carry and store food.

Through cultural evolution, human beings changed their environment in unprecedented ways, even as they adapted to its demands. By the domestication of animals, the mastery of agricultural practices, and the creation of densely populated settlements, human beings also generated new patterns of disease. The transition to new means of food production through farming and animal husbandry is known as the Neolithic Revolution. While archaeologists and anthropologists were once most concerned with the *when* and *where* of the emergence of an agricultural way of life, they are now more concerned with the *how* and *why*. Nineteenth-century cultural anthropologists tended to classify human cultures into a series of ascending stages marked by the types of tools manufactured and the means of food production. Since the 1960s new analytical techniques have made it possible to test hypotheses about environmental and climatic change and their probable effect on the availability of food sources. When the idea of progress is analyzed rather than accepted as inevitable, the causes of the Neolithic transformation are not as clear as previously assumed. Given the fact that the hunter-gatherer may enjoy a better diet and more leisure than the agriculturalist, prehistoric or modern, the advantages of a settled way of life are obvious only to those already happily settled.

Recent studies of the origins of agriculture suggest that it was almost universally adopted between 10,000 and 2000 years ago primarily in response to pressures generated by the growth of the human population. The revolutionary changes in physical and social environment associated with the transition from the way of life experienced by small mobile bands of hunters and gatherers to that of sedentary, relatively dense populations also allowed major shifts in patterns of disease. Settled communities change the environment through their activities; permanent dwellings, gardens, and fields provide convenient niches for parasites, insects, and rodents. Stored foods are subject to putrefaction, attract pests, and become contaminated with rodent excrement, insects, bacteria, molds, and toxins. Agricultural practices increase the number of calories that can be produced per unit of land, but a diet that overemphasizes grains and cereals may by deficient in protein, vitamins, and minerals. Lacking the mobility and diversity of resources enjoyed by hunters and gatherers, sedentary populations may be devastated by a crop failure. Migrations and invasions of neighboring or distant settlements triggered by local famines may carry parasites and pathogens to new territories and populations.

PALEOPATHOLOGY: METHODS AND PROBLEMS

Because direct evidence of disease among the first human beings is very limited, we will have to seek out a variety of indirect approaches in order to reach at least a tentative understanding of the prehistoric world. For example, studies of our closest relatives, the great apes and monkeys, have shown that living in a state of nature does not mean freedom from disease. Wild primates suffer from many disorders, including arthritis, malaria, hernia, parasitic worms, and impacted teeth. Our ancestors presumably experienced disorders and diseases similar to those found among modern primates.

In order to draw inferences about prehistoric patterns of disease, the paleopathologist must use a combination of primary and secondary evidence. The primary evidence includes bodies, bones, teeth, ashes, and charred or dried remains of bodies found at sites of accidental or intentional human burials. Secondary sources include the art, artifacts, and burial goods of preliterate peoples, and ancient documents that describe or suggest the existence of pathological conditions. The materials for such studies are very fragmentary, and the overrepresentation of the hard parts of bodies—bones and teeth—undoubtedly distorts our portrait of the past. Nevertheless, by combining a variety of classical and newly emerging techniques, scientists can use these fragments to gain insights into the patterns of ancient lives.

Archaeological chemistry, the analysis of inorganic and organic materials, provides many ways of reconstructing ancient human cultures from bits of bone, stone, tools, ceramics, textiles, paints, and so forth. Perhaps the most familiar aspect of archaeological chemistry is the carbon-14 method for dating ancient physical remains. This technique is especially valuable for studying physical remains from the last 10,000 years, the period during which the most profound changes in cultural evolution occurred. When combined with chemical analysis, microscopy can reveal information about the manufacture and use of human artifacts because such objects carry with them a "memory" of how they were manipulated in the past. Archaeological chemistry has been used in the discovery, dating, interpretation, and authentication of ancient remains. Multidisciplinary groups of scientists have combined their expertise in archaeology, chemistry, geophysics, imaging technology, and remote sensing as a means of guiding nondestructive investigations of sensitive archeological sites. As the techniques of immunology and molecular biology are adapted to the questions posed by paleopathologists, new kinds of information will undoubtedly be teased out of the surviving traces of proteins and nucleic acids found in some ancient materials. Despite the increasing sophistication of the analytical techniques employed in the service of paleopathology, many uncertainties remain, and the results must still be interpreted with caution.

Ancient bones may try to tell us many things, but the enemies of preservation mute their testimony and generate false clues, leading to pseudodiagnoses. Except for violent deaths in which a weapon remains in the body, ancient bones rarely disclose the cause of death. Even when the paleopathologist is confronted with a hole in the skull, making an unequivocal diagnosis is difficult. A "hole in the head" could be the result of a wound caused by an arrow or spear, the bite of a large carnivore, a ritual performed after death, or post-mortem damage due to burrowing beetles.

Funerary customs, such as cremation, can create severe warping and fragmentation of the remains. Added confusion arises from ritual mutilation of the body, the admixture of grave goods and gifts, which may include parts of animals or grieving relatives, and distortions due to natural or artificial mummification. Indeed the possibility of arriving at an unequivocal diagnosis is so small that some scholars suggest that the names of modern diseases should *never* be conferred upon ancient materials. Other experts have systematically catalogued Paleolithic ailments in terms of congenital abnormalities, injury, infection, degenerative conditions, cancers, deficiency diseases, and that all-too-large category, diseases of unknown etiology.

We tend to think of our bones as inert rods, but bones are malleable enough to adapt to continuous stresses. For example, a peculiarity of the ankle joint, known as a squatting facet, is found in people who spend much of their time in a squatting position. Thus, the absence of squatting facets distinguishes those who sat in chairs from those who did not. Certain tumors or cancers have been found in ancient human bones throughout the world. However, the pattern of malignant bone tumors in ancient times seems to be quite different from that in modern societies. Because hormones regulate the growth and development of all parts of the body, a malfunction of the endocrine glands may leave signs in the bones. Some peculiarities in ancient skeletal remains have been attributed to abnormalities of the pituitary and thyroid glands.

In rare instances, the soft parts of prehistoric bodies have been preserved because of favorable burial and climatic conditions or through human enterprise. Whether sophisticated or primitive, mummification techniques have much in common with the preservation of foods and animal hides. Especially well-preserved bodies have been recovered from the peat bogs of northwestern Europe. Peat has been used as a fuel for millennia, giving clumsy peat-gatherers a chance to sacrifice themselves for the enlightenment of paleopathologists. Some of the "bog bodies" were victims of a strange form of punishment or religious ritual. Sacrificial victims were apparently fed a ceremonial meal, stabbed in the heart, clobbered over the head, strangled with ropes left around their necks, and then pushed into the bog.

Mummies have also been found in the southwestern United States, Mexico, Alaska, and the Aleutian Islands. In the Western Hemisphere natural mummification was more common than was any artificial process, but the prehistoric people called the Basket-Makers deliberately dried cadavers in cists or caves, disarticulated the hips, wrapped the bodies in furs, and stuffed them into large baskets. Peruvian mummification techniques allowed the "living corpses" of chiefs, clan ancestors, and Incan rulers to be worshipped as gods. Such mummies provide suggestive evidence for the existence of tuberculosis, hookworm, and other diseases in pre-Columbian America.

Where conditions favor the preservation of organic matter, coprolites (desiccated human feces) may be found in or near prehistoric campsites and dwellings. For the dedicated paleopathologist, the contents of cesspools, latrine pits, and refuse piles are more precious than golden ornaments from a palace. Because certain parts of plants and animals are undigestible, information about diet, disease, seasonal activities, and cooking techniques can be inferred from the analysis of pollen grains, charcoal, seeds, hair, bits of bones or shells, feathers, insect parts, and the eggs or cysts of parasitic worms in coprolites. Moreover, the distribution of coprolites in and about ancient dwellings may reflect prevailing standards of sanitation.

Patterns of injury may provide clues to environment and occupation. Fractures of the leg bones were more common in Anglo-Saxon skeletons than were fractures of the forearm. These leg injuries are typically caused by tripping in rough terrain, especially if wearing clumsy footwear. The bones may also bear witness to acts of violence, mutilation, or cannibalism. The evidence concerning cannibalism remains highly controversial, but the ritualistic consumption of the ashes of departed relatives was practiced until recently by some tribes as a sign of respect for the dead. A disease known as *kuru*, caused by an agent known as a slow virus, has been linked to ritual cannibalism in New Guinea.

Evidence of infection has been found in the bones of prehistoric animals as well as humans, and infections of the soft tissues have been found in mummies. Schistosomiasis is of special interest because stagnant water, especially in irrigated fields, serves as a home for the snail that serves as the intermediate host for this disease. Therefore, the incidence of schistosomiasis in a population may reflect ancient agricultural and sanitary practices. Eggs of various parasitic worms have been found in mummies, coprolites, and latrine pits. These parasites cause a variety of disorders, including the gross enlargement of the legs and genitals called elephantiasis or pachydermia. Depictions of deformities suggesting elephantiasis are found in prehistoric artifacts. Some of the vitamin deficiency diseases, especially rickets and scurvy, leave characteristic signs in the skeleton. Osteomalacia, an adult form of rickets, can cause collapse of the bones of the pelvis, making childbirth a death sentence for mother and fetus.

A uniquely human source of pseudodiagnoses arises from the vagaries of fashion in the art world. Without knowledge of the conventions peculiar to specific art forms, it is impossible to tell whether some unnatural appearance represents pathology or deliberate distortion. Masks and pottery may depict abnormalities, artistic exaggeration, or the structural needs of the artifact, as in flat-footed and three-legged pots.

Striking abnormalities may be matters of convention or caricature. For example, the Paleolithic statues known as "Stone Venuses" or "fat female figurines" may be fertility symbols or examples of idiosyncratic ideas of beauty, rather than actual portrayals of gross obesity.

PALEOMEDICINE

Evidence of disease and injuries among ancient humans and other animals is incomplete for epidemiological purposes, but more than sufficient to establish the general notion of their abundance. Therefore, we would like to be able to determine when uniquely human responses to the suffering caused by disease and injury began. In other words, at what stage did human beings begin to practice medicine and surgery? Clues to the existence of paleomedicine must be evaluated even more cautiously than evidence of disease. For example, the "negative imprints" that appear to be tracings of mutilated hands found in Paleolithic cave paintings may record deliberate amputations, loss of fingers to frostbite, magical symbols of unknown significance, or even some kind of game. Early humans may have learned to splint fractured arms or legs to alleviate the pain caused by movement, but there is little evidence that they learned to reduce fractures. Moreover, well-healed fractures can be found among wild apes. Thus, the discovery of healed fractures and splints does not necessarily prove the existence of prehistoric orthopedic surgeons or bone-setters.

Perhaps the most striking proof of ancient surgical skill appeared in the form of the trepanned skulls discovered at Neolithic sites in Peru, Europe, Russia, and India. Although this operation is sometimes mistakenly referred to as "prehistoric brain surgery," trepanation consists of the removal of a disk of bone. When scientists first encountered such skulls, they assumed that the operation must have been performed after death for magical purposes. However, anthropologists have discovered that contemporary tribal healers perform trepanations for both magical and practical reasons. Prehistoric surgeons may also have had various reasons for carrying out this difficult and dangerous operation.

Several methods of trepanation were used by prehistoric surgeons. Boring a series of small holes to form a circle and then cutting out the "button" of bone with a sharp flint or obsidian knife was the most common and successful method. The patient could wear the disk as an amulet to ward off further misfortunes. Simple square or rectangular excisions may have been reserved for post-mortem rituals.

Peru was the major center of prehistoric skull surgery in pre-Columbian America. These trepanations were often associated with fractures apparently caused by weapons such as the bola and the star-headed mace; the operation presumably served the practical purpose of removing bone fragments and relieving pressure on the brain. Before the operation, both the patient and the surgeon chewed coca leaves. Presumably this provided both "mood elevation" and a crude "coca juice extract" used as a local anesthetic. The survival rate was quite impressive; many of the trepanned Peruvian skulls show signs of healing. Some individuals survived two or three independent operations.

Another prehistoric operation that left its mark on the skull is called "sincipital mutilation." In this case the "mark" is the scarring caused by cauterization (burning). Neolithic skulls with this peculiar lesion have been found in Europe, Peru, and India. In preparation for the application of the cauterizing agent, the surgeon made a T or L-shaped cut in the scalp. Cauterization was accomplished by applying boiling oil, or ropes of plant fibers soaked in boiling oil, to the exposed bone. In either case, permanent damage was done to the thick fibrous membrane covering the bone.

Most of the prehistoric victims of this operation were female, which might mean that the procedure had a ritualistic or punitive function rather than a therapeutic purpose. During the Middle Ages, this operation was prescribed to exorcise demons or relieve melancholy. Doubtless, the operation would dispel the apathy of even the most melancholic patient, or would give the hypochondriac a real focus for complaints.

In looking at the decorative motifs for which the human frame serves as substrate, objectivity is impossible. What is generally thought of as "cosmetic surgery" in our society—face-lifts, nose jobs, and liposuction—would be considered mutilation in societies that treasured double chins, majestic noses, and thunder thighs. While most of the cosmetic surgery of prehistoric times has disappeared along with the soft parts of the body, some decorative processes affected the bones and teeth. Ancient and widespread customs include "molding" the skulls of infants, and decorating or selectively removing the teeth. Tattooing and circumcision, of both males and females, were practiced in ancient times. Direct evidence can only be found in well-preserved mummies, but studies of cosmetic surgery among contemporary traditional societies can expand our understanding of the myriad possibilities for prehistoric cosmetic surgery.

NATURAL HISTORY OF INFECTIOUS DISEASE

Paleopathologists must make their deductions about the antiquity of infectious diseases with limited and ambiguous data; however, their conclusions must be consistent with modern medical knowledge. The impact of infectious diseases on human evolution is complex and subtle. Endemic and epidemic diseases may determine the density of populations, the dispersion of peoples, and the diffusion of genes, as well as the success or failure of battles and colonization. Thus, one way of testing hypotheses about disease in ancient times is to examine the pattern of disease among contemporary peoples whose culture entails features similar to those characteristic of prehistoric peoples.

Even if transistor radios, communication satellites, and television have turned the world into a "global village," it is still possible to find people who live in relative isolation, maintaining a way of life that seems little changed from the Old Stone Age. Until recently, anthropologists and historians generally referred to such people as "contemporary primitives." In terms of biological evolution, contemporary primitives are as far removed from Paleolithic peoples as any professor of anthropology, but their lives may be similar to those of the early hunter-gatherers, nomadic followers of semi-domesticated animals, or proto-agriculturalists. Because cultural patterns are a product of history, not biology, the term "traditional society" is now generally substituted for the term "primitive," which carries a rather pejorative connotation. The newer terminology, however, is somewhat confusing because of the various shades of meaning associated with the term "traditional." Where possible, we shall use the term "traditional society"; where necessary for clarity, we shall refer to "tribal societies" or "so-called primitives."

Many pathogens are species specific, but diseases like bubonic plague, malaria, yellow fever, and tuberculosis are formidable exceptions to this rule. Wild or domesticated animals can serve as reservoirs for diseases transmitted to humans directly or via insect vectors. The survival of pathogens that are species specific depends on the pathogen's virulence, the size and population density of the host group, the immune response mounted by the host, and the pathogen's ability to find new victims. Certain pathogens can only be transmitted during the acute phase of the disease, because the pathogen disappears upon recovery or death. When such an organism is introduced into a small group, virtually all individuals become infected and recover or die. Such diseases could not establish permanent residence among small bands of Stone Age peoples. New disease patterns became part of the price paid for living in large, densely populated, permanent towns and cities which, as Thomas Jefferson warned, were "pestilential to the morals, the health, and the liberties of man."

Pathogens that remain in the host during convalescence, persist in chronic lesions, or establish permanent residence in healthy carriers are likely to find new victims even among small bands of people. Other diseases are caused by commensal organisms—those that live harmlessly in or on their host until some disturbance triggers the onset of illness. Commensalism indicates a long period of mutual adaptation; thus, such diseases may be the most ancient. Variant forms of proteins and enzymes, such as sickle cell hemoglobin, may reflect evolutionary adaptations to ancient scourges like malaria.

It is often assumed that modern and so-called primitive peoples differ in their "susceptibility" and "resistance" to disease. However, comparisons of crude mortality rates for "moderns" and "primitives" are very misleading. Mortality rates during an epidemic may reflect the kind of care given to the sick rather than some mysterious quality called "resistance." During an explosive epidemic in a small, isolated population, there may be no healthy adults left to nurse the sick. Those who might have survived the disease may die because of the lack of food, water, and simple nursing care.

In general, the trait shared by all forms of so-called primitive medicine is a supernatural orientation, a belief in "magic." Magic, in this context, is not a trivial concept; it has influenced and shaped human behavior more deeply and extensively than the "scientific" or "rationalist" modes of thought, as we are pleased to call our own way of explaining the world. In societies where both magical and scientific beliefs coexist, one cannot predict which will appear stronger or more influential. Indeed, people may vacillate between alternative systems of medicine, depending on particular circumstances, perhaps relying on modern medicine for a broken arm and traditional medicine for arthritis.

Magic plays an important role in many cultures, it provides answers to questions that cannot be answered by existing "logical" or "rational" knowledge. Magic may be so closely related to religion that the borderline is difficult to define. The primary difference between a prayer and a spell is the assumption that magical practices, correctly performed, *must* bring about the desired reaction. A prayer, in contrast, requests aid from a supernatural being who has the power to grant or deny the request.

In primitive medicine, the supernatural is involved in all aspects of disease and healing. Because disease and misfortune are attributed to supernatural agents, magic is essential to the prevention, diagnosis, and treatment of disease. All events must have a cause, visible or invisible. Thus, diseases for which there are no obvious immediate causes must be due to ghosts, spirits, gods, sorcery, witchcraft, or the loss of one of the individual's special "souls." Illness calls for consultation with those who have the power to control the supernatural agents of disease: the shaman, medicine man, wise woman, diviner, witch-smeller, priest, chief, soul-catcher, or sorcerer. A close examination of the roles and powers assigned to such figures reveals many specific differences, but for our purposes the general term "healer" will generally suffice. However, we should note that most societies differentiate between healers and herbalists who dispense ordinary remedies and the shamans or priest-like healers who can intercede with the spirits that affect weather, harvests, hunting, warfare, conception, childbirth, disease, and misfortune.

Although the shaman performs magical acts, including deliberate deceptions, she or he is neither a fake nor a neurotic. The shaman is as sincere as any modern physician or psychiatrist in the performance of healing rituals. When sick, the shaman will undergo therapy with another shaman, despite knowledge of all the tricks of the trade.

For the shaman, the cause of the disorder is more significant than the symptoms because the cause determines the manner of treatment, be it penicillin or exorcism. Diagnostic aids may include a spirit medium, crystal gazing, and divination. Having performed the preliminary diagnostic tests, the healer conducts a complex ritual involving magic spells, incantations, the extraction of visible or invisible objects, or the capture and return of the patient's lost soul. To drive out or confuse evil spirits, the shaman may give the patient a special disguise or a new name, offer attractive substitute targets, or prescribe noxious medicines to transform the patient into an undesirable host.

The shaman may dispense powerful drugs, but it is the ritual, with its attempts to compel the cooperation of supernatural powers, that is of prime importance to healer, patient, and community. Outsiders may see the healing ritual in terms of "magical" and "practical" elements, but for healer and patient there is no separation between the magical and empirical aspects of therapy. In a society without writing or precise means of measuring drug concentrations and time, strict attention to ritual may provide a means of standardizing treatment, as well as a reassuring atmosphere. The shaman cannot isolate and "secularize" pharmacologically active drugs, because of the "holistic" nature of the healing ritual, but the problem of evaluating a remedy or procedure is more difficult than generally assumed.

Practitioners of "modern medicine" find it difficult to believe that the obvious "superiority" of scientific medicine has not caused the disappearance of all other systems. Nevertheless, traditional and alternative medicines continue to flourish from Africa and China to England and America. On the other hand, traditional medicine has been influenced by modern theory and practice. Today's shaman may dispense both penicillin and incantations to combat germs and evil spirits.

Ultimately, the success of any healing act depends on a combination of social, psychological, pharmacological, and biochemical factors. Where infant mortality is high and life expectancy low, the healer is unlikely to confront many cases of metabolic diseases among the young or the chronic degenerative diseases of the elderly. Many perceptive practitioners of the healing arts have acknowledged that, left to themselves, many diseases disappear without any treatment at all. Thus, if a healing ritual extends over a long enough period of time, the healer gets the credit for "curing" a "self-limited disease." Recovery is often a matter of the patient's triumph over both the disease and the doctor.

Because of the uncertainties involved in evaluating the treatment of disease, historians of medicine have often turned to the analysis of surgical operations as a more objective measure of therapeutic interventions. But even here there are difficulties in comparing practices carried out under greatly differing circumstances, by different kinds of practitioners, with different goals and objectives. One surprising aspect of so-called primitive surgery is the fact that operations for purely medical reasons may be rare or nonexistent in a particular tribe, although the practitioner may wield the knife with great skill and enthusiasm for ceremonial, decorative, or judicial purposes. Ritual scarification may signify caste, adulthood, or the "medicine marks" thought to provide immunization against disease, poisons, snakebites, and other dangers. Just how effective such protection might be is open to question, but there have been reports of African healers who impregnated "medicine cuts" with a mixture of snake heads and ant eggs. When twentieth-century scientists discovered how to detoxify toxins with formalin, which is present in ant eggs, the African ritual suddenly seemed less bizarre.

identification of species of origin. *Science* 220:1269–1271.

McEvedy, C., and Jones, R. (1978). *Atlas of World Population History*. New York: Penguin.

Moodie, R. L. (1923). *Paleopathology: An Introduction to the Study of the Ancient Evidences of Disease*. Urbana, IL: University of Illinois Press.

Ruspoli, Mario (1986). *The Cave of Lascaux*. New York: Harry N. Abrams.

Stead, I. M., Bourke, J. B., and Brothwell, Don (1986). *Lindow Man. The Body in the Bog*. Ithaca, NY: Cornell University Press.

Steinbock, R. Ted (1976). *Paleopathological Diagnosis and Interpretation: Bone Diseases in Ancient Human Populations*. Springfield, IL: Charles C. Thomas.

Steiner, Richard P., ed. (1988). *Folk Medicine. The Art and the Science*. Washington, DC: American Chemical Society.

Tambiah, Stanley J. (1990). *Magic, Science, Religion, and the Scope of Rationality*. Cambridge, England: Cambridge University Press.

Vogel, Virgil H. J. (1970). *American Indian Medicine*. Norman, OK: University of Oklahoma Press.

Wells, Calvin (1964). *Bones, Bodies, and Disease: Evidence of Disease and Abnormality in Early Man*. New York: Frederick A. Praeger.

MEDICINE IN ANCIENT CIVILIZATIONS: MESOPOTAMIA AND EGYPT

T he Greeks thought it easy to define "civilization": it referred to the qualities of citizens—free men living in cities. Today the concept is regarded as more complex, subtle, and problematic. The term "culture" is used to encompass all the ways of life and customary behaviors invented by human beings. Civilization is, therefore, a particular kind of culture, characterized by increasing complexity in social, economic, and political organization, a settled life, a food supply in excess of subsistence levels, occupational specialization, writing and reckoning, and innovations in the arts and sciences—all maintained by a large number of people over a significant period of time. The first civilizations developed in the period between about 3500 and 1500 B.C. in a few delimited areas of the world. Historians continue to pose questions about the nature of the factors that cause the development of civilizations and nurture their growth. No simple, definitive answer seems possible, but a variety of causes involving some complex balance between the bounties and challenges of geographic, climatic, and economic factors have been suggested. It has often been noted that four of the earliest civilizations developed in river valleys: the Nile River of Egypt, the Tigris-Euphrates in the Middle East, the Indus River in India, and the Yellow River in China.

Because the evidence from the earliest periods is ambiguous and fragmentary, the question of which civilization was the first to appear has been the subject of endless debate. We will, therefore, ignore these controversies and look instead at some of the major centers of civilization to see what they can tell us about health, disease, and ancient medicine.

MESOPOTAMIA

Mesopotamia, the land between the Tigris and Euphrates Rivers, was the arena of the growth and decay of many civilizations, including those known as Sumerian, Chaldean, Assyrian, and Babylonian. Although Egyptian civilization is better known, we will begin our survey of ancient civilizations with Sumer to emphasize the point that other, less well-known areas also became urban and literate at very remote dates.

Sumer flourished some 4000–5000 years ago, but by the first century A.D. its language had vanished and its writings, in the form of cuneiform script inscribed on clay tablets, were indecipherable. Most Sumerian tablets dealt with mundane economic and administrative transactions, but thousands of others record myths, fables, and ideas about science, mathematics, and medicine.

In Sumer, the mastery of agricultural techniques led to dramatic changes in population density and the establishment of the bureaucratic apparatus needed for planning, storage, and redistribution of crops. The great mass of people lived as peasants, but their productivity supported a small urban elite of priests, warriors, and noblemen. Because law and medicine were ascribed to divine origins, the priests also assumed the roles of judges, lawyers, and physicians.

The cuneiform texts pertaining to medicine can be divided into three categories: (a) therapeutic or "medical texts"; (b) omen collections or "symptom texts"; and (c) miscellaneous texts which incidentally provide information on diseases and medical practices. After deciphering cuneiform writings and studying numerous texts, scholars divided the medical traditions of Sumer into two categories, which have been called the "scientific" and the "practical" schools. According to this scheme, the scientific practitioners were the authors and users of the "symptom texts." In contrast, members of the practical school concentrated on empirical medical techniques and were the authors and users of the "medical texts."

The medical texts of the practical school followed a formal arrangement typical of Mesopotamian scribal practice. Each tablet was composed of a sequence of units following the general format: "If a man is sick (and has the following symptoms) . . ." or "If a man suffers from (such and such) pain in (wherever it was) . . ." The healer was provided with instructions for the medicines needed, their preparation, the timing, and means of administration. The physician "discovered" significant symptoms by listening to the patient's account of the illness, not by performing a direct physical examination. Although most units conclude with the comforting promise that the patient would get well, certain symptoms presaged a fatal outcome.

In contrast, the "conjurer," "diviner," or "priest-healer" looked at the patient's symptoms and circumstances as omens that identified the disorder and predicted the outcome of the disease. Unlike his "practical" counterpart, the diviner performed a direct physical examination in order to discover signs and omens. Clearly the gods were at work if a snake fell onto the patient's bed because this omen indicated that the prognosis was favorable, but wine-colored urine was a portent of further deterioration, chronic illness, and great pain. If the priest could not wrest sufficient information from his direct examination of the patient, he could find signs in the viscera of sacrificial animals. Omens provided by animal livers were applied to the patient, whose liver was inaccessible.

Although there are many uncertainties in interpreting ancient texts, tentative diagnoses of some of the disorders discussed in Mesopotamian writings are possible. Mesopotamian physicians were probably familiar with a wide range of diseases, including schistosomiasis, dysentery, pneumonia, and epilepsy. Malnutrition would obviously correlate with the periodic famines alluded to in various texts, but even when food supplies were adequate in quantity, the daily diet was probably monotonous and unbalanced. Descriptions of eye disorders, paralysis, swollen bellies, and the "stinking disease" are consistent with various vitamin deficiency diseases. A chronic combination of malnutrition and infestation with various parasites greatly amplifies the effects of other diseases and retards the growth of children.

Because illness was regarded as a divine punishment for sins committed by the patient, healing required the spiritual and physical catharsis obtained by combining confession and exorcism with purgative drugs. Sumerian prescriptions include about 250 vegetable and 120 mineral drugs, as well as alcoholic beverages, fats and oils, parts and products of animals, honey, wax, and various kinds of milk thought to have medical virtues. Medical texts, like almost all Mesopotamian literature, were anonymous, but some medical tablets provide enthusiastic personal endorsements and testimonials for particular remedies. Medications are said to have been tested or discovered by unimpeachable authorities, such as sages and experts. Some remedies were praised for their antiquity or exclusivity. Of special interest is a small cuneiform tablet containing about a dozen recipes recorded by a Sumerian physician about 4000 years ago. This tablet appears to be the oldest written collection of prescriptions.

The separation of magical and empirical aspects of medicine is a very recent development. Thus, it should not be surprising that Mesopotamian patients considered it prudent to attack disease with a combination of magic and medicine. A healer who was both priest and physician could increase the efficacy of drugs by reciting appropriate incantations. Although the healer needed some knowledge of anatomy and drug lore, precise knowledge of magical rituals was more important because errors in this department could alienate the gods.

Hordes of demons and devils were thought to cause disease and misfortune; each evil spirit tended to cause a particular disorder. As in the case of folk medicine and so-called primitive medicine, Mesopotamian practitioners also attempted to rid their patients of disease-causing demons by the administration of remedies containing noxious ingredients. Enveloped in the aroma of burning feathers, and liberally dosed with dog dung and pig's gall, the patient hardly seemed an inviting abode for a discriminating demon. The magician might also try to transfer the demon into an animal or a magical figure. Sometimes the priest engaged the demon in a formal dialogue, as in the conversation between the priest and the "tooth worm" recorded about 2250 B.C. While "The Worm and the Toothache" hardly sounds like the title of a major epic, it is a rich source of Mesopotamian cosmological concepts and creation myths.

Mesopotamian pharmaceutical texts reflect familiarity with fairly elaborate chemical operations for the purification of crude plant, animal, and mineral components. Plants and herbs were so important to ancient medicine that the terms for "medicine" and "herbs" were essentially equivalent. Drugs made from seeds, bark, and other parts of plants were dissolved in beer or milk and administered by mouth, or mixed with wine, honey, and fats and applied externally. In retrospect, it is logical to assume that the wine used in wound dressings provided some benefit as an antiseptic. Whether red or white, wine is a better antiseptic than 10% alcohol.

According to the Mesopotamian legend known as the Gilgamesh Epic, human beings lost possession of the most powerful, life-giving herb in creation because of the Mesopotamian superhero Gilgamesh, a being two-thirds god and one-third human. When his friend Enkidu was stricken with illness, Gilgamesh swore that he would never give up hope of saving Enkidu until "a worm fell out of his nose" (a striking omen of death). After many trials and tribulations, Gilgamesh learned the secret of the herb of life and swam to the bottom of the waters where the marvelous plant grew. Gilgamesh planned to take the herb back to the city of Uruk, but, exhausted by his exertions, he stopped to rest. While Gilgamesh slept, a serpent ate the herb of life. As a result, the snake shed its old skin and was instantly rejuvenated while Gilgamesh wept for himself and all mankind.

When Herodotus visited Babylonia in the fifth century B.C., he reached the conclusion that the Babylonians had no doctors. The sick, he said, were taken to the marketplace to seek advice from those who had experienced similar illnesses. This story proves only that we should not take the tales told by tourists too seriously. As we have seen, Mesopotamia had a complex medical tradition. Both the empirical and the magical approach to healing were well established in Mesopotamia, but the balance of power tended to tilt in favor of the magician. Evidence about the various kinds of healers who practiced the art in the region can be extracted from the most complete account of Babylonian law, the Code of Hammurabi.

Hammurabi, King of Babylon, is of more interest now for the code of laws bearing his name than for his military and political triumphs. Toward the end of his reign, Hammurabi commissioned the creation of a great stele portraying the king receiving the insignia of kingship and justice from the gods. Below this portrait were inscribed the 282 clauses or case laws now referred to as the *Code of Hammurabi*. The Code governs criminal and civil matters such as the administration of justice, ownership of property, trade and commerce, and professional conduct.

Criminal penalties were based on the concept of *lex talionis*, literally, the "law of the claw," that is, a demand that retribution or punishment should fit the crime. The penalties specified by the laws fell with different degrees of severity on the three classes that made up Babylonian society: gentlemen, or seigniors; commoners, or plebians; and slaves, whose lowly status was indicated by a physical mark. Slaves seem to have carried a 30-day warranty against certain disorders. The law stated that if a slave was attacked by epilepsy within one month of purchase the seller must reclaim that slave and return the purchase price.

The laws of special interest to the history of medicine—those pertaining to surgeons, veterinarians, midwives, and wet nurses—follow the laws dealing with assault. Nine paragraphs are devoted to the regulation of medical fees and specifications concerning the relationship between the status of the patient and the appropriate fees and penalties. The severe penalties set forth for failures suggest that practitioners would be very cautious in accepting clients and would shun those that looked hopeless or litigious. The laws also reflect a profound distinction between medicine and surgery. The physicians, who dealt with problems that would today be called "internal medicine," were of the priestly class, and their professional conduct was not governed by the criminal laws pertaining to assault and malpractice.

Because internal disorders were caused by supernatural agents, those who wrestled with such diseases were accountable to the gods. Wounds were due to direct human error or aggression; thus, those who wielded the "bronze knife" were accountable to earthly authorities. Fees and penalties for surgical operations were substantial. If a doctor performed a major operation and saved the life or the eyesight of a seignior, his fee was 10 shekels of silver. The fee was reduced by half for operating on a commoner, and was only two shekels when the patient was a slave. However, if the surgeon performed such an operation and caused the death of a seignior, or destroyed his eye, the doctor's hand should be cut off. If the physician caused the death of a slave, he had to provide a replacement. If he destroyed the eye of a slave, he had to pay the owner one-half his value in silver.

Just what operation was involved in "opening the eye-socket" or "curing" the eye is a matter of some dispute. The operation could have been the couching of a cataract or merely the lancing of an abscess of the tear duct. While such an abscess causes intense pain, it does not affect vision, whereas cataracts lead to blindness. Probing or lancing might help in the case of an abscess, but if poorly done could cause blindness. Presumably eye surgery was only twice as difficult as setting a broken bone or healing a sprain, because the fee for such services was five shekels of silver for a seignior, three for a commoner, and two for a slave. The veterinarian, also called the "doctor of an ox or an ass," carried out various surgical operations, including castration of domesticated animals.

Women served as midwives, surgeons, and even palace physicians in Mesopotamia, but the Code of Hammurabi does not specifically mention female doctors. However, the laws did cover women who served as wetnurses. If a seignior gave his son to a nurse and the child died, her breast could be cut off if she had taken in other infants without informing the parents. Obviously, such a woman would never commit that offense again.

In excavating the remains of ancient Mesopotamian cities, archaeologists continue to unearth thousands of cuneiform tablets. Most refer to mundane business transactions and political matters, but as more texts are painstakingly translated, and new information appears, our picture of the civilizations of Mesopotamia may undergo profound changes.

EGYPT

Egyptian civilization has fascinated travelers and scholars since Herodotus initiated the tradition of Nile travelogues. Collecting Egyptian antiquities was already fashionable in Roman times, but modern Egyptology begins with the discovery of the Rosetta Stone, a slab of black basalt inscribed with a message in three forms of writing: hieroglyphic Egyptian, demotic Egyptian, and Greek. Formal hieroglyphs, "the god's words," were not only a way of writing, but also a form of artistic expression. Egyptian scribes developed a simplified script known as demotic, but by the fifth century A.D. other forms of writing were adopted and the ancient writings became indecipherable.

Ancient Greek writers from Homer to Herodotus praised the physicians of Egypt for their wisdom and skill, but the Greeks also knew Egypt as the "mother country of diseases." Certainly, ancient Egyptian skeletons, portraits, writings, and, above all, mummies provide ample evidence of the crushing burden of disease in the ancient world. Although mummified bodies have been found in many parts of the world, for most people the term "mummy" conjures up the Egyptian mummy, as seen in museums and late-night horror shows. The word comes from a Persian word for bitumen (natural asphalt), reflecting the mistaken notion that ancient Egyptian bodies had been preserved and blackened by soaking in pitch.

For the ancient Egyptians, life after death was of paramount importance, but success in the afterlife depended on preserving the body so that the soul would have a place to dwell. Within their tombs, wealthy Egyptians were surrounded by grave goods meant to provide for their comforts in the next world. In addition to the treasures that lured grave robbers to even the most well-protected tombs, mummies were accompanied by "texts" painted on the walls of their tombs and coffins and written texts known as the Book of the Dead. These "books" contained collections of spells and maps to guide the departed along the path taken by the dead.

In predynastic Egypt (before 3100 B.C.) bodies were wrapped in skins or linen and interred in shallow graves in the desert. If the body was not discovered by jackals, the hot dry sand would draw out the moisture from the soft tissues, leaving the body looking rather like tanned leather, but still recognizable after a period of thousands

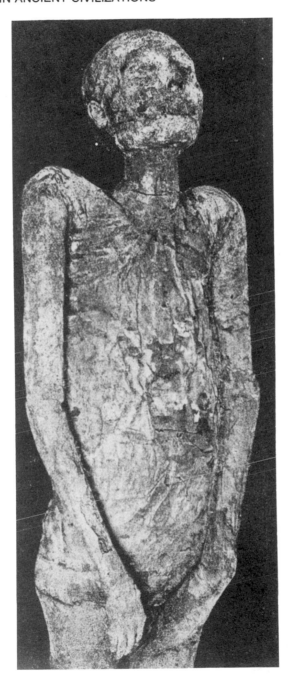

An Egyptian mummy

of years. Simple sand burials continued to be the norm for peasants, but during the Dynastic Period, the pharaohs and other notable individuals fashioned more elaborate burial chambers for themselves. Unfortunately, putting bodies in relatively cool, damp, underground tombs allowed the forces of putrefaction to prevail. If the pharaoh were to enjoy both an elegant resting place and a well-preserved body, new methods of preparing the corpse were essential.

Much has been made of the "mysteries" of Egyptian mummification, but the basic steps are simple: removing the viscera, thoroughly drying the cadaver, and wrapping the desiccated corpse. Over the course of almost 3000 years, the methods and quality of workmanship of the embalmers varied, but the basic principles remained the same.

Desiccation could have been achieved by techniques used to preserve food and hides, such as salting fish or pickling vegetables. Perhaps there was some aesthetic obstacle to preserving a pharaoh like a pickle. A secret and mysterious procedure would provide a better bridge to eternity. In place of hot, dry sand or a vinegar brine, embalmers used natron, a naturally occurring mixture of sodium salts, as a drying agent and removed the organs most susceptible to rapid decay. The heart, which was regarded as the "seat of the mind," was left inside the body.

Herodotus left the best known account of embalming, but his discussion contains much doubtful material and represents a late, probably degenerate, state of the art. According to Herodotus, there were three methods of mummification which varied in thoroughness and price. For the "first class" procedure, the embalmers drew out the brain through the nose with an iron hook. The intestines were removed through a cut made along the flank and the abdominal cavity was washed with palm wine and aromatics before the belly was filled with exotic spices. According to Herodotus, the body was kept in natron for 70 days. Other sources, however, indicate that the entire embalming procedure took 70 days, of which 40 were used for dehydrating the body by packing it, inside and out, with bags of natron. When embalming was completed, the corpse was washed, wrapped in bandages of fine linen, smeared with gum, and enclosed in a wooden case shaped like a man.

If the embalmers were asked to follow a more economical course, they would omit the removal of the brain and the incision into the abdominal cavity. Instead, they injected cedar oil into the belly through the anus and embalmed the body in natron. Seventy days later they removed the plug from the anus and allowed the oil and dissolved bowels to escape. The cadaver, now reduced to skin and bones, was returned to the relatives. Poorer people could only expect a simple purge to cleanse the belly and 70 days of embalming.

Sometimes the embalmers resorted to simplified procedures, neglecting evisceration and employing onions and garlic in place of the proper aromatic preservatives. Poor workmanship and outright fraud are manifest in mummy packs where the viscera were badly mutilated, bones broken or lost, and animal remains or pieces of wood were used to fill out the form.

Paleopathologists have subjected mummies to increasingly sophisticated methods of investigation such as X-ray examination, computerized tomography (CT) scanning, electron microscopy, chemical analyses, immunological evaluations, and other analytical techniques that provide significant data with minimal damage. Biochemical techniques can be used to detect malaria, various forms of anemia, and parasitic diseases. Well-preserved mummies offer information about parasitic diseases, trauma, infections, and metabolic and genetic defects. For example, biochemical studies of the mummy of a man who died about 1500 B.C. provided evidence for what is probably the earliest known case of alkaptonuria, a metabolic disease due to the absence of an enzyme needed to break down the amino acids phenylalanine and tyrosine.

The first lessons from autopsy and radiography of mummies concern the health hazards associated with the life-giving Nile; the fertile soil and irrigation ditches fed by the Nile River harbored hordes of parasitic worms. Calcified eggs in liver and kidney tissues reflect the prevalence of schistosomiasis in ancient Egypt. The snail in which the worm completes an essential stage of its life cycle flourishes in stagnant irrigation canals. Although schistosomiasis does not kill outright, the chronic irritation caused by the worm and its eggs leads to increasing mental and physical deterioration throughout the victim's life.

Winds blowing in from the desert carried fine particles of sand that lodged in the lungs to cause sand pneumoconiosis, a disorder similar to the black lung disease found among coal miners. Sand pneumoconiosis can be detected by electron microscopy of mummified lung tissue, but because only the elite were mummified, it is not possible to tell how common this disorder was among the masses of peasants. Another disorder associated with sand is a severe form of dental attrition caused by the abrasive action of sand particles found in bread and other foods. Carbon deposits in the lung, a condition known as anthrocosis, reflect the use of wood fires for warmth. Other disorders found in mummies include tuberculosis, hardening of the arteries, and arthritis. Worn down by these ever-present hazards, helpless in the face of disease and traumatic accidents, even the most privileged were unlikely to attain a life span greater than 40 years. Probably few of those who died as adults actually resembled the idealized portraits that adorned their coffins and tombs.

Before the introduction of modern techniques for determining the age of ancient materials, Egyptologists depended on indirect methods, such as evaluating the decorations on the coffin and the name and grave goods of the deceased person. But identifications were generally tentative and sometimes incorrect because many mummies had been mutilated by grave robbers. Egyptian priests rescued and rewrapped many royal mummies, but the bodies often ended up in mismatched coffins with new identities.

Carbon-14 dating can be used to estimate the age of mummies, if uncontaminated samples of tissue are used, but impurities from the mummification materials are hard to remove from samples of flesh and rather large parts of the body must be sacrificed to use bone collagen. X-ray analysis can provide valuable data about medical and dental diseases, estimates of age at death, and morphological variations. It can also save modern scholars from the embarrassing mistakes that sometimes occurred when nineteenth century archaeologists, trying to enliven their lectures, unwrapped the mummy of some great Egyptian prince only to find the body of a princess or, worse yet, a baboon. Modern medical techniques have also been used to "cure" mummies suffering from "museum ailments" caused by display, storage, and the attacks of insects, fungi, and bacteria.

The abundance of diseases that flourished in Egypt provides a rationale for Herodotus' observation that the whole country swarmed with highly specialized physicians dedicated to care of the eyes, head, teeth, stomach, and obscure ailments. Not all Egyptian physicians were specialists, but there is evidence that specialists, lay physicians, priests, and magicians worked in harmony and referred patients to each other as appropriate. One specialist called Iri, Shepherd of the Anus (or Keeper of the Bottom), held a place of honor among the court physicians. Often referred to as the first proctologist, the Keeper of the Royal Rectum might have served primarily as the pharoah's enema-maker. According to Egyptian mythology, the enema itself had a noble origin; it was invented by the god Thot.

Medical specialization in ancient Egypt reflected the religious doctrine that no part of the body was without its own god. Like the gods they served, priest-physicians tended to specialize in a particular organ or disease. Pharmacists traced the origin of their art to Isis, who had imparted the secrets of remedies to her son Horus. All who participated in the medical work of the Houses of Life attached to the temples, as well as the embalming establishments, claimed the god Anepu as their patron. However, responsibility for the "necessary art" as a whole was eventually ascribed to Imhotep, the first real physician known to us by name.

A prodigy and master of all fields of learning, Imhotep designed and built the famous Step Pyramid of Sakkara and served the Pharaoh Zoser as Vizier, Minister of State, Architect, Chief Priest, Sage, Scribe, Magician-Physician, and Astronomer. Imhotep, no less than Asclepius, the Greek god of medicine, is a powerful symbol and true ancestral god of the healing profession. Imhotep's career as a healer can be divided into three phases: first, as a physician in the court of Zoser (ca. 2980 B.C.); second, as a medical demigod (ca. 2850–525 B.C.); and third, much later, as a major deity (ca. 525 B.C.–550 A.D.).

When Imhotep died, the sick flocked to the temple that had been built over his grave. The cult of Imhotep eventually spread from Memphis throughout Egypt. Excavations of the temples of Imhotep suggest that "temple sleep," or therapeutic incubation, so much associated with the Greeks, was really of Egyptian origin. Priests carefully tended to the sick and encouraged their expectation that the god would appear and effect miraculous cures. The priests used "holy water," baths, isolation, silence, suggestion, and therapeutic dreams in their healing rituals. As a god who healed the sick, promoted the fertility of barren women, protected against misfortune, and gave

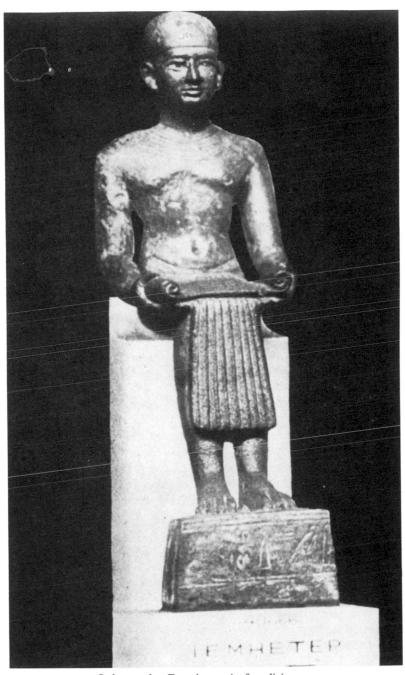

Imhotep, the Egyptian god of medicine

life to all, Imhotep understandably became one of the most popular deities. Although worship of Imhotep sharply declined by the end of the second century A.D., he remained a major deity in Memphis into the fourth century.

Some scholars have argued that magic was the motive force behind almost all the achievements of the Egyptians, but others have defended the ancients against the charge that their medicine was little more than superstition and magic. Operating within the context of ancient society, physician and patient expected incantations and charms to increase the efficacy of treatment; certainly they would do no harm. Spells and stories about the healing acts of the gods were a source of comfort and hope which accompanied the administration of a remedy or the treatment of a wound.

Many aspects of the evolution of the medical profession in ancient Egypt remain obscure; even the etymology of the word for *physician* is unclear. Some scholars interpret the hieroglyph for physician—an arrow, a pot, and a seated man—as "the man of the drugs and lancet" or "opener of the body," while others suggest "man of pain" or "the dealer with disease." Worse yet, the same term was also used for the "tax valuer."

Priest-physicians were expected to conduct a detailed examination of the patient in order to observe symptoms and elicit signs. The physician noted general appearance, expression, color, swellings, stiffness, movement, odors, respiration, perspiration, excretions, and listened to the patient's account of the history of the illness. The physician was allowed to touch the patient to study the quality of the pulse, abdomen, tumors, and wounds. Functional tests, such as having the patient move in particular ways, were conducted to elicit information, follow the course of the disease, and evaluate the success of treatment.

Not all of the Egyptian healers were priests; lay physicians and magicians also offered their special services to the sick. The priest-physician enjoyed the highest status, but some individuals acquired qualifications in two or three categories. Physicians and surgeons were assisted by specialists in the art of bandaging, a skill that had its origin in mummy wrapping. The government paid lay physicians to oversee public works, armies, burial grounds, the sacred domains, and the royal palace. Despite uncertainty about the precise role played by the institutions known as the Houses of Life, they seem to have functioned along the lines of an "open college" rather than a formal school or temple. Unfortunately, the collections of papyrus scrolls that were stored at the Houses of Life have not survived.

A woman physician known as Peseshet held the title "Lady Director of Lady Physicians," indicating that she supervised a group of women practitioners. An interesting group of women surgeons used flint chisels and stick drills with which they worked at a patient until blood was drawn. Such treatments were especially recommended for headache. Many Egyptian queens were well versed in medicine and pharmacology, including Mentuhetep (ca. 2300 B.C.), Hatsheput (ca. 1500 B.C.), and Cleopatra (60–30 B.C.). At the Temple of Sais, near the Rosetta Mouth of the Nile, there was a medical school where women professors taught obstetrics and

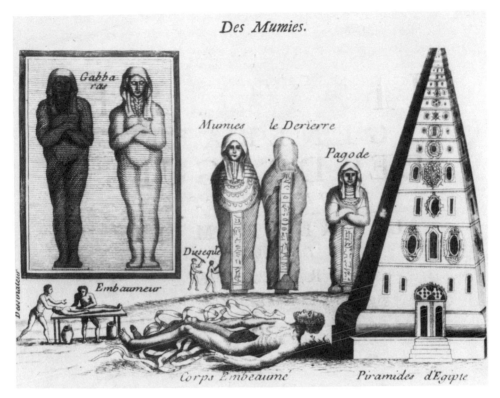

Des Mumies.

Egyptian mummies, pyramids, and the embalming process as depicted in a seventeenth-century French engraving.

gynecology to female students; women may have studied at the medical school at Heliopolis.

According to Egyptian medical theory, human beings were born healthy, but were innately susceptible to disorders caused by intestinal putrefaction, visible or occult external entities, and strong emotions, such as sorrow, unrequited love, and homesickness. The body was threatened by ''winds'' that originated with changes in the weather, spirits or ghosts, and poisoned breaths added to the air by witchcraft. Worms and insects represented exogenous causes of disease; the term ''worms'' included both real and imaginary agents, or a misperception of bits of tissue, mucus, or blood clots that appeared in feces and wounds. Whether disease was due to visible or occult causes, cure required forcing the morbid agents from the body by purging or exorcism. Healer and patient would expect to see signs of the departing invader in the excretions and secretions of the patient.

Many threats to health were avoidable, intermittent, or random, but intestinal decay was a constant and inescapable danger. Obviously, food was needed to sustain life, but as it passed through the intestinal tract it was subject to the same putrid processes that could be observed in rotting foods, wounds, and unembalmed corpses. If the products of decay were strictly confined to the intestines, eating would not be so dangerous, but putrid intestinal materials often contaminated the system of channels that carried blood, mucus, urine, semen, water, tears, and air throughout the body, causing localized lesions and systemic diseases. Health could only be maintained by frequent use of emetics and laxatives to purge the body of intestinal putrefaction. Convinced that the rectum was a particularly dangerous center of decay, the Egyptians relied on remedies designed to soothe and refresh the orifice and keep it from twisting or slipping. Thus, the Keeper of the Royal Rectum truly deserved the honors due to a specialist with primary responsibility for the health of the pharoah.

Herodotus noted the Egyptian concern with internal sources of decay and reported that 3 days each month were set aside for purging the body with emetics and enemas. These prophylactic purges were not the only preventive measures taken by the Egyptians in their pursuit of health. Cleanliness of body was even more valued by the Egyptians than by the Greeks. Rules for the disinfection of dwellings and proper burial of the dead sprang from a combination of hygienic and religious motives. Fear of exacerbating intestinal putrefaction by the ingestion of impure foods and drink encouraged protective food inspection and dietary restrictions. Despite the preoccupation with diet and health, overeating, drunkenness, and disorders due to unwholesome foods were not uncommon.

Popular accounts of Egyptian medicine have presented it as either "mere superstition" or a mysteriously advanced science, but neither extreme is correct. The ancient Egyptians could distinguish between magic and medicine as separate activities, but they expected the effects of the combination to be synergistic. The efficacy of magic rested upon the spell, the rite, and the character of the practitioner. Words used in a spell were so powerful in both their written and spoken forms that objects over which an incantation had been spoken became protective amulets. Spells were recited over a mixture of drugs before giving the remedy to the patient. Many remedies were noxious substances meant to make the patient too repulsive an abode for disease-causing demons. Ritual acts or gestures added power to words. Rituals varied from simple symbolic acts such as tying knots in a thread to bind up the agents of disease to elaborate ceremonies combining music, dance, drugs, and divination. Other magical methods were based on the principle of transfer. For example, to cure migraine, the affected side of the head should be rubbed with a fried fish.

Unfortunately, except for a few fragmentary "medical papyri," the texts used for teaching the art of medicine in the Houses of Life have been lost. The eight surviving medical papyri were composed between about 1900 and 1100 B.C., but they are probably compilations and copies of older texts. In modern translations, the surviving medical papyri constitute only about 200 printed pages.

Remedies and case histories taken from the Ebers, Smith, and Kahun papyri provide the most significant insights into ancient Egyptian ideas about health and disease, anatomy and physiology, magic and medicine. The other medical paypyri include collections of remedies, aphrodisiacs, incantations against disease, descriptions of fertility tests, and spells for the safety of pregnant women and infants.

The Ebers papyrus, which was probably written about 1500 B.C., is the longest, most complete and most famous of the medical papyri. It is named after Georg Ebers, who obtained the papyrus in 1873 and published a facsimile and partial translation 2 years later. It is an encyclopedic collection of prescriptions, extracts of medical texts on diseases and surgery, and incantations, based on at least 40 older sources. The Ebers papyrus was apparently planned as a guide for three kinds of healers: those who dealt with internal and external remedies, surgeons who treated wounds and fractures, and sorcerers or exorcists who wrestled with the demons of disease.

Although the ancients did not see any reason for a strict separation between natural and supernatural diseases, there was a tendency for what might be called "realistic prescriptions" to be grouped together with diseases that could be treated; incurable disorders are generally clustered together with more magically oriented practices. Healers were warned against causing additional suffering by attempting radical treatments in hopeless cases.

Many recipes call for incomprehensible, exotic, or seemingly impossible ingredients, like Thot's feather and heaven's eye, which may have been secret names (like patent medicines) or picturesque names for simple plants. No doubt Egyptian pharmacists would have ridiculed prescriptions calling for "fox's gloves" (digitalis), "pretty lady" (belladonna), or "male duck" (mandrake).

About 700 drugs, made up into more than 800 formulas, are found in the Ebers papyrus. Drugs were administered as pills, ointments, poultices, fumigations, inhalations, gargles, suppositories, enemas, and so forth. Physicians apparently relied on specialized assistants and drug collectors, but sometimes they prepared their own remedies. In contrast to Mesopotamian custom, Egyptian prescriptions were precise about quantities. Generally, components were measured by volume rather than by weight. However, balances have been found along with mortars, mills, and sieves used in preparing drugs.

Remedies fortified by spells were said to open and close the bowels, induce vomiting, expel worms and demons, cure fevers, rheumatism, cough, bloody urine, and a plethora of other diseases. Hemorrhages, wounds, and crocodile bites could be dressed with a mixture of oil, honey, and roasted barley, and covered with fresh meat; other prescriptions called for crocodile dung, human urine, natron, and ostrich eggs.

Gold, silver, and precious stones were identified with the flesh and limbs of gods; thus, they were used in amulets and talismans to ward off disease. Less exotic minerals such as sulfur, natron, and various salts of the heavy metals were commonly associated with skin diseases, but one interesting ointment called for burnt frog in oil. Minerals were used either in their native form or as powders recycled from broken pottery, bricks, and millstones.

Diseases of the eye were apparently as much a problem in ancient Egypt as they are today in many parts of the Middle East, India, and Africa. Blindness was not uncommon, as indicated by various documents and paintings. For a disorder which was probably night blindness (a condition generally due to vitamin A deficiency), roasted ox liver was enthusiastically recommended. On the other hand, a mixture of honey, red ochre, and the humor of a pig's eye poured into the patient's ear was supposed to improve vision.

Rheumatism is the diagnosis suggested by descriptions of chronic aches and pains in the neck, limbs, and joints. Treatment for this painful condition included massages with clay or mud and ointments made of herbs, animal fat, ox spleen, honey, wine dregs, natron, and various obscure materials. The recommendation that certain remedies be applied to the big toe suggests that gout appeared among the various forms of rheumatism.

Not all prescriptions in the medical papyri were for life-threatening conditions. The medical papyri also provide recipes for cosmetics and hair restoratives, such as a mixture of burnt hedgehog quills mixed with oil. Another ingenious recipe could be applied to the head of a woman one hated in order to make her hair fall out. Cosmetics generally reflect only vanity and the tyranny of fashion, but cleansing unguents, perfumes, and pigments probably had valuable astringent and antiseptic properties.

Another example of the lighter side of ancient medicine comes from the study of masticatories or quids, materials which are chewed but not swallowed. The masticatory favored by the Egyptians was the stem of the papyrus plant. The Greeks thought the Egyptian habit of chewing papyrus stems and spitting out the residue was ludicrous and squalid, until they too took up the custom. Resin-based pellets and balls of natron and frankincense were chewed to purify and sweeten the breath. Other masticatories were said to prevent disorders of the teeth and gums.

The Kahun papyrus consists of fragments dealing with gynecology and veterinary medicine, including methods for detecting pregnancy, predicting the sex of the fetus, and preventing conception. One of the contraceptives was basically a pessary containing crocodile dung. Other prescriptions call for a plug (rather like a contraceptive sponge) made with honey and natron, extract of the acacia plant, and an obscure gum-like material. Later contraceptive prescriptions kept the spirit of the Egyptian recipe, but substituted elephant dung for that of the crocodile. Greek observers noted that the ancient Egyptians were able to regulate the size of their families without infanticide. This suggests that even the most noxious and bizarre pessaries might work if they functioned as mechanical barriers or spermicides or caused a total lack of interest in sexual intercourse. Prolonged lactation, which tends to suppress ovulation, and a 3-year interval between births were considered essential for the health of mother and child.

Although midwives were probably the main childbirth attendants, physicians were acquainted with various gynecological disorders, including prolapse of the uterus, cancer, leukorrhea, dysmenorrhea, amenorrhea, and menopause. Many complex and noxious mixtures were recommended for disorders of the uterus, abnormal delivery, and miscarriage. Such remedies were said to warm the breasts, cool the womb, regulate menstruation, and increase milk production. Generally, these medicines were taken as fumigants, douches, or suppositories, but in some cases the woman simply sat on the remedy. Fertility tests were based on the assumption that in fertile women free passages existed between the genital tract and the rest of the body. Therefore, when the woman sat on test substances, such as date flour mixed with beer, vomiting proved that conception could occur and the number of vomits corresponded to the number of future children. Once pregnancy was established, the physician studied the effect of the patient's urine on the germination and growth of wheat and barley in order to make a prediction about the sex of the child.

While pediatrics, a field based on the age of the patient rather than the parts of the body, does not seem to have been recognized as a specialty, there were specific remedies and spells for the health of infants and the cure of various obscure childhood diseases, bed-wetting, retention of urine, cough, and teething. For example, chewing on a fried mouse was recommended to ease the pain of cutting teeth and an old letter boiled in oil was used for retention of urine. Since the child was commonly breast-fed for 3 years, remedies could be given to the mother or wet nurse.

Since the Egyptians made mummies of humans and other animals, they had the opportunity to study comparative anatomy. Nevertheless, despite centuries of experience with mummification, their anatomical concepts remained rudimentary. The embalmers, who belonged to a special guild of craftsmen, were not practicing physicians or disinterested scientists. Even the embalmers seem to have been ambivalent about the task of opening the abdomen. As part of the ritual for this act, a man called the scribe drew a mark along the flank; the man who actually made the incision was symbolically abused and driven away with stones and curses.

Haruspicy, divination through the study of animal organs, offered another source of anatomical information. Since the structure, size, and shape of organs used for divination were important omens, haruspicy probably provided a greater impetus to anatomical study than mummification. Support for this hypothesis is found in the animal-like hieroglyphic signs used for human organs. Egyptologists have catalogued names for over 100 anatomical entities; many names apply to parts of the all-important alimentary canal. The nerves, arteries, and veins were poorly understood and undifferentiated.

Physiological and pathological phenomena were explained in terms of the movement of fluids in a system of "channels" that brought nourishment to the body just as the flooding of the Nile brought nourishment to the land. A complicated system of vessels carried blood, mucus, water, air, semen, urine, and tears. The heart, the "seat of the mind," was clearly regarded as a major gathering place for the vessels, but there was another confluence of channels in the vicinity of the anus. Because the anus was also associated with dangerous decaying matter, the arrangement of the vessels exposed the entire system to potential contamination with the products of internal decay.

As a sign of its special significance, the heart was left in the body during mummification. "Weighing the heart" was an important step in the judgment of the dead by the gods. Afraid that their hearts might not measure up, the Egyptians carefully fortified their tombs with magical amulets to secure successful judgments. By weighing the hearts of the dead, the gods could measure their moral worth. In the living, the physician measured health by placing his fingers on the pulses of head, neck, stomach, and limbs, because the heart spoke out through the vessels of the body. Indeed, knowledge of the heart and its movements was called the "physician's secret."

In 1862 Edwin Smith (1822–1906), a pioneer Egyptologist, purchased a papyrus scroll found in a grave near Luxor. When James Henry Breasted translated this document he revolutionized ideas about the relative weight of magic, empiricism, and surgery in Egyptian medicine. Breasted viewed the Smith papyrus as a document in a class by itself, because it was a systematic collection of case histories that offered the physician important anatomical and physiological information. Sections of the Smith papyrus were copied from texts so ancient that the idioms and concepts were incomprehensible. Therefore, the scribe had to include explanations to make the text useful to his contemporaries.

The 48 cases preserved in the Edwin Smith papyrus were arranged systematically from head to foot in order of severity. Each case consists of a title, instructions to the physician, the probable prognosis, and the proper treatment. Ailments were divided into three categories: (a) those that were almost definitely curable; (b) those that were treatable, but uncertain; and (c) incurable disorders for which no treatment should be attempted.

The section called the "book of wounds" describes treatments for fractures, dislocations, bites, tumors, ulcers, and abscesses. Broken bones were set in splints made from ox bones, supported by bandages soaked in quick-setting resin. Recognizing the poor prognosis for compound or open fractures (fractures in which the broken ends of the bone have pierced the skin), the practitioner who was prepared to "contend with" simple or closed fractures considered an open fracture an ailment beyond treatment. Plasters or adhesive bandages were generally used to close wounds, but some injuries called for sutures. The Egyptian surgeon used a variety of bandages, adhesive plasters, splints, braces, drains, plugs, cleansers, and cauteries.

Although the Egyptians were familiar with the sedative effects of opium and henbane, there is no direct evidence of their use as surgical anesthethics. A scene depicting circumcision accompanied by a text that states: "This is to render it agreeable," has been interpreted as evidence of anesthesia, but another inscription found with a similar depiction of this operation says: "Hold him so that he does not fall.'' Since circumcision was a religious ritual, it fell within the province of the priest and would not be discussed in a medical treatise.

Unfortunately, the "books of wounds" is incomplete; the scribe stopped writing in the middle of an interesting account of afflictions of the spine and left the rest of that "page" blank. When he resumed work, he apparently turned to another source and copied out recipes to "transform an old man into a youth of twenty" and incantations against "the wind of the pest of the year." This abrupt transition may be symptomatic of the gradual transformation of priorities in Egyptian culture over the millennia.

SUGGESTED READINGS

Andrews, Carol (1978). *Egyptian Mummies*. Cambridge, MA: Harvard University Press.

Breasted, J. H. (1930). *The Edwin Smith Surgical Papyrus*, 2 vols. Chicago: University of Chicago Press.

Brothwell, D. R., and Chiarelli, B. A., eds. (1973). *Population Biology of the Ancient Egyptians*. New York: Academic Press.

Bucaille, Maurice (1991). *Mummies of the Pharaohs. Modern Medical Investigation.*, (Trans. by Alastair D. Pannell and Maurice Bucaille). New York: St. Martin's Press.

Budge, E. A. Wallis (1960). *The Book of the Dead. The Hieroglyphic Transcript of the Papyrus ANI*. New York: University Books.

Budge, E. A. W. (1928). *The Divine Origin of the Craft of the Herbalist*. London: The Society of Herbalists.

Budge, E. A. W. (1913). *Syrian Anatomy, Pathology and Therapeutics or "The Book of Medicines,"* 2 vols. London: Oxford University Press.

Childe, V. Gordon (1951). *Man Makes Himself*. New York: Mentor.

Cockburn, Aidan, and Cockburn, Eve, eds. (1980). *Mummies, Disease, and Ancient Cultures*. Cambridge, England: Cambridge University Press.

Darby, William J., and Ghalioungui, Paul (1977). *Food: The Gift of Osiris*. New York: Academic Press.

David, Rosalie, ed. (1970). *Mysteries of the Mummies. The Story of the Unwrapping of a 2000-Year-Old Mummy by a Team of Experts*. New York: Scribner.

Dawson, Warren Royal (1930). *The Beginnings. Egypt and Assyria*. Clio Medica Series. New York: Hoeber.

Dijk, Jan van, Hussey, Mary I., and Goetze, Albrecht (1975). *Early Mesopotamian Incantations and Rituals*. New Haven, CT: Yale University Press.

Ebbell, B. (1937). *The Papyrus Ebers. The Greatest Egyptian Medical Document*. Copenhagen: Levin & Munksgaard.

Elliot Smith, G., and Dawson, W. R. (1924). *Egyptian Mummies*. New York: Dial Press.

Estes, J. Worth (1990). *The Medical Skills of Ancient Egypt*. Canton, MA: Science History Publications.

Fleming, Stuart (1980). *The Egyptian Mummy: Secrets and Science*. Philadelphia: The University Museum, University of Pennsylvania.

Gardner, John, and Maier, John, trans. (1984). *Gilgamesh*. New York: Knopf.

Ghalioungui, Paul, and Dawakhly, Z. (1965). *Health and Healing in Ancient Egypt*. Cairo: Organization of Translation and Authorship.

Ghalioungui, Paul (1973). *The House of Life: Magic and Medical Science in Ancient Egypt*. Amsterdam: B.M. Israel.

Ghalioungui, Paul (1983). *The Physicians of Pharaonic Egypt*. Cairo: Al-Ahram Center for Scientific Translations.

Harris, James E., and Wente, Edward F. (1980). *An X-Ray Atlas of the Royal Mummies*. Chicago: University Chicago Press.

Himes, Norman (1970). *Medical History of Contraception*. New York: Schocken.

Hurry, Jamieson Boyd (1928). *Imhotep: The Vizier and Physician of King Zoser and Afterwards the Egyptian God of Medicine*, 2nd ed., London: Oxford University Press.

Kramer, S. N. (1981). *History Begins at Sumer*. Philadelphia, PA: University Pennsylvania Press.

Leichty, Erle (1988). "Guaranteed to Cure." In Erle Leichty, Maria de J. Ellis, and Pamela Gerardi, eds. *A Scientific Humanist: Studies in Memory of Abraham Sachs*. Occasional publications of the Samuel Noah Kramer Fund, No. 9, Philadelphia, 1988.

Majno, Guido (1975). *The Healing Hand. Man and Wound in the Ancient World*. Cambridge, MA: Harvard University Press.

Pritchard, James B., ed. (1958). *The Ancient Near East. An Anthology of Texts and Pictures*, 2 vols. Princeton, NJ: Princeton University Press.

Saggs, H. W. F. (1989). *Civilization Before Greece and Rome*. New Haven, CT: Yale University Press.

Saunders, J. B. de C. M. (1963). *The Transition from Ancient Egyptian to Greek Medicine*. Lawrence, KS: University of Kansas Press.

Schmandt-Besserat, Denise (1978). The Earliest Precursor of Writing. *Scientific American* 238: 50–59.

Sigerist, H. E. (1951). *A History of Medicine*. Vol. I. *Primitive and Archaic Medicine*. New York: Oxford University Press.

Steuer, Robert O., and Saunders, J. B. de C. M. (1959). *Ancient Egyptian and Cnidian Medicine. The Relationship of Their Aetiological Concepts of Disease*. Berkeley: University of California Press.

Thompson, Reginald Campbell (1924). *The Assyrian Herbal*. London: Luzac.

THE GREAT MEDICAL TRADITIONS OF INDIA AND CHINA

I n surveys of the history of medicine, the invention of science and "rational med-icine" is generally credited to the Greek natural philosophers who lived during the sixth century B.C. Accustomed to tracing the roots of Western culture back to Greece, with some slight concessions to those civilizations mentioned in the Bible, European scholars generally ignored the development of medicine, science, and philosophy in India and China. This gargantuan omission is especially unfortunate because, unlike the medical traditions of Mesopotamia and Egypt, those of India and China are still very much alive.

INDIA

Densely populated, with a mixture of races, languages, cultures, and religions, the Indian subcontinent is a world of bewildering complexity. In the 1920s, our understanding of Indian history was transformed by the discovery of the wonders of Mohenjo-daro and Harappa, two major cities that were part of the forgotten Indus River Civilization that had flourished from about 2700 to 1500 B.C.

Memories of centuries of growth, turmoil, and decay survived in the form of four collections known as the *Vedas*, which are revered by Hindus as sacred books of divinely inspired knowledge. The *Vedas* are accompanied by later commentaries known as the *Brahmanas* and the *Upanishads,* which explain the older texts and speculate about the nature of the universe and the human condition.

Many aspects of Indian history are vague until the fourth and third centuries B.C. when the Indus valley region was conquered first by the Persians and then by the forces of Alexander the Great (356–323 B.C.). Although Alexander spent less than 2 years in India, the invasion led to cultural exchanges between the Greak-speaking world and the peoples of India. During the turmoil that followed the death of Alexander, Chandragupta Maurya was able to drive out the remaining Macedonian officials and establish his own empire. His grandson, Asoka, who reigned from about 273 to 232 B.C., was able to bring most of India under the domination of the Maurya Dynasty. The *Artha Sastra*, or science of politics and administration, is said to have been written for Chandragupta. It contains many laws that are of interest to the history of medicine, such as those regulating medical practitioners, midwives, nurses, drugs and poisons, prostitution, sanitation, and public health. The judicial mutilations prescribed for improper behaviors would have provided gruesome employment for surgeons. For example, the penalty for a person who had insulted his parents or teachers was amputation of the tongue.

Initially regarded as a cruel despot, King Asoka became so overwhelmed with remorse over the bloodshed and misery he had caused that he renounced warfare and became a Buddhist. Buddhism originated in India in the sixth century B.C. in the teachings of Buddha, "The Enlightened One" (ca. 563–483), and developed as a protest against the strict stratification of Hindu society and the religious rituals controlled by the Brahmanic priests. Buddha's teachings emphasized universal love, service, and the peace of mind brought about by the abandonment of desire. According to the great stone edicts posted throughout his empire, Asoka devoted himself to peace and righteousness through good deeds, compassion, religious tolerance, and purity. Giving up the sport of hunting and the eating of flesh, Asoka offered animals as well as humans his protection and established rest houses, facilities for the care of the sick, and other charitable institutions.

Although the edicts of Asoka suggest that free hospitals and dispensaries were widely distributed throughout ancient India, other lines of evidence are ambiguous. One fifth-century Chinese traveler described Indian hospitals that cared for the poor and the sick, but noted that these institutions were privately endowed rather than state supported. Other observers commented on rest houses sponsored by the king where travelers and the poor could find physicians and medicines, as well as food and drink. Medical aid was apparently available at some temples and schools. Charitable hospitals seem to have been more characteristic of neighboring countries that imported Buddhism and Ayurvedic medicine from India. Later visitors to India were amazed to find hospitals for animals and asserted that charity and mercy were more likely to be given to cows and dogs than to human beings.

During the reign of Asoka, Buddhist monks held the great "Council of Patna" (250 B.C.) to determine which texts should be regarded as authentic tenets of their religion and how its members should be organized. Buddhist missionaries traveled to Syria, Egypt, Greece, Tibet, and China. Although Buddhism became well established in other parts of the world, in India the ancient Vedic traditions eventually reasserted themselves. After the reign of Asoka, the history of India become a series of assassinations, betrayals, and invasions by Greeks, Scythians, Muslims, Mongols, and Europeans. Independence from Great Britain in 1947 led to riots, mass migrations, and massacres waged between Hindus and Muslims. In 1950, India became a sovereign democratic republic; Pakistan became a separate Islamic republic in 1956.

Thus, although Buddhism exerted a profound impact in many of the countries that imported both Buddhism and Indian medicine, Ayurvedic medicine remained intimately linked to the Hindu religion. The universe portrayed by Indian religions was of immense size and antiquity, undergoing a continuous process of development and decay. Human beings were enmeshed in this universal cycle by the process of reincarnation into positions higher or lower in the complex caste system. As interpreted by the Brahmanic priests, India's caste system was a reflection of the order of nature found in the hymn of creation in the *Rigveda*. From the sacrifice that created the world, the *brahmans* (priest) appeared from the head, the *kshatriyas* (warriors and nobles) from the arms, the *vaisyas* (farmers, merchants, craftsmen) from the thighs, and the *sudras* (laborers, servants, slaves) from the feet. The four major castes gave rise to more than 3000 subcastes and the "untouchables."

Growing within and beyond the boundaries of the mythic lore and epic battles of gods, conquerors, and castes, Indian medicine developed in a series of distinct phases: (a) prehistoric or pre-Vedic, (b) Vedic, and (c) Ayurvedic. According to Hindu mythology, Brahma, the First Teacher of the Universe, was the author of the *Ayurveda*, or *The Science of Life*, an epic consisting of 100,000 hymns and the source of all knowledge pertaining to drugs and medicines. The divine sage Dhanvantari, who arose from the cosmic ocean bearing the miraculous potion that conferred immortality on the gods, taught Ayurvedic lore to a long line of sages before it was finally committed to writing. The texts that have survived are said to be only shadows of the lost *Ayurveda* composed by Brahma.

While the authorship and time of composition of the *Vedas* cannot be determined with any precision, the *Rigveda* is said to represent materials from the period 4500 to 2000 B.C. and the *Atharvaveda* is a collection of materials from the period 1500 to 1000 B.C. In Vedic hymns and legends, gods and healers wrestled with demonic forces and performed rites that consecrated mysterious remedies against disease and pestilence. All medicines, including more than 1000 healing herbs, were said to be derived from heaven, earth, and water. The Vedas contain many references to medical lore, anatomy, wounds, diseases, healers, demons, drugs, charms, and spells.

Because disease was the result of sin or the work of demons, cure required confession, spells, incantations, and exorcism. Vedic healers prepared herbal remedies and charms against the demons that caused fevers, fractures, wounds, and venomous bites. Specific remedies and surgical techniques could only be therapeutic when combined with the appropriate ritual, but the roles of magicians, physicians,

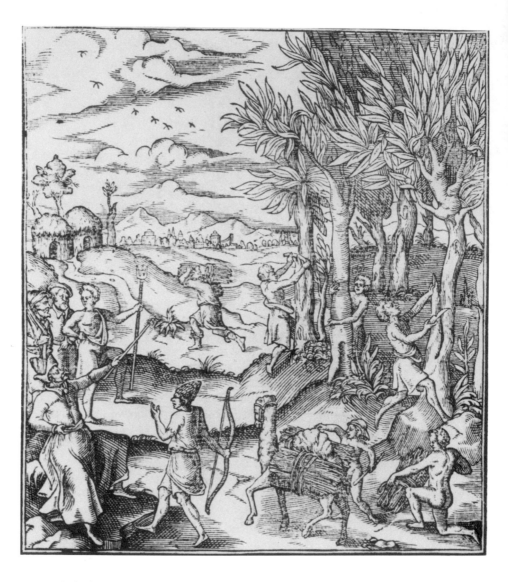

Gathering cinnamon bark in India as depicted in a sixteenth-century woodcut.

and surgeons were differentiated to some extent. Surgeons treated wounds and snake bites, removed injured eyes, extracted arrows, amputated limbs, and fitted patients with artificial legs. If the skulls discovered at two Harappan sites are representative of a lost tradition, Indian surgeons also practiced trepanation.

Additional insights into the practice of Indian medicine and surgery can be gleaned from ancient laws, monuments, inscriptions, surgical instruments, artwork, and the stories told by travelers, pilgrims, and foreign invaders. A study of the present folk customs and the work of traditional healers may also throw light on ancient practices. However, the most direct literary guide to ancient Indian medicine is found in the classics of Ayurvedic medicine. These texts are fundamental sources for a civilization in which the oral tradition remained a dominant force, but they must be regarded as portraits of the *ideal physician* rather than the *typical healer*.

AYURVEDIC MEDICINE, THE SCIENCE OF LIFE

Ayurveda, the learned system that forms the basis of the traditional medicine widely practiced in India today, is known as "the science of life." The practitioner who has come to understand the science of life is known as the *vaidya*. The physician, the medicine, the attendant, and the patient constitute the four pillars of Ayurvedic medicine. The task of the physician was to exercise good judgment about his duties, the attendant was expected to prepare medicines and perform nursing duties, and the patient's role was to provide an accurate history of the disease and follow the physician's orders. It was important for the physician to assess his patient and his assistant carefully, because when therapy was unsuccessful only the physician's competence would be questioned.

Properly speaking, Ayurveda is composed of eight branches: internal medicine, diseases of the head, surgery, toxicology, demonic diseases, pediatrics, rejuvenation, and aphrodisiacs. The primary objective of the science of life was the maintenance of health, rather than the treatment of disease. Health was not simply the absence of disease, but a state attained and enjoyed only by vigorous pursuit of an elaborate, individualized program of prophylactic measures prescribed by the Ayurvedic doctor. The origin of Ayurvedic theory is uncertain, but its materia medica may have evolved from Vedic or even prehistoric drug lore.

Caraka, Susruta, and Vagbhata, the semi-legendary authors of the classic texts that illuminate the eight branches of Ayurvedic medicine, are honored as the "Triad of Ancients." Although many colorful stories have become associated with these sages, there is little definitive biographical information about any of them. Traditionally, Caraka is said to have lived in the period of 1000 to 800 B.C., but Western scholars have placed him as late as the first century A.D. In any case, the *Caraka Samhita* probably reached its present form in the first century A.D. Honored as the first great treatise of Indian medicine, the text describes hundreds of drugs and classifies them in terms of the diseases for which they are useful. Susruta is said to have lived about

600 B.C. While the *Susruta Samhita* might be considered more systematic in its treatment of pharmacology, its emphasis on the art of surgery is of particular interest. Because Vagabhata's text mentions both Caraka and Susruta, he is obviously the most recent author, but his biography is similarly obscure.

Caraka taught that the attainment and maintenance of health and happiness was a necessary and noble pursuit. Diseases obstructed the attainment of humanity's highest goals, but Ayurveda, the most sacred of the sciences, benefited human beings in their present and future lives. The text provides a guide to the three forms of medicine: (a) mantras and religious acts; (b) diet and drugs; and (c) psychic therapy, or subjection of the mind.

Both Caraka and Susruta devoted considerable attention to the characteristics that distinguish the good physician from pretenders to the art. Understanding the anatomy, physiology, and development of the human body, as well as the origin and evolution of the universe, a wise physician was never in doubt about the etiology of disease, recognized the earliest and most subtle signs and symptoms, and knew which diseases were easily cured and which were incurable.

Because physicians were members of a professional group rather than a specific caste, a practitioner could accept students from the three upper castes. Students were expected to live with and serve their teacher until the master was satisfied that their training was complete. Access to the classics could only be obtained by listening to a master physician read and explain the texts. It was the student's duty to memorize the sacred texts and demonstrate competence in medicine and surgery. Using fruits, vegetables, meats, and manikins, the apprentice developed his surgical skills before operating on patients. For example, he learned to make incisions by operating on cucumbers and practiced venesection on the veins of dead animals or lotus stems.

The good physician exhibited four primary qualifications: theoretical knowledge, clarity of reasoning, wide practical experience, and personal skill. Sympathetic and kind to all patients, the physician devoted himself to those who could be cured while maintaining a sense of detachment towards those who would die. The surgeon must have courage, steady hands, sharp instruments, a calm demeanor, unshakable self-confidence, and the services of strong-nerved assistants. Although the physician must never desert or injure a patient, he was not obligated to accept patients who were known criminals, nor those suffering from incurable diseases. Yet the ideal doctor would strive with all his might to cure his patient even if he placed his own life at risk.

According to Ayurvedic physiology, bodily functions could be explained in terms of the three *dosas*, the primary humors, fluids, or principles—*Vata*, *Pitta*, and *Kapha* —which are usually translated as wind, bile, and phlegm. Although the basic principles of Indian humoral pathology are similar to those of Greek medicine, the Ayurvedic system provides additional complications. The three Ayurvedic humors, in combination with blood, determined all vital functions. The body was composed of a combination of the five elements—earth, water, fire, wind, empty space—and the seven basic tissues. Bodily functions were also dependent on five separate winds, the vital soul, and the inmost soul.

Health was the result of a delicate and harmonious balance among the primary humors that was easily disturbed by stress, wounds, accidents, and demonic possession. Thus, an imbalance among wind, bile, and phlegm was the fundamental cause of disease; the degree of derangement determined whether the disease would be minor, major, or incurable. Except for a few perfectly balanced individuals, each person was born with some degree of discord among the three humors that created a predisposition to particular diseases. Discord among the three humors produced a disturbance in the blood. Therefore, in addition to restoring balance through proper diet, the physician had to remove ''bad blood'' by venesection or leeching.

Diagnosis was a formidable task because more than 1000 ''diseases'' were alluded to in the ancient texts. ''Fever'' was given pride of place as the ''king of all bodily diseases.'' When the fever was intermittent, the intervals between the peak periods of fever provided the key to prognosis. This interest in the intervals between episodes of fever is also found in Greek medicine.

Accurate diagnosis was the key to selecting the proper treatment for curable disease. After listening closely to the patient's narrative concerning the illness, the physician studied the patient's general appearance, blood, body fluids, and excretions. The physician employed palpation and auscultation, elicited latent symptoms by using drugs as therapeutic tests, and assessed the odor and taste of secretions and discharges. If a physician did not want to taste the secretions himself he could assign this task to his students, or feed them to insects and observe their reactions. The most famous diagnostic taste text was for the ''honey urine disease'' (diabetes).

Almost 1000 drugs derived from plant sources are referred to in the major medical classics, but many are unidentifiable materials or ''divine drugs'' such as ''soma.'' Vedic myths say that Brahma created soma to prevent old age and death, but the identity of this ''king of plants'' was a mystery to later sages. Minerals and animal products, such as honey, milk, snake skin, and excrements, are also well represented.

For diseases involving corruption of the bodily humors the proper remedies included internal cleansing, external cleansing, and surgery. Diseases caused by improper diet called for remedies that accomplished internal cleansing, but physicians often began treatment with a 7-day fast. Some patients recovered during this period and needed no other remedies; presumably some died and also needed no further remedies.

Perhaps the most striking aspect of ancient Indian healers was their mastery of surgical skills. Vedic myths speak of remarkable operations on men and gods, such as a cure for impotence achieved by transplanting the testes of a ram to the afflicted god Indra. Ayurvedic texts describe more prosaic but still challenging operations such as cesarean section, lithotomy, couching the cataract, tonsillectomy, amputations, and plastic surgery.

While the therapeutic use of the knife was accepted in India, use of the knife on the dead and contact with cadavers were prohibited by custom and religion. Nevertheless, Susruta taught that physicians and surgeons must study the human body by direct observation in order to gain knowledge of its parts. While acknowledging religious prohibitions against contact with dead bodies, Susruta justified the study of anatomy, or the "science of being," as a form of knowledge linked to higher phenomena, including the relationship between humans and gods. Ingeniously working his way around the prohibition against the use of the knife on dead bodies, Susruta proposed an unusual form of anatomical investigation. If a body was complete in all its parts, neither too old nor too young, and if death had not been caused by protracted illness or poison, it was suitable for study. After removing the excrements from the intestines, the anatomist should cover the body with grasses, place it in a cage of fine mesh, and leave it to steep in a quiet pond. Seven days later the anatomist could gradually remove successive layers of skin and muscle by gently rubbing the body with soft brushes. According to Susruta, this process rendered the most minute parts of the body distinct and palpable. There is, however, little evidence that teachers of Ayurvedic medicine followed Susruta's prescription for human dissection.

One aspect of human anatomy that all students were expected to master was the complex system of "vital points," or "marmas," distributed throughout the body. These vital points seem to be sites where major veins, arteries, ligaments, joints, and muscles unite and where injuries are likely to be incapacitating or fatal. The classical system included 107 points, each of which was assigned a special name.

When examining an injured patient, the physician's first task was to determine whether a wound corresponded to one of the marmas. If injury to a marma would lead to death, the surgeon might amputate the limb at an auspicious site above the marma. In venesection or any form of surgical intervention, the surgeon had to avoid damage to the marmas.

Bleeding and cauterization were among the most routine surgical operations. Cauterization was the method of choice for treating hemorrhages and diseases that resisted medicinal remedies. Susruta believed that the healing properties of the actual cautery (red-hot irons) were far superior to those of the potential cautery (chemically induced burns). Blood-letting was considered a sovereign remedy, but bleeding had to be done with caution because blood was the source of strength, vitality, and longevity. Leeching was recommended as the gentlest form of bleeding because leeches instinctively discriminated between vitiated blood and healthy blood.

Preparations for any surgical operation were exacting, involving special attention to the patient, the operating room, and the "one hundred and one" surgical instruments. One reason for the large number of surgical tools was the preference for instruments resembling various animals. If the lion-mouth forceps did not fit the task, the surgeon could try the hawk, heron, or crocodile-mouth version. Surgeons also needed tables of different shapes and sizes for particular operations and a "fracture-bed" for stretching fractured or dislocated limbs. Above all, the surgeon must see to it that the room used for surgery was carefully prepared to ensure cleanliness and comfort.

Medical care of pregnant women encompassed efforts to ensure male offspring, management of diet, easing the pains of labor, delivery, and the postnatal care of mother and child. Normally childbirth was managed by midwives, but in difficult deliveries, a surgeon might be needed to perform operations in which the fetus was turned, flexed, mutilated, or destroyed. If natural delivery was impossible, or if the mother died in childbirth, Susruta recommended cesarean section. Certain signs foretold the outcome of pregnancy. For example, if the mother was violent and bad-tempered, the child would be epileptic, while the child of an alcoholic woman would suffer from weak memory and constant thirst. If the wishes of a pregnant woman were not gratified, the child might be born hunchbacked, lame, or mute. A malformed child might also be the result of misdeeds in a prior life, physical or emotional injury to the mother, or an aggravated condition of the three humors.

Indian surgeons seem to have developed techniques for dealing with the major problems of surgery: pain and infection. Fumigation of the sickroom and the wound before surgery in the pursuit of an idealized standard of cleanliness might have reduced the dangers of infection, but the effectiveness of such techniques is an open question. Claims that the ancients discovered potent anesthetic agents are likely to be somewhat exaggerated, since both Caraka and Susruta recommended wine before surgery to prevent fainting and afterwards to deaden pain. In some cases the doctor was told to have the patient bound hand and foot. The narcotic effect of the fumes of burning Indian hemp were apparently understood, but references to drugs called "the producer of unconsciousness" and "the restorer of life" remain obscure.

The *Susruta Samhita* describes many difficult operations, such as couching the cataract, lithotomy (removal of bladder stones), opening the chest to drain pus, and the repair of torn bellies and intestines. Various kinds of threads and needles were used for closing wounds, but when the intestines were torn, large black ants were recommended as wound clips.

Plastic surgery, especially the art of reconstructing noses, lips, and ears, was probably the most remarkable aspect of the Indian doctor's achievements. Noses and ears were at risk among Indian warriors, who worked without helmets, and among the general run of sinners and criminals, because, in India, as in Mesopotamia, justice was meted out by mutilation and amputation. More prosaic cases resulted from the destruction of earlobes stretched beyond endurance by the large, heavy earrings thought to ward off misfortune.

Repairs of noses, lips, and ears were made with the "sensible skin-flap" technique. For example, using a leaf as his template, the surgeon would slice a patch of "living flesh" (now called a pedicle flap) from the cheek or forehead in order to create a new nose. After scarifying the patch, the physician quickly attached it to the site of the severed nose and covered the wound with an aesthetically pleasing bandage. Because a pedicle flap used as a graft must remain attached to its original site, the free end can only be sewn to an area within easy reach. After the graft had grown attached to the new site, the base of the flap was cut free. If the surgeon had superb skill, steady hands, and sharp razors, the operation could be completed in less than 2 hours.

During the nineteenth century, the British colonial experience gave Western doctors the opportunity to investigate traditional Indian medical and surgical practices. While working at the Madras Ophthalmic Hospital in the 1910s, Dr. Robert Henry Elliot assembled a collection of 54 eyeballs in a study of the Indian operation of couching the cataract. He detected many complications, but since all the eyes were taken from blind patients, these cases represented only the failures of traditional surgeons.

Unfortunately, Elliot never observed a traditional practitioner at work, but his informants claimed that practitioners often told the patient that surgery was unnecessary. Then, while pretending to examine the eye, the operator suddenly pushed a needle through the cornea and quickly detached the lens. Immediately after the operation, the surgeon tested the patient's vision, bandaged the eyes, and advised the patient to rest for at least 24 hours. Elliot noted that this would allow the operator time to disappear before the outcome of the case could be ascertained.

While cleanliness was a major precept for Susruta and Caraka, Elliot claimed that it was of no concern to contemporary practitioners. Moreover, unscrupulous practitioners operated on patients suffering from optic atrophy or glaucoma rather than cataract. Twentieth-century Indian practitioners might give us some insight into the surgical procedures of the followers of Susruta, but these accounts cannot be directly related to the ancient Indian science of life. The wandering empiric, crudely performing a specific operation in the shadows of colonial power, had only the most tenuous links to the scholarly practitioner envisioned by Susruta and Caraka.

Although modern science and medicine have won a place in India, Ayurvedic medicine still brings comfort to millions of people. Instead of dismissing Ayurveda as "mere superstition," scholars in India are finding valuable medical insights and inspiration in the ancient writings. Like students of traditional Chinese medicine, followers of Ayurveda see their ancient traditions as a treasure-house of remedies and medical practices.

CHINESE MEDICINE: CLASSICAL, TRADITIONAL, AND MODERN

Until recently, Western historians of science generally ignored China, except for a few exotic items and inventions that could be rationalized as crude precursors of technologies brought to fruition in the West, such as gunpowder and printing. Fortunately, the work of Joseph Needham, Nathan Sivin, Paul Unschuld, and others has helped redefine the place of Asian studies in the global history of science.

More than any other culture, China has maintained its traditional medicine not only in folk remedies, but in mature and respected forms. In part, this unique stability can be attributed to a profound reverence for the past, religious beliefs based on ancestor worship, and a system of writing perhaps 6000 years old. Although many scholars have discounted the earliest chapters in Chinese "recorded history," recent archaeological and archival discoveries will doubtless transform much "mythology" into history and much "history" into mythology. Since the 1970s, Chinese archaeologists have experienced a "golden age" of discovery. Ancient tombs are yielding treasures ranging from panels of magnificent wall paintings and manuscripts written on bamboo or silk, to well-preserved bodies, skeletons, and hordes of life-sized pottery figures of warriors complete with weapons and horses from the Ch'in Dynasty (221-206 B.C.).

Much of China's history is obscured by warfare and chaos until the Ch'in unification in 221 B.C. To enforce the Dynasty's goal of reorganization, the Emperor Shih Huang-ti ordered the destruction of all surviving manuscripts to erase unacceptable historical traditions. Exceptions were made only for texts dealing with medicine, drugs, divination, agriculture, and forestry. During the centuries of conflict, scholars as well as peasants assimilated the concepts that formed the framework of classical Chinese medicine: belief in the unity of nature, the yin-yang dualism, the theory of the five phases, and a medical practice based on the theory of systematic correspondences.

Some elements of this system can be traced back to China's Bronze Age, the period of the Shang Dynasty, which was already flourishing by the fifteenth century B.C. Scholars once consigned the Shang Dynasty to the realm of legend, but excavations begun in the 1930s have provided evidence that the Shang era served as the formative period of Chinese culture. For our purposes, the Shang "oracle bones," inscribed with an archaic but essentially mature form of written Chinese, are of special importance.

"Oracle bones" were used in divination ceremonies dating back to about 1300 B.C. Various materials, including the shoulder blades of oxen, goats, and sheep, turtle shells, antlers, and even human cranial bones were used as oracles. According to Shang beliefs, the well-being of the living was dependent on the will of the ancestral spirits that ruled the world. If the ancestors were displeased, their curse could cause disease, poor harvests, and military defeats. To communicate with the spirits, appropriate bones or shells were carefully prepared for the king and his diviners. Oracle bones answered questions about weather, harvests, hunting expeditions, battles, illness, and epidemics. During the ceremony, pairs of antithetical questions were addressed to the spirits; for example, "Will the king recover from his illness?" and "Will the king not recover from his illness?" Heat was applied to the oracle bone with a heated bronze rod, a burning stick, or a glowing piece of charcoal. If the bones had been properly prepared, they would produce a pair of cracks resembling the written character "pu," a vertical line joined about midpoint from the right by a perpendicular line (⊢). If the angle between the lines was close to the perpendicular, the answer was yes; if not, the answer was no.

Shang writing and divination were essentially forgotten until the end of the nineteenth-century even though "oracles" could be found in almost every traditional Chinese apothecary shop. When physicians included "dragon bones" in their prescriptions for disorders ranging from lung diseases to anxiety and nocturnal emissions, apothecaries used bits of ancient bones and shells, including many that had served as oracles. Since nineteenth century fossil hunters discovered that collections of "dragon bones" often contained valuable fossils, hundreds of thousands of oracle bones have been collected; how many were pounded into medicines over the centuries can only be imagined.

History yields to mythology in accounts of the Three Celestial Emperors, revered as the founders of Chinese civilization. Fu Hsi, who is said to have reigned about 2000 B.C., is the legendary founder of China's first dynasty; his most important inventions include writing, painting, music, the original eight mystic trigrams, and the yin-yang concept. The *I Ching*, or *Canon of Changes*, honored as the most ancient of Chinese books, is ascribed to Fu Hsi.

Shen Nung, the second Celestial Emperor, is said to have introduced the fundamental techniques of agriculture and animal husbandry. When the "Divine Peasant" saw his people suffering from illness and poisoning, he taught them to sow the five kinds of grain and personally investigated 1000 herbs so that the people would know which were therapeutic and which were toxic. In his experiments on poisons and antidotes, Shen Nung is said to have taken as many as 70 different poisons in one day. Having collected many remedies in the first great treatise on herbal medicine while setting a magnificent example of unselfish devotion to medical research, the Emperor died after an unsuccessful experiment.

During his 100-year reign, Huang Ti, last of the Celestial Emperors, gave his people the wheel, the magnet, an astonomical observatory, the calendar, and the *Nei Ching* (*The Yellow Emperor's Classic of Internal Medicine*), a text that has inspired and guided Chinese medical thought for over 2500 years. Like many ancient texts, the *Nei Ching* has been corrupted over the centuries by additions, excisions, and misprints. Other medical texts have sometimes overshadowed it, but most of the classics of Chinese medicine may be considered interpretations, commentaries, and supplements to the Yellow Emperor's *Canon*.

As it exists today, the *Nei Ching* is a collection of sometimes contradictory ideas and interpretations forced into a supposedly integrated conceptual system. The *Nei Ching* is cast in the form of a dialogue between Huang Ti and Ch'i Po, his Minister of Health and Healing. Together, Emperor and Minister explore a medical philosophy based on the balance of the *yang* and *yin*, the five phases (also called the five elements), and the correlations found among them and almost every conceivable entity impinging on human life, from family and food to climate and geography. The terms yin and yang are generally taken to represent all the pairs of opposites which express the dualism of the cosmos. Thus, whereas yin is characterized as female, dark, cold, soft, earth, night, empty, yang represents male, light, warm, firm, heaven, day, full, and so forth. Yin and yang, however, should be understood as "relational concepts," that is, not firm or soft, per se, but only in comparison to other states or entities.

The original meaning of the characters for yin and yang are obscure; they seem to suggest the two banks of a river, one in shade and the other in the sun, or the shady side and the sunny side of a hill. In any case, "light" and "shade" appear to be fundamental components. Applying these concepts to the human body, the outside is relatively yang, the inside is relatively yin, and specific internal organs are associated with yang or yin. Huang Ti taught that the principle of yin-yang is the basis of everything in creation, the cause of all transformations, and the origin of life and death. Yin and yang generate the five phases: wood, fire, earth, metal, and water.

Because the terms yang and yin were essentially untranslatable, they have been directly adopted into many languages. But the same lack of meaningful correspondence applies to the *wu-hsing*, a term that was usually translated as "five elements" because of a false analogy with the four elements of the Greeks. The Chinese term actually implies "passage," "transition," or "phase," rather than stable, homogeneous chemical constituents. In recent years, scholars have invented new terms, such as "five conventional values" and "five evolutive phases" to convey a more precise meaning. For the sake of simplicity, we shall use the term "five phases."

Chinese philosophers and scientists created an elaborate system to rationalize the relationships of the five elements to almost everything else. Thus, the sequences of creation and destruction among the five elements provided a foundation for classical concepts of human physiology.

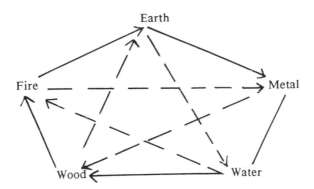

The five phases. As individual names or labels for the finer ramifications of yin and yang, the five phases represent aspects in the cycle of changes. The five phases are linked by relationships of generation and destruction. Patterns of destruction may be summarized as follows: water puts out fire; fire melts metal; a metal ax will cut wood; a wooden plow will turn the earth; an earthen dam will stop the flow of water. The cycle of generation proceeds as water produces the wood of trees; wood produces fire; fire creates ash, or earth; earth is the source of metal; when metals are heated they flow like water.

One aspect of Chinese medicine that is likely to seem especially peculiar to the modern reader is the classical approach to human anatomy and physiology. However, if Chinese anatomy is properly thought of in terms of function rather than structure, distinctions between "anatomy" and "physiology" become irrelevant. Anatomy, in the Western sense, did not form the basis of classical Chinese medical theory or practice. Western anatomists study the body as if dealing with an assemblage of bits and pieces belonging to a machine. In contrast, classical Chinese anatomy is concerned with the dynamic interplay of "functional systems" rather than "organs." Because of this emphasis on *function* rather than *structure*, Chinese anatomy can incorporate "organs" that have no physical substrate, such as the "triple-warmer." Rather like the *id*, *ego*, and *superego* in psychiatry, the triple-warmer has functions, but no specific location. Thus, for the learned physician the term "liver" does not mean the substance used to create pâté, but the functional sphere within the body that corresponds to wood, spring, morning, quickening, and germination.

The yin and yang, and the five phases, are closely related to the five "firm organs" (heart, spleen, lungs, liver, kidneys) and the five "hollow organs" (gall bladder, bladder, stomach, large intestines, small intestines). Residing deep within the body, the five firm organs, or viscera, are classified as yin and function as storage facilities, reservoirs, or depots. Located relatively close to the exterior of the body, the five hollow organs, or bowels, are classified as yang, and assumed the functions of elimination. Interactions among the various organs were made possible by linking them through a system of conduits rather like irrigation channels.

Because of the vital importance of irrigation to agriculture in China, the functions of the conduits in the body were often compared to the hydraulic works maintained by the government. For example, the "triple-warmer" was analogous to officials who were charged with planning the construction of ditches and sluices. The organs, like the officials of the state, must dutifully assist one another. Thus, when the system functioned harmoniously, the heart acted with insight and understanding like the king's minister, while the liver acted like the military leader responsible for strategic planning.

The system of fivefold correspondences could have created an embarrassing discrepancy between medical philosophy and medical practice, because acupuncture and moxibustion had become standardized around a system of six pair of conduits or acupuncture tracts. The problem was resolved by adding the "pericardium" or heart-enclosing network and the triple-warmer to the list of firm and hollow organs, respectively.

Despite considerable debate about various details, there is little argument about the fact that Chinese scholars accepted the relationship between the heart and pulse and the circulation of the blood long before these concepts were incorporated into Western science and medicine by William Harvey (1578–1657) in the seventeenth century. Westerners generally coped with the challenge to Harveian originality by dismissing Chinese concepts of the circulation as obscure mysticism "improved" by loose translation. Philosophical arguments, rather than dissection, presumably led Chinese physicians to the concept of the ceaseless, circular movements of blood and "energy" within the body's network of channels. Although the *Nei Ching* assumes that the movement of blood is controlled by the heart and the movement of energy by the lungs, scholars disagree as to the meaning and the implications of the terms that are generally translated as blood and energy. In any case, in contrast to Western doctors, Chinese physicians rejected the practice of bloodletting, which was an important component of Western medicine up to the early twentieth century.

Within this philosophical system, disease was basically ascribed to an imbalance of yin and yang, resulting in a disorder of one of the five phases, expressed as a dysfunction of the corresponding organ and the organs controlled by the injured organ. Therefore, all therapies were directed towards restoration of the state of harmony. In accordance with the fivefold system, the *Nei Ching* described five methods of treatment: curing the spirit by living in harmony with the universe, dietary management, acupuncture, drugs, and treatment of the bowels and viscera, blood and breath. In prescribing any preventive or therapeutic regimen, the physician had to carefully consider the influence of geography, climate, and local customs.

According to the Yellow Emperor and his Minister, in a previous golden age, human beings practiced temperance and lived in harmony with nature for over 100 vigorous years. Later, people disregarded the ways of nature and became feeble, short-lived, and subject to many diseases. For example, the people of the East ate fish and craved salt; this diet injured the blood and caused ulcers. Winds, or "noxious airs," caused much illness because they disturbed the harmony of yin and yang in the body. Generally, winds caused chills and fevers, but specific winds associated with the changing seasons were linked to particular dangers. Disturbances of the harmonious relationship between mind and body could also cause illness.

For diagnosis and prognosis, the Chinese physician relied on *sphygmology*, a very complicated examination of the pulse. Because of the intimate connection between the tracts and vessels through which yang and yin flowed, the study of yin in the blood could reveal problems of yang in the tracts. Thus, by listening to the waves of blood generated by the heartbeat, the physician could detect disease in various parts of the body. The physician was expected to study some 50 pulses, recognize more than 200 variations, and know those that indicated the imminence of death. Pulses could be sharp as a hook, fine as a hair, dead as a rock, deep as a well, soft as a feather. The volume, strength, weakness, regularity, or irregularity of the pulse revealed the nature of the disease, whether it was chronic or acute, its cause and duration, and the prospects for death or recovery. Sphygmology revealed incipient illness and allowed the physician to prescribe preventive measures or manage the course of therapy. Other kinds of diagnostic clues might be necessary, especially when dealing with children. Through close inspection of the patient, the physician could find diagnostic clues in the sounds made by the patient when talking, moaning, laughing, or weeping, and the colors of various parts of the body. For example, inspection of the tongue could reveal 30 different shades of color that provided evidence of disease or the possibility of death.

Physicians also had to recognize various types of difficult and skeptical patients, such as those who were arrogant, miserly, addicted to overeating and dissipations, and those who had more faith in magicians and quacks than physicians. According to the teachings of Huang Ti, the great sages of ancient times did not treat those who were already ill. Instead, they gave the benefit of their instruction to those who were healthy, because seeking remedies after diseases had already developed was as foolish as waiting until a war broke out to cast weapons. In theory, superior physicians guided the healthy patient; inferior physicians treated the sick. While the scholar practiced preventive medicine and took no fee for his work, hordes of healers without scholarly pretensions—surgeons, apothecaries, magicians, fortunetellers, peddlers, and assorted quacks—were eager to collect fees and quite willing to serve sick and stupid patients. The typical practitioner was more interested in fees and favors than theories and philosophy.

Although the education and activities of physicians in the Imperial Service are hardly typical of the general practice of medicine in China, many interesting innovations are associated with the evolution of this institution. For example, the Institutions of the Chou indicate that during the Chou Dynasty (ca. 1122–255 B.C.) the government conducted yearly examinations of those who wished to practice medicine. Schools of medicine were established in almost every province, but most practitioners were trained by apprenticeship, and lower class healers were largely self-taught. For the Imperial Service, the salaries of successful applicants were determined by how well they had placed in the examinations. Rank and salary for physicians serving the government were determined by an analysis of their success rate. Physicians who cured all of their patients were ranked first class; the lowest grade contained those who could not cure more than 60% of their patients. This took into account the belief that half the patients would probably have recovered without any treatment at all. Veterinarians were also ranked according to their rate of successful treatments. The Chou Imperial Service included Food Physicians, Physicians for Simple Diseases, Ulcer Physicians (surgeons), Physicians for Animals, and the Chief-of-Physicians who supervised the others. Physicians for Simple Diseases were assigned the simple task of testing the five kinds of breaths, the five kinds of sounds, and the five colors to determine whether the patient was dead or alive.

The Imperial College of Medicine consisted of about 30 physicians attached to the Imperial palaces. Physician-scholars of the highest rank gave lectures on the classics to junior colleagues. These physicians had access to the Imperial Library's collection of 12,000 works on medicine and the natural sciences. Obviously, very few Chinese were served by the sages. Lowly practitioners of "public medicine" and "street medicine" far outnumbered those involved in "court medicine." A rather diffuse system of public assistance may have existed in theory, but it was never sufficiently funded to have a significant impact on the medical needs of the populace.

Patients who were more worried about demons and spirits than the five phases found their medical practitioners on street corners, along with astrologers, geomancers, and fortune-tellers, or made their way to monasteries where healers dispensed medical advice and amulets with equal enthusiasm. Protective measures for dealing with magical forces included charms, prayers, exorcisms, incantations, amulets, and talismans. A talisman might resemble an official Imperial document, except that the named official was a high ranking demon who ordered demons lower in the hierarchy to cease and desist from causing illness and misfortune.

Driving out demons might require drugs compounded from powerful poisons or highly odoriferous materials. To prevent the poison from killing the patient, the prescription or drug could be worn as a charm or burned as a fumigant. A worm spirit, known as the *ku*, figured prominently among the demon diseases described in both scholarly literature and folklore. Elaborate beliefs developed about the *ku* spirit, including the belief that the only way for the original victim to rid himself of the *ku* was to provide another host. *Ku* antidotes included prayers, charms, drugs, and centipedes because centipedes consume worms. Law codes show that belief in *ku* magic survived into the nineteenth century. The penalties for *ku* magic were quite severe, including bizarre methods of executing the criminal and his whole family.

Physicians with scholarly training or aspirations tried to separate their profession from magic and sorcery, but sometimes compromised by offering prescriptions that combined medicine with magic. One example of a "mixed prescription" used in treating digestive complaints consisted of magic characters written on thick, yellow paper with medicinal pigments. The prescription was burnt down to a powdery ash, which was added to hot water and taken as a medicinal tea.

Drug lore, herbal medicine, and magical practices are essentially universal aspects of traditional and ancient medical systems. Chinese medicine is unique in the development of the techniques known as *acupuncture* and *moxibustion* and the sophisticated rationalizations that justified these very ancient practices. Both acupuncture and moxibustion could be used to restore the free flow of yin and yang that was essential to health. For at least 2500 years, acupuncture, the art of inserting needles at specific points on the surface of the body, has been a part of Chinese medicine. Moxa or moxibustion, a related technique in which burning tinder made from the powdered leaves of *Artemisia vulgaris* (mugwort or wormwood) is applied to specific points on the skin, may be even older than the art of needling. Acupuncture has attained considerable notoriety, and a degree of acceptance in the West, whereas moxibustion has been largely ignored. Although moxibustion may produce burns and scars, practitioners claim that the pain is not an "unpleasant pain." Skeptics find it difficult to imagine a burn associated with a "pleasant pain."

The goddesses Scarlet and White are said to have given the secret of acupuncture to the Yellow Emperor, who then devised nine kinds of needles from flint and bone. According to obscure and fragmentary references to the use of pointed stones to open abscesses and cure disease in China's semi-legendary past, marvelous needle-like stones were found at the foot of a jade-crowned mountain. Unfortunately, the series of steps leading from opening abscesses with sharp stones to the sophisticated system described in the *Nei Ching* remains obscure.

In the *Nei Ching*, the total number of acupuncture points is said to be 365. However, Huang Ti seems to name only about 160 acu-points. The number 365 may represent a theoretically perfect system symbolically correlating the number of degrees in the celestial circle, the days in the year, and the number of parts in the human body. In its mature form, the acupuncture system consists of 12 main tracts, each of which carries the name of the solid or hollow organ with which it is primarily associated. The system also accommodates various auxiliary tracts and organs. For outside observers, the most disconcerting thing about the system is probably the lack of any obvious relationship between the organ or disorder being treated and the site of the therapeutic acu-point.

Theoretically, acupuncture provides access to the system of tracts which distribute "energy" by allowing the practitioner to insert needles into specific points where the tracts are close to the surface. The idea that the acupuncturist can extract, purge, or drain "energy" by needling points on the tracts might be analogous to the empirical foundations of the system, i.e. draining pus or blood from an abscess. Certain sensations are supposed to occur when the needling is effective. These include warmth, numbness, and a feeling that the sensation is traveling slowly up or down the limbs or trunk. If the points are the primeval basis of the system, it is possible that the subjective sensation of a response traveling through the body gave rise to the idea of the acu-tracts. Much ink has been spilled in Western writings as to whether the tracts enjoy a true physical existence. While the existence of the tracts remains a fundamental principle of classical Chinese medicine, it is possible that the system of vessels is a mnemonic device by which physicians learned to associate physiological phenomena with empirically determined points.

According to scholar-physicians, the most dangerous aspect of the acupuncture system is the possibility of misuse by ignorant practitioners. The system includes a number of "forbidden points"; needling at forbidden points could cause serious derangements or death. Such points are reminiscent of the Indian system of marmas.

Aspiring physicians could learn the art of acupuncture from illustrated manuals or by practicing on bronze models or wooden dolls. Ultimately, the practitioner had to leave behind idealized models and work with patients who were large or small, fat or thin, male or female, old or young. Acupuncture was especially recommended for all disorders involving an excess of yang; moxibustion was thought preferable when yin was in excess. However, the relationships among yin and yang, the five phases, and the organs are so complex that use of either method could be justified.

Moxa was generally recommended for chronic conditions, such as tuberculosis, bronchitis, and general weakness, but it was also used for toothache, headache, gout, diarrhea, and some psychological disorders. Pao Ku, wife of the alchemist Ko Hung (254–334), was famous for treating skin diseases with moxibustion. Officials of seventh-century China would not undertake a journey unless protected against foreign diseases and snake bites by moxa. In China today physicians are experimenting with moxa for influenza, chronic bronchitis, and infections of the respiratory tract.

Today there are professional acupuncturists in Russia, Europe, and North and South America, as well Asia. Nevertheless, the legal status of practitioners in some countries remains ambiguous. Until the 1970s, the legal status of acupuncture was of no interest to the American medical community. Traditional Chinese medicine was dismissed as pure quackery. What could be more bizarre than killing pain by sticking needles into people? (Unless, of course, the needles were hypodermics full of narcotics.) However, Westerners already on the "fringes" of science eagerly welcomed acupuncturists into the fold.

As acupuncturists increasingly gained both notoriety and clients, the medical profession began to pay attention. The American Medical Association took the position that acupuncture was "folklore," not science, but that it could only be performed by licensed physicians because needling was an invasive procedure. In 1975, Nevada became the first state to establish a state Board of Chinese Medicine and require that physicians and nonphysicians pass an examination to qualify as licensed acupuncturists. Although other states have established licensing procedures, conditions governing the practice of Chinese medicine remain chaotic.

DRUG LORE AND DIETETICS

According to the *Nei Ching*, a diet balanced in accordance with the fivefold system of correspondences would promote health and longevity, strengthen the body, and drive out disease. Indeed, the first remedies were found among the herbs, trees, plants, and animals that served as foods. On the other hand, medical theory and folklore taught that normally harmless foods could be dangerous under special circumstances, such as pregnancy. For example, if a pregnant woman consumed hare meat, the child would be mute and lack an upper lip; eating mule meat would cause a difficult birth. Dietary physicians also warned against eating foods that were spoiled, meat that moved by itself, and apricots with two pits.

The use of tea illustrates the overlap between "foods" and "drugs." For about 6000 years, the Chinese have been making a beverage from the leaves of the tea shrub. Tea contains small amounts of nutrients, but it is rich in physiologically active alkaloids, including caffeine, theobromine, and theophylline. Perhaps the most important health aspect of tea drinking is the use of vigorously boiling water.

Where dietary measures were insufficient, physicians could turn to a large collection of drugs. However, because the nature of drugs was often violent, scholars warned against recklessly prescribing or consuming them. Nevertheless, when brought together in the proper proportions, drugs could accomplish wonderful effects. With about 5000 native plants in common use as medicinal herbs, Chinese scientists today are attempting to isolate specific active ingredients from traditional remedies. For guidance in this quest, they often turn to the *Pen-ts'ao kang mu*, an encyclopedic study of medicine, pharmacology, botany, and zoology, compiled by Li Shih-Chen (1518–1593), China's "prince of pharmacists." Published by his sons in 1596, Li's great work included close to 2000 drugs from the animal, vegetable, and mineral kingdoms, more than 8000 prescriptions, references to over 900 other texts, and more than 1000 illustrations.

The three classes of drugs—vegetable, animal, and mineral—were said to correspond to heaven, man, and earth. Animal organs were highly regarded as sources of remarkable "vital principles," such as tiger liver for courage and snake flesh for endurance. Among the more prosaic and presumably effective remedies were sea horse powder and seaweed, which are good sources of iodine and iron, for goiter and chronic fatigue, and ephedra for lung diseases and asthma. Generally, the Chinese exhibited admirable skepticism about foreign "wonder drugs," but expeditions were launched in response to rumors that Indian physicians had discovered the "herb of immortality." Many Chinese regarded ginseng, the "queen of medicinal herbs," as little short of the Indian wonder drug.

Medical therapy can take two general forms: healers can attempt to strengthen the body so that it can heal and defend itself, or they can attack the agents of disease directly. The primary goal of Chinese medicine is to enhance the regulatory effectiveness of the body's "executive center" and restore the normal "balance of energy." The reverence inspired by ginseng illustrates the classical Chinese approach to healing. Ginseng has been used as a tonic, rejuvenator, and aphrodisiac. Modern researchers have called it an "adaptogen," a substance that increases resistance to all forms of stress, from disease to misfortune. Li Shih-Chen described an ingenious experiment to demonstrate the effect of ginseng: select two men of about the same size and have both run a certain distance after giving ginseng to one of the runners. At the end of the test, the man given ginseng would not be fatigued, whereas the other man would suffer shortness of breath. The same test could be used to determine whether a given specimen was genuine ginseng.

The gathering and preparation of ginseng was surrounded by a rich body of folklore, ritual, and myth. Because metal implements would destroy the virtues of a ginseng root, only wooden knives and earthenware pots could be used in its preparation. Wild ginseng was said to assume a luminous glow and walk about at night disguised as a bird or a child who lured ginseng hunters to their death. China's emperors established ginseng monopolies, appointed their own gatherers, and kept the best roots for themselves.

Classical sources describe ginseng as a tonic for the five viscera; it opens the heart, quiets fears, expels evil effluvia, improves the understanding, invigorates the body, and prolongs life. Ginseng is prescribed for fatigue, anemia, insomnia, arthritis, disorders of the nerves, lungs, and stomach, impotence, tuberculosis, and so forth. Ginseng is sometimes marketed as an aphrodisiac, but herbalists claim that it increases stamina and allows even very elderly men to become fathers, in addition to preventing graying, baldness, wrinkles, and age spots.

The Chinese materia medica also included typical examples of "dreckapothecary"—remedies made of noxious and repulsive ingredients such as dried salamander, donkey skin, medicinal urines, and human parts and products. Smallpox inoculation can be considered an example of a "medicine derived from man." To provide protection against 40 forms of the "heavenly blossom disease," doctors collected the crusts from pustules of a mild case of smallpox. The powdered material was blown into the nostrils; males snorted the powder through the left nostril and females via the right side.

A different approach to human health was developed by Chinese alchemists. Alchemy generally conjures up the image of mystics vainly attempting to turn lead into gold. Alchemists were, however, also associated with the search for the "elixir of life." Chinese alchemists were obsessed with both the theoretical aspects of gold-making (and gold-faking) and "macrobiotics," the search for the great drugs of well-being and immortality. Ko Hung (ca. 300 A.D.), an eminent alchemist, Taoist adept, and physician, taught that minor elixirs could provide protection from ghosts, wild animals, and digestive disorders. More powerful elixirs could restore those who had just died, while superior elixirs would confer immortality.

In contrast to India, surgery generally remained outside the domain of China's scholarly medicine. Presumably, reluctance to mutilate the body and the lack of dissection-based anatomy inhibited the development of surgery in China, but such obstacles are not necessarily insurmountable. Indeed, forensic medicine reached a high level of sophistication in China. When confronted with this line of inquiry, Chinese scholars contended that the efficacy of their preventive and therapeutic medicine obviated the need for surgical interventions. Nevertheless, Chinese history provides accounts of remarkable physicians who performed miraculous operations. Interactions between China and India during the transmission of Buddhism may have inspired such stories, although they did not lead to the integration of surgery into classical Chinese medical traditions.

The most famous Chinese surgeon, Hua T'o (ca.145–208), was credited with the invention of anesthetic drugs, medicinal baths, hydrotherapy, and medical gymnastics. Master of acupuncture and a brilliant diagnostician, Hua T'o could cure migraine headaches with one acupuncture needle. One of his most ususual cases involved a patient suffering from a painful tumor between the eyes. When the physician skillfully opened the tumor, a canary flew out and the patient was completely cured. Although canary-filled tumors may be a rarity in medical practice, headaches and chronic pains are not, and Hua T'o usually treated such disorders with acupuncture. Perhaps he had discovered the principle of acupuncture anesthesia. Unfortunately, when consulted by the Emperor Ts'ao Ts'ao, the surgeon recommended trepanation as a treatment for his intractable headaches. Ts'ao Ts'ao suspected an assassination plot and ordered Hua T'o's execution.

According to tradition, of all the operations invented by Hua T'o the only one to survive and enjoy considerable usage was his technique for castration, which was needed to provide the eunuchs favored as civil servants and palace attendants. The lost secrets of Hua T'o supposedly included ointments which prevented and cured infection as well as his miraculous anesthetics.

Although the nations surrounding China were heavily influenced by Chinese philosophy, the direction of exchange is sometimes obscure. Shared medical traditions have different creation myths among the peoples who fell within the Chinese cultural sphere. For example, in Korea the invention of moxa and stone acupuncture needles was attributed to Tan Gun, the legendary founder of that nation. During the Edo period (1603–1868), European surgery flourished in Japan, while Europeans were fascinated with acupuncture, moxa, and Oriental drug lore.

MEDICAL PRACTICE IN MODERN CHINA

When the People's Republic of China was founded in 1949, Chairman Mao Zedong declared that Chinese medicine and pharmacology constituted a great treasure-house that must be explored and improved. Mao's call for the use of both traditional and Western-trained doctors was a pragmatic response to China's desperate need to expand the pool of health-care workers to serve 540 million people, typically living in impoverished, rural areas without public health, sanitary, or medical facilities. Circumstances impelled China into a unique experiment in the integration of past and present, East and West. The revival of traditional medicine was launched with the ''Great Leap Forward'' (1958–59), gained momentum during the Cultural Revolution (1966–69), and peaked in the aftermath of this ideological frenzy.

China's new health-care system is committed to dealing with common and recurrent diseases, public health work, and the eradication of major endemic disorders. The motto of the Chinese medical system is: ''Extinguish the four pests!'' The official four pests are rats, flies, mosquitoes, and bedbugs, but cockroaches, fleas, lice, and snails were also targeted for eradication.

By the 1980s, China had firmly established a health-care system that is generally conceded to be a model for other developing countries. Sensitive measures of health in Shanghai in 1980, such as infant mortality and life expectancy at birth, compared favorably with New York City. Western visitors have been impressed by Chinese experiments in medical education and restructuring of medical practice which obliged the physician to share diagnositic and therapeutic responsibilities with a newly empowered array of lay and paramedical personnel. Preventive medicine and basic primary health care is provided by legions of ''barefoot doctors,'' midwives, and nurses. The use of herbal remedies, acupuncture, and moxibustion remain the core of medical practice, but traditional doctors also study microbiology and pharmacology. China's colleges of Western medicine include training in traditional medicine.

The development of acupuncture anesthesia has been hailed in China as another great leap forward. Inspired by the thoughts of Chairman Mao, hospital workers began to wonder whether the pain-relieving effects of needling that had long been exploited in the treatment of postsurgical distress might be used in place of chemical anesthetics during surgery. Even in China the prospect of acupuncture anesthesia was greeted with some skepticism, but in the 1960s acupuncture anesthesia was being used in about 60% of all surgical operations in China. Modern acupuncturists argue that, in contrast to chemical anesthesia, needling allows the body to mobilize all its defense mechanisms while maintaining normal physiological functions.

The revival of interest in acupuncture and herbalism has not been accompanied by commensurate attention to the theoretical basis of traditional medicine. Separated from its theoretical framework, Chinese medicine could become merely a hodge-podge of empirical remedies, rather than a philosophical system capable of providing guidance and inspiration for both patients and practitioners. However, Chinese philosophy and medicine have always demonstrated a remarkable capacity for syncretism and adaptation. China is a living civilization, in which the traditional arts are intimately linked to their modern counterparts. Perhaps the thoughts of both Huang Ti and Chairman Mao will be integrated into a new synthesis of Chinese medical thought, still reflecting the goals of the Three Celestial Emperors for the perfection of Chinese medicine as a source of peace of mind, health, strength, and long life.

SUGGESTED READINGS

Asthana, Shashi (1985). *Pre-Harappan Cultures of India and the Borderlands*. New Delhi: Books and Books.

Bag, A. K. (1985). *Science and Civilization in India*. Vol. 1: Harappan Period. New Delhi: Navrang.

Bannerman, Robert H., Burton, John, and Ch'en Wen-Chieh, eds. (1983). *Traditional Medicine and Health Care Coverage: A Reader for Health Administrators and Practitioners*. Geneva: World Health Organization.

Basham, A. L. (1955). *The Wonder That Was India: A Survey of the Culture of the Indian Sub-continent Before the Coming of the Muslims*. New York: Evergreen.

Bhatia, S. L. (1972). *Medical Science in Ancient India*. Bangalore, India: Bangalore University.

Bishagratna, Kaviraj Kunja Lal, trans. and ed. (1907–1911). *An English Translation of the Sushruta Samhita*. 3 vols. India: Chowkhamba Sanskrit Series Office, repr. 1963.

Bowers, John Z. (1981). *When the Twain Meet: The Rise of Western Medicine in Japan*. Baltimore, MD: Johns Hopkins University Press.

Bowers, John Z., Hess, J. W., and Sivin, Nathan, eds. (1989). *Science and Medicine in Twentieth-Century China*. Research and Education. Ann Arbor, MI: University of Michigan Press.

Caraka (1976). *Agnivesa's Caraka Samhita.* (Text with English translation and critical exposition by Dr. Ram Karan Sharma and Vaidya Bhagwan Dash.) Varanasi, India: Chowkhamba Sanskrit Series Office.

Chang, Kwang-chih (1987). *The Archaeology of Ancient China.* New Haven, CT: Yale University Press.

Chang, Kwang-chih, ed. (1977). *Food in Chinese Culture: Anthropological and Historical Perspectives.* New Haven, CT: Yale University Press.

Chopra, Ram Nath (1933). *Indigenous Drugs of India, Their Medical and Economic Aspects.* Calcutta: Art Press.

Chopra, Ram Nath, Nayer, S. L., and Chopra, I. C. (1956). *Glossary of Indian Medicinal Plants.* New Delhi: Council of Scientific and Industrial Research.

Eliot, Robert Henry (1918). *The Indian Operation of Couching for Cataract.* New York: Paul B. Hoeber.

Epler, D. C. (1980). Bloodletting in Early Chinese Medicine and Its Relation to the Origin of Acupuncture. *Bulletin of the History of Medicine* 54: 337–367.

Filliozat, Jean (1964). *The Classical Doctrine of Indian Medicine.* Delhi: Munshi Ram Manohar Lal Oriental Publishers.

Fu Wei-Kang (1972). The Development of Acupuncture in China. In *Acupuncture Anesthesia.* Peking: Foreign Languages Press, pp. 20–26.

Gupta, Nagendra Nath Sen (1901–1907). *The Ayurvedic System of Medicine,* 3 vols. Calcutta: K. R. Chatterjee.

Hall, A. J. (1974). A Lady from China's Past. *National Geographic Magazine* 145(5): 660–681.

Ho, Ping-Ti (1976). *The Cradle of the East. An Inquiry into the Indigenous Origins of Techniques and Ideas of Neolithic and Early Historic China, 5000–1000 B.C.* Chicago: University of Chicago Press.

Hoernle, August F. R. (1907). *Studies in the Medicine of Ancient India.* Oxford, England: Clarendon Press.

Horn, Joshua S. (1969). *Away With All Pests. An English Surgeon in People's China: 1954–1969.* New York: Monthly Review Press.

Hsiao, Yang (1976). The Making of a Peasant Doctor. Peking: Foreign Languages Press.

Hu, Shiu-ying (1980). *An Enumeration of Chinese Materia Medica.* Seattle: University of Washington Press.

Huard, P., and Wong, M. (1968). *Chinese Medicine.* New York: McGraw-Hill Book Co.

Jaggi, O. P. (1980). *Western Medicine in India: Social Impact.* History of Science, Technology, and Medicine in India, vol. 15. Delhi: Atma Ram & Sons.

Jeffery, Roger (1988). *The Politics of Health in India.* University California Press.

Keightley, David N. (1985). *Sources of Shang History: The Oracle-Bone Inscriptions of Bronze Age China.* Berkeley, CA: University of California Press.

Keswani, Nandkumar H. (1970). Medical Education in India Since Ancient Times, in C.D. O'Malley, ed. *The History of Medical Education.* Berkeley, CA: University of California Press.

Kleinman, Arthur (1980). *Patients and Healers in the Context of Culture.* Berkeley, CA: University of California Press.

Krippner, Stanley, and Rubin, Daniel, eds. (1972). *Galaxies of Life: The Human Aura in Acupuncture and Kirlian Photography*. New York: An Interface Book.

Kutumbiah, Pudipeddy (1962). *Ancient Indian Medicine*. Bombay: Orient Longmans.

Leslie, Charles, ed. (1976). *Asian Medical Systems. A Comparative Study*. Berkeley: University of California Press.

Li Shih-Chen (1973). *Chinese Medical Herbs*. (Trans. by F. Porter Smith and G. A. Stuart.) San Francisco: Georgetown Press.

Li, C. P. (1974). *Chinese Herbal Medicine*. National Institutes of Health, Washington, DC: Department of Health, Education, and Welfare Publication No. NIH 75-732.

Liu, Yanchi (1988). *The Essential Book of Traditional Chinese Medicine*. Vol. 1: Theory. Vol. 2: Clinical Practice. New York: Columbia University Press.

Lu, Gwei-Djen, and Needham, Joseph (1980). *Celestial Lancets. A History and Rationale of Acupuncture and Moxa*. Cambridge, England: Cambridge University Press.

Marshall, Sir John (1931). *Mohenjo Daro and the Indus Civilisation*. 3 vols. London: Arthur Probsthain, Ltd, for the Archaeological Survey of India.

McCormick, James P. and Parascandola, John (1982). Dragon Bones and Drugstores. The Interaction of Pharmacy and Paleontology in the Search for Early Man in China. *Pharmacy in History* 23(2): 55-70.

McDowell, F. (1969). Ancient Ear Lobe and Rhinoplastic Operations in India. *Plastic and Reconstructive Surgery* 43(5): 515-522.

McKnight, Brian E. (1981). *The Washing Away of Wrongs: Forensic Medicine in Thirteenth-Century China*. Ann Arbor, MI: University of Michigan Press.

Mehta, Dharma Deva (1974). *Positive Sciences in the Vedas*. India: Arnold Heinemann Publishers.

Meulenbeld, G. J. and Wujastyk, D., eds. (1987). *Studies on Indian Medical History*. Groningen, Sweden: Egbert Forsten Publ.

Mukhopadhyaya, Girindranath N. (1913-14). *The Surgical Instruments of the Hindus*. 2 vols. Calcutta: University of Calcutta Press.

Mukhopadhyaya, Girindranath N. (1923-9). *History of Indian Medicine*. 3 vols. Calcutta: University of Calcutta Press (reprinted New Delhi, 1974).

Nakayama, Shigeru and Sivin, N., eds. (1973). *Chinese Science: Explorations of an Ancient Tradition*. Cambridge, MA: MIT Press.

Needham, Joseph (1954-). *Science and Civilization in China*. Cambridge, England: Cambridge University Press.

Needham, Joseph (1981). *Science in Traditional China: A Comparative Perspective*. Cambridge, MA: Harvard University Press.

Porkert, M. (1974). *The Theoretical Foundations of Chinese Medicine: System of Correspondence*. Cambridge, MA: MIT Press.

Porkert, Manfred, with Ullmann, Christian (1988). *Chinese Medicine: Its History, Philosophy and Practice, and Why it May One Day Dominate the Medicine of the West*. New York: William Morrow.

Ramachandra Rao, S. K., ed. (1985) *Encyclopaedia of Indian Medicine*. Bombay: Popular Prakashan.

Ray, P., Gupta, H., and Roy, Mira (1980). *Susruta Samhita: A Scientific Synopsis*. New Delhi: Indian National Science Academy.

Reddy, D. V. Subba (1966). *Glimpses of Health and Medicine in Mauryan Empire.* Hyderabad: Osmania Medical College.

Rinpoche, R. (1976). *Tibetan Medicine.* Berkeley, CA: University of California Press.

Rosenthal, Marilynn M. (1987). *Health Care in the People's Republic of China: Moving Toward Modernization.* Boulder, CO: Westview.

Salmon, Warren J., ed. (1984). *Alternative Medicines, Popular and Policy Perspectives.* New York: Tavistock Publications.

Schafer, Edward (1985). *The Golden Peaches of Samarkand: A Study of T'ang Exotics.* Berkeley, CA: University of California Press.

Sidel, V. W. and Sidel, R. (1974). *Serve the People: Observations on Medicine and Mental Health in the People's Republic of China.* Boston: Beacon.

Singhal, G. D. and Guru, L. V., eds. (1973). *Anatomical and Obstetric Considerations in Ancient Indian Surgery* (Ancient Indian Surgery Series. G. D. Singhal, general editor). Varanasi, India: Bharata Manisha.

Sivin, Nathan, ed. (1987). *Traditional Medicine in Contemporary China.* Ann Arbor, MI: University of Michigan Center for Chinese Studies.

Tamba, Yasuyori (1986). *The Essentials of Medicine in Ancient China and Japan.* Yasuyori Tamba's *Ishimpo* (trans., intro., and annotations by Emil Ch.H. Hsia, Ilza Veith, and Robert H. Geertsma). Leiden: E.J. Brill.

Unschuld, Paul U. (1979). The Chinese reception of Indian medicine in the first millennium A.D. *Bulletin of the History of Medicine* 53: 329–345.

Unschuld, Paul U. (1985). *Medicine in China. A History of Ideas.* Berkeley, CA: University of California Press.

Unschuld, Paul U. (1985). *Medicine in China. A History of Pharmaceutics.* Berkeley, CA: University of California Press.

Unschuld, Paul U. (1986). *Nan-Ching: Classic of Difficult Issues* (trans. and annotated by Paul U. Unschuld). Berkeley, CA: University of California Press.

Veith, I. (1972). *The Yellow Emperor's Classic of Internal Medicine* (introduction and trans. by Ilza Veith). Berkeley: University of California Press.

Wasson, R. G. (1968). *Soma, Divine Mushroom of Immortality.* New York: Harcourt, Brace & World.

Wheeler, Mortimer (1966). *Civilizations of the Indus Valley and Beyond.* London: Thames and Hudson.

Woodroffe, Sir John (Arthur Avalon) (1918). *The Serpent Power. Two Works on Laya-yoga.* (trans. from Sanskrit). New York: Dover, (reprinted 1974).

Zimmermann, Francis (1988). *The Jungle and the Aroma of Meats. An Ecological Theme in Hindu Medicine.* Berkeley, CA: University of California Press.

Zysk, Kenneth G. (1985). *Religious Healing in the Vedas.* Philadelphia, PA: The American Philosophical Society.

GRECO-ROMAN MEDICINE

I n contrast to the gradual evolution found in Egyptian, Indian, and Chinese history, Greek civilization seems to have emerged suddenly, much like Athena from the head of Zeus. Although this impression is certainly false, it is difficult to correct because of the paucity of material from the earliest stages of Greek history. Whatever their origins, the intellectual traditions established in ancient Greece provided the foundations of Western philosophy, science, and medicine. The early history of Greece can be divided into two periods: the Mycenaean, from about 1500 to the catastrophic fall of Mycenaean civilization about 1100 B.C., and the so-called Dark Ages from about 1100 to 800 B.C. Very little information from the latter period has survived, nor is it clear what forces led to the collapse of the early phase of Greek civilization. As in India, the chaos of invasions, internal unrest, and warfare was remembered in the form of myths and legends transmitted by means of poems and songs. Much of this material was gathered into great epic cycles by poets of the ninth century B.C. Two great epics known as the *Illiad* and the *Odyssey* have survived; they are traditionally attributed to the ninth-century poet known as Homer. Deep within these great stories of life and death, gods and heroes, strange lands, home, and family, are encoded ancient concepts of epidemic disease, the vital functions of the body, the treatment of wounds, and the roles played by physicians, surgeons, priests, and gods.

Greek medicine, as portrayed by Homer, was already an ancient and noble art. Apollo appears as the most powerful of the god-physicians; he could cause epidemic disease as a form of punishment and revive and heal the wounded. Priests, seers, and dream readers dealt with the mysterious plagues and pestilences attributed to the gods. When angered, the gods could cause physical and mental disorders, but they might also provide sedatives and antidotes to save those they favored. In the *Iliad*, the skillful physician is praised as a man more valuable than many others; indeed, the skills of the physician were as praiseworthy as those of the seer or the maker of weapons. Given the large number of war injuries so poignantly described by Homer, skillful doctors were desperately needed. In some instances, however, warriors treated their comrades or bravely extracted arrows from their own limbs. Wound infection, traumatic fever, and deaths due to secondary hemorrhage were probably uncommon, because the wounded rarely lingered long enough to develop complications. The mortality rate among the wounded was close to 80%.

Medical treatment in the *Iliad* was generally free of magical practices, but when medicine failed, healers might resort to magical practices such as reciting an incantation to stop a hemorrhage. Sometimes the surgeon would suck the site of a wound, perhaps as an attempt to draw out poisons or some ''evil influence'' in the blood. After washing the wound with warm water, physicians applied soothing drugs and consoled or distracted the patient with wine, pleasant stories, or songs. Unfortunately for the Greek warriors, their physicians did not know the secret of Helen's famous Egyptian potion, *nepenthe*, which could dispel pain and strife and erase the memory of disease and sorrow. Indeed, the specific identities of most of the drugs referred to by Homer are obscure, although various sources suggest that the soothing agents, secret potions, and fumigants used by the healers and priests of this time period probably included warm water, wine, oil, honey, sulfur, saffron, resins, and opium.

In the *Iliad*, Asclepius, who was said to be the son of Apollo, appears as heroic warrior and ''blameless physician.'' According to Homer, Chiron, the wise and noble centaur, taught Asclepius the secret of the drugs that relieve pain and stop bleeding. The sons of Asclepius were also warriors and healers; their special talents presage the future division of the healing art into medicine and surgery. The cunning hands of Machaon could heal all kinds of wounds, but it was Podalirius who understood hidden diseases and their cure. When Machaon was wounded, his wound was simply washed and sprinkled with grated goat cheese and barley meal. The methods Machaon used to cure the hero Menelaus were only slightly more complicated. After extracting the arrow that had pierced the hero's belt, Machaon sucked out the blood and sprinkled the wound with soothing remedies that Chiron had given to Asclepius.

The magical and shamanistic practices that once flourished in Greece left their traces in myths, poems, and ceremonial practices, such as the annual festival held in honor of Melampus, founder of a long line of seers, who had acquired knowledge of divination from Egypt. Combining elements of purification and ''psychotherapy'' with strong purgative drugs, Melampus was able to cure disorders ranging from impotence to insanity. Melampus is also said to have taught Orpheus how to use healing drugs.

The Orpheus myth incorporates the shamanistic elements of the healer who enters the underworld in pursuit of a departed soul, and the dismemberment and reconstitution of the shaman. As the son of the muse Calliope, Orpheus possessed skill in healing and supernatural musical gifts. When his beloved wife Eurydice died, Orpheus descended into Hades where he charmed the gods of the underworld into allowing him to bring back her soul. However, contrary to the explicit instructions he had received from the gods, Orpheus turned to look at Eurydice before she had completed the journey from Hades back to the earth. Once again, Orpheus had lost Eurydice. Orpheus was later torn to pieces by wine-crazed followers of Dionysus, but his spirit continued to sing as his head floated to Lesbos.

Shamanistic, religious, and empirical approaches to healing are, as we have seen, universal aspects of the history of medicine. Where Greek medicine appears to be unique is in the development of a body of medical theory associated with natural philosophy, that is, a strong secular tradition of free enquiry, or what would now be called science. Unlike previous civilizations, the Greeks were not primarily organized around agriculture and a strong central government or priesthood. The city-state became their unit of organization, and because Greece was relatively overpopulated in relation to cultivatable land, trade, colonization, industry, and shipping were encouraged. The earliest Greek natural philosophers were profoundly interested in the natural world and the search for explanations of how and why the world and human beings came to be formed and organized as they were. Natural philosophy developed first, not in the Athens of Socrates, Plato, and Aristotle, but on the Aegean fringes of the mainland of Asia Minor. By the sixth century B.C., Greek philosophers were attempting to explain the workings of the universe in terms of everyday experience and by analogies with craft processes rather than divine interventions and supernatural agencies.

Many of these early philosophers are known only through a few fragments of their work, but enough has survived to reveal their ingenious theories as the seed crystals that were to stimulate the subsequent development of our concepts of physics, astronomy, biology, and medicine.

Pythagoras of Samos (ca. 530 B.C.) is said to have been the first Greek philosopher with a special interest in medical subjects. Although the Pythagorean concept of a universe composed of opposite qualities is reminiscent of Chinese yin-yang philosophy, the Pythagorean approach was apparently inspired by mathematical inquiries. Just as numbers formed the two categories "odd" and "even," so could all things be divided into pairs of opposites. The harmony, or balancing of pairs of qualities, such as hot and cold, moist and dry, was especially important in matters of health and disease.

Although the medical theories of Alcmaeon of Croton (ca. 500 B.C.) have much in common with those of Pythagoras, the exact relationship between them is uncertain. Both Alcmaeon and Pythagoras believed that pairs of opposites were the first principles of existence. Alcmaeon taught that health was a harmonious blending of each of the qualities with its appropriate opposite. Disease occurs when one member of a pair appears in excess; an excess of heat causes fever, an excess of cold causes chills. Alcmaeon is said to have formulated the idea that the systematic dissection of animals would provide a means of understanding the nature of living beings.

A paradoxical blend of philosophy and mysticism is part of the legacy of Empedocles (ca. 500–430 B.C.). Echoing themes common to shamanism, Empedocles boasted that he could heal the sick, rejuvenate the aged, raise the dead, and control wind and weather. Numerous references to him in later medical writings suggest great fame and success as a healer, but it was his theory of the four elements that became a major theme in the history of medicine. According to Empedocles, all things were composed of various mixtures of four primary and eternal elements: air, earth, water, and fire. Changes and transformations in the cosmos and the human body were simply reflections of the mixing and unmixing of the eternal elements.

HIPPOCRATES AND THE HIPPOCRATIC TRADITION

Many of the early Greek philosophers and medical writers have been largely forgotten, but the name Hippocrates has become synonymous with the phrase "Father of Medicine." The establishment of medicine as an art, a science, and a profession of profound value and dignity has been associated with the life and work of the physician who is said to have lived from about 460 to 361 B.C. Yet surprisingly little is known about his life. Indeed, some historians argue that Hippocrates was neither the author of the Hippocratic collection nor even a real person. For the sake of simplicity, we shall use the name Hippocrates for the historical person and for any of the authors of the collection of medical works known as the Hippocratic collection; physicians who practiced medicine in accordance with the principles ascribed to Hippocrates will be referred to as Hippocratic physicians.

Although Hippocrates was widely praised and respected in antiquity, many of the most fascinating biographical details were supplied several centuries after his death. According to ancient biographers, Hippocrates was born on the island of Cos, lived a long, exemplary life, and died in Larissa when 95 or 110 years old. In genealogical tables constructed by his later admirers, Hippocrates traced his ancestry back to Asclepius on his father's side and to Hercules on the maternal side. Plato and Aristotle speak of Hippocrates with respect, despite the fact that he taught medicine for a fee. Not all ancient writers praised Hippocrates; the great healer was accused of burning down the medical library at Cos in order to eliminate competing medical traditions. An even more unflattering story accused Hippocrates of plagiarizing the prescriptions of Asclepius before destroying the god's temple and claiming clinical medicine as his

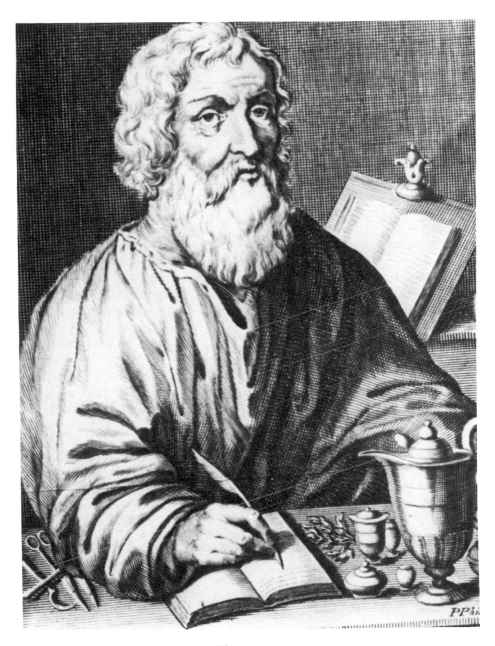

Hippocrates

own invention. Another legend says that the great doctor never thought about collecting fees and was always ready to admit his errors.

Whatever uncertainty there may be about Hippocrates himself, the collection of 50–70 essays and texts attributed to him is undoubtedly the foundation of Western medicine. Ironically, as scholars gained more information about the writings of the ancients, they had to admit to less and less certainty about distinctions between the "genuine" and the "spurious" works of Hippocrates. Nevertheless, throughout the centuries of Greek, Roman, and medieval times, the texts that had made their way into the Hippocratic collection remained authoritative and worthy of study, interpretation, and commentary. In Western history, Hippocratic medicine is revered for its emphasis on the patient instead of the disease, observation rather than theory, respect for facts and experience rather than philosophical systems, "expectative therapy," as opposed to "active intervention," and the Hippocratic motto: "At least do no harm."

One of the most important and characteristic expressions of Hippocratic medicine is the text *On Ancient Medicine*. A major thesis of this work is that nature itself has strong healing forces. The purpose of the physician, therefore, was to cultivate techniques that would work in harmony with natural healing forces to restore the body to a harmonious balance. Other characteristics of the Hippocratic texts are perceptive descriptions of the symptoms of various diseases, insights into medical geography and anthropology, and explorations of the idea that health and disease can be affected by climate, social institutions, religion, and government.

By assigning explanations for the phenomena of health and disease to nature and reason, the Hippocratic physician rejected superstition, divination, and magic. In other words, if the world was uniform and natural, all phenomena were equally part of nature. If the gods were responsible for any particular phenomenon, they were equally responsible for all phenomena. Thus, Nature was everywhere both natural and divine. While Hippocrates ridiculed the deceptions practiced in the name of religious healing, he was not opposed to prayer and piety. "Prayer indeed is good," Hippocrates conceded, "but while calling on the gods one must oneself lend a hand." Skepticism was also appropriate with respect to the claims of philosophers, because, according to Hippocrates, one could learn more about Nature through the proper study of medicine than from philosophy alone.

The true physician understood that disease was a natural process, not the result of possession, supernatural agents, or punishment sent by the gods. Disease could be interpreted as punishment only in the sense that one could be punished for transgressing against nature by improper behaviors. Thus, to care for his patient, the physician must understand the individual constitution and determine how health was related to food, drink, and mode of life.

In a fundamental sense, *dietetics* was the basis of the art of healing. According to Hippocrates, human beings could not consume the rough food suitable for other animals; thus, the first cook was the first physician. From such crude beginnings, the craft of medicine developed as people empirically discovered which diets and regimens were appropriate in sickness and in health. As medicine became more sophisticated, physicians became skilled and knowledgeable craftsmen. As knowledge about human beings and nature accumulated, philosophers propounded theories about the nature of human life and derived therapeutic systems from their theories. Medicine and philosophy interacted to their mutual benefit, but Hippocrates refused to be bound by any rigid medical dogma, or therapeutic system, such as treatment by "similars" or "opposites." The experienced physician knew that some diseases were cured by the use of opposites and others by the use of similars. That is, some "hot" diseases might be cured by cooling medicine, but others might require warming remedies.

While the physician must not be bound by philosophical systems, neither should a practitioner of the art ever act as an unthinking technician. The true physician understood the principles guiding his course of action in each case, as related to the nature of man, disease, diagnosis, remedies, and treatment. Moreover, this display of medical knowledge and proper behavior helped win the trust of the patient. In the absence of legally recognized professional qualifications and standards, virtually anyone could claim to be a physician. Thus, to compete with quacks and magicians, the physician had to prove that medicine was an art and science that could promote health and heal the sick. Complaints about ignorant physicians and outright quacks appear in many Hippocratic texts, suggesting that the profession was already plagued by impostors who were bringing disrepute to the art.

The related problems of professional recognition, standards, and ethical obligations are addressed by several Hippocratic texts. However, the brief text known as the "Hippocratic Oath" which has made the name Hippocrates part of popular discourse may have been composed and popularized long after the death of Hippocrates. There are many uncertainties about the origins, usage, purpose, and meaning of the Oath, but there is considerable evidence to suggest that the document honored as the nucleus of Western medical ethics was actually a "neo-Pythagorean manifesto." Moreover, the Oath seems to have had a very limited influence until it proved to be a suitable bridge between antiquity and Christianity.

Although the Oath includes the promise to practice medicine for the benefit of the patient, a prohibition against giving anyone a lethal drug, or using medicine to cause the sick any danger or injury, it is primarily a private contract between the new physician and his teacher, not, as commonly assumed, a promise from practitioner to patient. Moreover, the Greeks had no official medical practice act to enforce such contracts. Presumably, it was love of the art, joined with love of man and fear of dishonor, more than the swearing of oaths that made the Hippocratic physician conform to the highest standards of medical etiquette.

The fact that the Hippocratic Oath prohibits prescribing a "destructive pessary" may be the best evidence that the Oath represents the precepts of the Pythagoreans rather than physicians in general, because this prohibition was essentially unique to that sect. The ancients generally accepted abortion and infanticide as means of population control. Surgical abortions were condemned because they were more dangerous than childbirth; moreover, unwanted infants could be "exposed." Midwives dealt with normal childbirth, abortion, and assorted "female complaints," but the physician could prescribe appropriate fumigations, fomentations, washes, and pessaries.

Within the ethical framework of antiquity, very different patterns of medical treatment were considered appropriate to the rich and the poor. For the rich, the aesthetic pursuit of health was far more significant than the mere absence of disease. Striving for optimum health required a complex, time-consuming regimen and presupposed that the patient could assign complete control over food, drink, exercise, rest, and other aspects of life to the most skillful physician. Patients who were free but poor could expect an intermediate kind of medical care. The poor must either recover quickly and resume their work or die and so be relieved of all further troubles. The Hippocratic texts indicate that the physician did not necessarily refuse to treat slaves, or to adapt dietetic therapy to the needs of the poor. But various sources suggest that, for the most part, the treatment of slaves was rather like veterinary medicine and was carried out by the doctor's servants.

Ideally, the Hippocratic physician did not practice medicine merely for the sake of money, but like other craftsmen who had perfected their skills, the physician was entitled to a fee for his services. The ethical physician was expected to consider the status of the patient in determining the size of the fee. He was not to argue about fees before treating a patient, especially in acute illnesses, because extra worries might interfere with the patient's recovery. Patients without money who hoped to find the ideal physician described in the texts were well advised to remember the Greek proverb: "There is no skill where there is no reward."

Many noble sentiments about the practice of medicine and the relief of suffering are found in the Hippocratic texts, but the limits of the art were sharply defined. Knowing that it was impossible to cure all patients, the Hippocratic physician had to determine which patients would die, in order to avoid blame. Unlike the temple priest, who had the authority of the gods to protect and excuse him, the secular physician was in a peculiar, highly vulnerable position. Only skill, success, and a rigorous committment to the ethical standards of the profession protected the physician. The physician was a craftsman, judged by his patients, not by a peer review committee, according to the results of his art.

The modern physician and patient are especially eager for a precise *diagnosis*—the ceremonial naming of the disease—but this was of little importance to the Hippocratic physician. His main preoccupation was *prognosis*, which meant not only predicting the future course of the disease, but also providing a history of the illness. This recital of past and future was a factor in impressing the patient and family with the knowledge and skill of the physician. It also was essential in predicting crises and deaths so that no blame would be attached to the physician when they occurred.

THE NATURE OF DISEASE AND THE DOCTRINE OF THE FOUR HUMORS

For Hippocrates, disease was not a localized phenomenon, but a disturbance affecting the whole person through some imbalance in the four humors. The four humors—blood, phlegm, black bile, and yellow bile—and the four associated qualities—hot, cold, moist, and dry—in the *microcosm* or small world of the human body reflect the four elements—earth, air, fire, and water—that make up the *macrocosm* or universe. Various texts in the Hippocratic collection offer observations and theoretical rationalizations concerning the relationship between health and disease and the humors, qualities, and elements; sometimes these explanations are obscure and inconsistent.

Health is the result of the harmonious balance and blending of the four humors. An excess of one of the humors results in a *dyscrasia*, or abnormal mixture. Particular

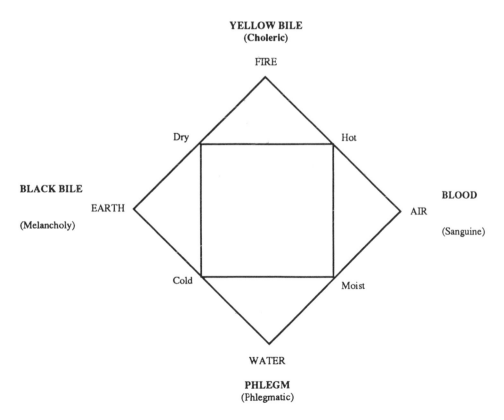

The four humors and four elements

temperaments were associated with a relative abundance of each humor; the sanguine, phlegmatic, choleric (or bilious), and melancholic temperaments are roughly equivalent to different personality types, and suggest vulnerability to characteristic disorders.

Although the four humors are theoretically related to the four elements, the physician could also justify their existence in term of certain common observations. It is important to remember that until very recent times the only ''analytic laboratory'' available to the physician was that made up of the five senses; in other words, the nose was the first chemist. All of the patient's excretions, secretions, and effluvia had to be studied directly by sense perception. As a ''thought experiment'' we might reflect upon the condition of clotted blood in terms of the theory of the four humors: the darkest part of the clot corresponds to black bile, the serum above the clot is apparently yellow bile, and the light material at the top is phlegm. Alternatively, phlegm is equivalent to mucus, yellow bile is the bitter fluid stored in the gall bladder, and black bile is the dark material sometimes found in vomit, urine, and excrement (a sign of internal bleeding).

According to Hippocratic theory, the processes by which the body fought off disease were essentially exaggerated forms of normal physiological functions. Disease was a state in which the organism experienced a greater degree of difficulty in mastering the environment. Restoration of humoral equilibrium proceeded through stages in which the crude or morbid matter in the humors ripened sufficiently to be eliminated through secretions, excretions, or hemorrhages during a *crisis*, which might end in recovery or death. In acute diseases, the elimination of morbid matter generally occurred on certain ''critical days.'' Charting the course of a disease by means of the ''critical days'' and characteristic patterns of signs and symptoms, the physician could expedite the process with proper treatments.

Humoral pathology provided a natural explanation for even the most feared and dreaded mental as well as physical illnesses. Indeed, no treatise in the Hippocratic collection provides a more powerful and timeless attack on ignorance and superstition than *On the Sacred Disease*. Hippocrates declared that even the Sacred Disease, which we know as epilepsy, was no more sacred or divine than any other illness; like any disease, it arose from a natural cause. But, frightened by the specter of recurrent, unpredictable seizures in otherwise healthy individuals, ignorant people attributed the disease to the gods. Those who ''cured'' the disease by magical means supported the false belief in its ''sacred'' nature. Prescribing purifications, incantations, and bizarre rituals, quacks were quick to claim credit when the patient seemed to recover. When the patient relapsed or died, they blamed their failures on the gods. The Hippocratic physician regarded such deceptive practices as impious and unholy.

Humoral theory could explain epilepsy, just as it explained any other disease. (Indeed, one of the problems with this theory is the ease with which it explains *everything*.) Hippocrates suggested that a child could be born with epilepsy if both father and mother were phlegmatic, because excess phlegm might accumulate during gestation and injure the fetal brain. Many ancient philosophers considered the heart to be the seat of consciousness, but Hippocrates assigned that role to the brain. Therefore, it followed that afflictions of the brain produced the most dangerous diseases. Attitudes towards epilepsy can be seen as a sort of litmus test for the achievement of enlightened attitudes towards the sick. Unfortunately, Hippocratic medicine was no match for the prejudice and fear surrounding epilepsy and other supposedly mysterious afflictions. Throughout history, remedies for epilepsy have included magical and superstitious practices, as well as dangerous and futile treatments ranging from bleeding and cauterization to trephination and hysterectomy.

Humoral theory rationalized a therapeutic regimen designed to assist the natural healing tendency, by bleeding, purging, and regulating the diet in order to remove morbid humors and prevent the formation of additional bad humors. Given the dangers thought to lurk in most foods, the physician might allow no foods stronger than barley water, hydromel (honey and water), or oxymel (vinegar, honey, and water). Despite the Hippocratric preference for mild and simple remedies, Greek physicians could prescribe a wide array of drugs which were administered in many forms, including poultices, ointments, pessaries, pills, and suppositories. Remedies might contain pleasant ingredients like cinnamon and saffron, but a diuretic for dropsical patients included three cantharides beetles, minus the heads, feet, and wings. ("Spanish fly" or "blistering beetle" has long been used as a diuretic or putative aphrodisiac when taken internally and as a skin irritant when applied externally.)

Some cases called for stronger methods such as cupping, scarification, venesection, cauterization, and other forms of surgery. For the most part, "surgery" meant the treatment of wounds, fractures, dislocations, and other traumatic injuries. In such cases, the practitioner's experience and acquired skills were all important because Hippocratic physicians did not perform postmortems. Thus, only observations on injured patients and general knowledge of animal anatomy illuminated the "black box" that was the human body. In managing wounds and ulcers, simple remedies and cleanliness allowed healing to proceed with a minimum of inflammation and pus. Various kinds of herbs, boiled in water or mixed with wine, were used as cleansing agents and wound dressings. Remedies containing certain minerals, such as salts or oxides of copper and lead, were used to dry and soothe wounds.

When necessary, the physician could suture wounds, trephine the skull, perform artificial pneumothorax (collapsing the lung), and insert tents and tubes into the chest cavity to drain pus, as recorded in various case histories presented in *On Disease* and *On Wounds*. However, when wounds became gangrenous, the physician was reluctant to intervene, because amputation could lead to death from shock and bleeding. Similarly, the physician preferred to treat abscesses with medicines that would encourage them to discharge spontaneously rather than open them with the knife.

Whatever success the Hippocratic physician may have had in caring for individual patients, the plague that struck Athens in 430 B.C. during the Peloponnesian War demonstrated that his skills were no match for epidemic disease. The most vivid portrait of the plague was recorded not by a physician, but by the Athenian general Thucydides. The general felt well qualified to write about the plague, because he had survived the disease and had seen many cases.

After a year relatively free of disease, the plague attacked Athens so suddenly that at first the people thought that the wells had been poisoned. Healthy people were seized with headaches, sneezing, hoarseness, pain in the chest, coughing, vomiting, and spasms. Although the body was not very hot to the touch, it became reddish and livid, with the eruption of blisters and ulcers. Death usually occurred on the seventh or ninth day, but in those who lingered on, the disease descended into the bowels, where it led to ulceration, diarrhea, and death.

The most terrible feature of the disease, according to Thucydides, was the depression that fell upon the afflicted and the general abandonment of morality and custom. Only those who had survived an attack of the disease were willing to nurse the sick, because the same person was never stricken twice. Despite Thucydides' vivid description, the exact nature of the disease is obscure. Among the diagnoses that have been offered are typhus, scarlet fever, bubonic plague, smallpox, measles, and anthrax. Whatever this pestilence may have been, it provides a striking example of the recurrent theme of social disintegration linked to war and epidemic disease.

Physicians were also challenged by endemic diseases such as malaria that insidiously attacked the Mediterranean region. The causative agent and mechanism of transmission for malaria were not discovered until the late nineteenth century, but the association between marshes and malarial fevers was suspected by the time of Hippocrates. When first introduced into a region, malaria may cause deadly epidemics, but the disease generally becomes stubbornly endemic. Instead of killing or immunizing its victims, malaria makes them more susceptible to further attacks and to other diseases. People learn to associate seasonal activity and all forms of exertion with attacks of fever. The chronic loss of agricultural productivity leads to malnutrition, famine, and further susceptibility to disease. Malaria has been called the greatest killer in all of human history and a major factor in the decline of Greek science, art, and literature.

THE CULT OF ASCLEPIUS

Although Hippocrates is the dominant figure in modern accounts of Greek medicine, in antiquity the good doctor shared the stage with the healer who began his career as the "blameless physician" in the *Iliad*. It was during the age of Hippocrates, not the age of Homer, that Asclepius was elevated to the status of a god. As we have seen in our discussions of other ancient civilizations, what we call modern scientific medicine has not totally displaced traditional, folk, or religious approaches to healing. Thus, it should not be surprising that what we call rational Hippocratic medicine did not totally displace religious medicine in the ancient world. For chronic, episodic, and unpredictable conditions, such as arthritis, gout, migraine headache, epilepsy, malaria, impotence, and infertility, when patients felt that the physician was ineffective, magicians and priests could always offer them hope and even the illusion of cure during the intervals between attacks. For some conditions, improvement or cure might indeed result from the combination of rest, fresh air, good diet, and suggestion encountered at the temples of Asclepius.

Over several centuries, while Greek science rose and fell, the cult of Asclepius spread throughout the Greek world, established itself in Rome, and only gradually gave ground to Christianity as arbiter of the meaning of disease and healing. Served by priests calling themselves Asclepiads (descendants of Asclepius), Asclepian temples were built at Cos, Cnidus, Epidaurus, and other sites blessed with springs of pure water and magnificent views. The god was often portrayed as accompanied by his daughters, Hygeia (hygiene) and Panacea (cure-all), and Telesphorus, the god of convalescence. Like Lourdes today, the temples were places for hopeful pilgrimages and miraculous cures. Information about temple medicine has come from studies of archaeological remains, votive tablets which record the stories of satisfied patients, models dipicting the organs healed at the temples, and references to temple magic in literary sources. Skeptics ridiculed the testimonies as deliberate forgeries or the ravings of hypochondriacs and noted that there would have been many more tablets if those who were not cured had made dedications.

Among the ruins of the temple at Epidaurus is a shrine dedicated to Hygeia, who may have been the original Greek goddess of health. Like the Chinese sages who would not treat the sick, Hygeia taught people to achieve health and longevity by proper behavior. Her independent cult was eventually subsumed by that of Asclepius, and her status was reduced from independent practitioner to physician's assistant.

In contrast to the Mesopotamian hero Gilgamesh, who lost the herb of healing to a snake, Asclepius received it from a sacred serpent. Thus, Aslepius was often portrayed with a snake coiled about his staff. The caduceus, the sign of the modern physician, which contains two snakes intertwined on a winged staff, seems to suggest increased snake-power, but it is actually closer to the magic wand of Mercury, the messenger of the gods and patron of thieves and merchants.

The Asclepiads boasted that all who entered the sanctuary were cured. Presumably, they achieved a perfect record by carefully selecting their patients. Temporary remissions and spontaneous recovery from psychosomatic complaints and self-limited diseases provide all medical systems with a large measure of success. The most important part of temple medicine was called "incubation," or temple sleep. Incubation was part of the ancient practice of seeking divine dreams of guidance after preliminary rites which might include fasting, prolonged isolation, and self-mutilation. Sleeping on an animal skin in front of an image of Asclepius was a rather mild form of this nearly universal ritual. Some patients reported instantaneous cures after being touched by the god, or licked by the sacred snakes and holy dogs that guarded the temple. Sometimes the god recommended simple remedies, such as vegetables for constipation, but he might also direct the patient to smear his eyes with blood or swim in icy rivers. Hope, rest, fresh air, and the power of suggestion probably cured many psychosomatic complaints, while religious rituals provided comfort where cure was impossible.

Women were not allowed to give birth within the grounds of the temple, but Asclepius accepted various obstetrical and gynecological challenges, especially infertility. As demonstrated by the testimonial of Ithmonice who asked the god if she could become pregnant with a daughter, supplicants had to be very careful in framing their requests. Asclepius asked Ithmonice whether she wanted anything else, but she could not imagine wanting more. After carrying the child in her womb for three years, Ithmonice came again to Asclepius. The god reminded her that she had only requested conception and had not mentioned delivery. However, he graciously granted her this new favor, and after she left the sacred precincts her daughter was born.

Patients praised the god for curing headaches, paralysis, general debility, and blindness. A man who claimed to have swallowed leeches and a woman who thought she had a worm in her belly testified to being cut open by the god, who removed the infestation and stitched up the incision. Even relatively minor problems might receive the god's attention. One man came to the temple for help because his neighbors made fun of his bald head. During temple sleep, the god anointed him with a drug that caused the growth of thick black hair.

THE AGE OF ALEXANDER

In the ancient world, Alexandria, the city in Egypt named for Alexander the Great (356–323 B.C.), represented wealth and stability, a fusion of the ancient lore of Egypt and the most dynamic elements of Greek civilization. Among the greatest treasures of the city were its museum and library. The scholars who worked at the museum and library, under the sponsorship of the rulers of Alexandria, participated in an unprecedented intellectual experiment. According to some estimates, the Alexandrian Library contained at least 700,000 manuscripts. The librarians collected, confiscated, copied, and edited many manuscripts, including the texts now known as the Hippocratic collection. The magnificent facilities of the museum are said to have included a luxurious promenade, observatory, zoological and botanical gardens, lecture halls, and rooms for research. To encourage the exchange of ideas, the scholars took their meals together at the great hall of the museum; the meals were free and the salaries of the professors were tax exempt.

Many sciences flourished at Alexandria, although research was primarily oriented towards fields with practical applications, such as medicine and engineering. Medical

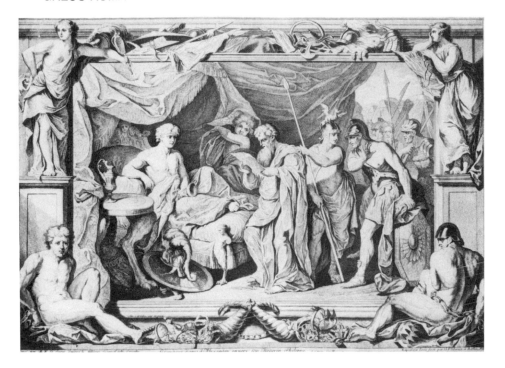

Alexander the Great and his physician

experts were expected to supervise city and army sanitation and train military doctors. Most important, for a brief and rare interval, the practice of human dissection was not only tolerated, but actively encouraged. Alexandrian scientists helped establish two of the major themes of Western medical theory: first, that systematic dissection provides essential information about structure and function; second, that this knowledge is valuable in and of itself, even if it provides little or nothing of immediate practical value to clinical medicine, patient care, or public health. Unfortunately, so little direct information about the Alexandrian era has been preserved that the exact relationship of its best known anatomists to the city of Alexandria, the museum, and each other remains obscure and controversial.

For medical science, the Hellenistic period (roughly the time between the death of Alexander the Great to about 30 B.C., when the Romans annexed Egypt) is most notable for the work of Herophilis and Erasistratus. Both were skillful anatomists who eagerly exploited the opportunity to conduct studies of human bodies. However, it is not clear whether the anatomists of this era performed some of their studies on living human beings or confined themselves to post-mortems. The vivisection question remains unanswered because the writings of the Hellenistic anatomists have not survived. Accusations made hundreds of years later cannot be taken as definitive proof, but there is no particular reason to believe that the authorities would have prohibited this form of death and dissection, especially if the victims were criminals or prisoners of war. Certainly, the atrocities committed in the twentieth century provide no evidence that "civilized" human beings have lost the capacity for cruelty. Nevertheless, even though conditions during the Hellenistic era made systematic anatomical research possible, human dissection was still offensive to prevailing standards, evoked superstitious dread, and created an evil reputation for Herophilus and Erasistratus.

Little is known about the life of Herophilus, who is said to have flourished about 300 B.C., except that he was a student of Praxagoras and the author of many lost medical treatises. There is no direct evidence that Herophilus was a member of the museum, or that he did his dissections and research at the museum. Nevertheless, his access to human cadavers, and perhaps live prisoners, was probably the result of governmental intervention. Herophilus had a special interest in the arteries and their pulsations. In addition to describing the pulse in terms of size, strength, rate, and rhythm, Herophilus attempted to measure pulse rate with an improved water clock invented by Alexandrian scientists. In his studies of the nervous system, Herophilus far surpassed all his predecessors and vigorously disputed Aristotle's claim that the heart was the most important organ of the body and the seat of intelligence. In place of the four humors, Herophilus seems to have favored a theory of four life-guarding faculties: a nourishing faculty in the liver and digestive organs; a warming power in the heart; a sensitive or perceptive faculty in the nerves; and a rational or intellectual faculty in the brain.

For Herophilus, health was the greatest good. The aphorism, "Wisdom and art, strength and wealth, all are useless without health," is attributed to him; so too is: "The best physician is the one who is able to differentiate the possible from the impossible." He urged physicians to be familiar with dietetics, gymnastics, drugs, surgery, and obstetrics. As practitioners, his followers favored bleeding and the aggressive use of complex drug mixtures.

The most unusual of Herophilus' pupils was said to be the Athenian woman Agnodice. Distressed by the suffering of women who would rather die than be examined by a male physician, Agnodice disguised herself as a man in order to study and practice medicine. When her subterfuge was discovered, she was prosecuted for violating laws that prohibited women from studying medicine. Her loyal patients are said to have warned her male prosecutors that they would by seen as the cruel enemies of womankind if they condemned to death their only female physician. Agnodice's semi-legendary story has been used for hundreds of years to rally support for the education of medical women. Indeed, in writing about the diseases of women, Hippocrates had pointed to the problem epitomized in the story of Agnodice; women were often so reluctant to discuss their problems with male physicians that simple illnesses became incurable.

Like Hippocrates, Erasistratus (ca. 310–250 B.C.) was born into a medical family. Little is known of his life, other than his decision to give up medical practice to devote himself to the study of anatomy and physiology. In a fragment preserved by Galen, Erasistratus spoke of the joys of research that made the investigator ready to devote day and night to solving every aspect of a scientific problem. Erasistratus may have carried out his research at the court of Antiochus in Seleucia, rather than at Alexandria, but the research interests of Herophilus and Erasistratus were strikingly similar.

Ancient sources credit Erasistratus with over 50 books, including specialized texts on fevers, bloodletting, paralysis, drugs, poisons, and dietetics. Skeptical of many standard therapeutic methods and Hippocratic humorology, Erasistratus invoked a mechanical, localized concept of physiological and pathological phenomena based on the atomic theory of Democritus. Erasistratus saw the body tissues as a network of veins, arteries, and nerves. Having traced the veins, arteries, and nerves to the finest subdivisions visible to the naked eye, Erasistratus postulated further ramifications beyond the limits of vision. Erasistratus invented the concept of *parenchyma* (material poured in between the network of vessels) to complete his picture of the fine structure of the body.

Erasistratus supported the traditional idea that the function of the arteries was to carry *pneuma* (air) rather than blood. The veins and arteries were thought to be separate systems with the arteries originating from the heart and the veins from the liver. However, some rationalization was needed to account for the fact that blood spurted from torn arteries. Erasistratus argued that although the veins and arteries were separate in healthy, uninjured individuals, there were tiny collapsed or closed connections between them. When an artery was damaged, air escaped and venous blood was forced through the connections between the veins and arteries, because nature abhorred a vacuum.

According to Erasistratus, disease was due to *plethora*, an excess of blood from undigested foods which tended to become putrid. When local excesses of blood accumulated in the veins, the tissues were damaged and blood spilled over from the veins into the arteries. Given this theoretical framework, the logical objective of therapy was to diminish the plethora of blood. In addition to emetics, diuretics, massage, hot baths, and general starvation, Erasistratus ingeniously induced ''local starvation'' by tying tight bandages around the limbs to trap blood until the diseased part had used up its plethora.

A story concerning Erasistratus as a medical practitioner demonstrates his powers of observation and insight into the relationship between afflictions of mind and body. When Seleucus, one of Alexander's generals, married a woman named Stratonice, his son Antiochus fell in love with his stepmother. Desperately trying to hide his feelings, the young man fell ill and seemed close to death. Many physicians had failed to help him when Erasistratus determined that an affliction of the mind had weakened the body through sympathetic relationships. Erasistratus decided to observe his patient's physiological reactions to the people who visited him. The stammering, blushing, palpitations, and pallor that followed each visit by Stratonice revealed the source of his illness. Erasistratus reasoned that although we can consciously conceal our thoughts, their influence on the body cannot be controlled. This story was retold many times for its literary merit, but the medical insights were largely ignored. Similar incidents appear in the biographies of other great physicians, including Galen and Avicenna, and were often cited in the extensive medieval and Renaissance literature concerning love-sickness.

For 200 years, the Museum of Alexandria enjoyed a high level of creativity in science, technology, and medicine, and trained physicians, engineers, geographers, astronomers, and mathematicians. Although it is difficult to assess the vitality of such a complex institution, there is some evidence that medical science was already slipping into a state of decline during the time of Herophilus and Erasistratus. Much of the deterioration of scientific research during the Hellenistic era can be blamed on the tumultuous political climate, but scientists and scholars seem to have been undermining the structural supports of their own houses of learning by attacking rival schools of thought, or by leaving Alexandria to establish new schools elsewhere.

The decline of the Alexandrian tradition was not limited to medical science. Little of the work at the museum or library survived. The first major episode in the destruction of the library occurred in 48 B.C. during the riots sparked by the arrival of Julius Caesar and some 3000 legionnaires. Later, Christian leaders encouraged the destruction of the Temple of Muses and other pagan institutions. According to tradition, in 395 A.D., the last scholar at the museum, a woman philosopher and mathematician named Hypatia, was dragged out of the museum by Christian mobs and beaten to death. The Muslim conquest of the city in the seventh century (642–646) resulted in the final destruction of the library and the loss of its precious manuscripts.

MEDICINE IN THE ROMAN WORLD

The Roman Empire was a complex and vigorous combination of Greek and Roman cultural elements forged through centuries of war. Originally a republic of yeoman farmers, rather than merchants and adventurers like the Greeks, the Romans retained a preference for the practical over the abstract and a tendency to idealize the pastoral life even as they constructed cities unprecedented in size and complexity. They excelled in the arts of warfare and administration, as well as architecture, engineering, public health and hygiene. Roman writers boasted that their ancestors had lived without physicians, though not without medicine, being well endowed with folk remedies, healing deities, and diviners. Presumably, the remarkable sanitary engineering achievements that are associated with Republican and Imperial Rome played an important, if unacknowledged, role in maintaining the public health as well as the "good life." When comparing Rome to Greece, critics characterized the Romans as a people without art, literature, science, or philosophy. However, they certainly could not be called a people without gods.

Like the Egyptians, the Romans accumulated deities for all major organs and functions of the body. Nevertheless, they still had room in their hearts for new gods, especially when the old ones seemed unwilling or unable to do their duty. In 293 B.C., when the indigenous gods were unable to stop a pestilence decimating Rome, the elders consulted Asclepius at the Temple of Epidaurus. While the Asclepiads conferred with the Roman delegation, a sacred snake emerged from the temple and boarded the Roman ship; this was taken as a omen that the Greek god intended to go to the aid of the Romans. Thus, in 292 B.C. the cult of Asclepius was established in Rome; an Asclepian temple was constructed on a site selected by the snake and the epidemic ended. Greek physicians were as eager to come to the aid of Rome as the sacred snake, but the reception they received was not always quite as warm as that given to Asclepius.

The Romans did not condemn the practice of medicine, but they regarded it as unethical to charge fees for treating the sick. Cato the Elder (234–149 B.C.) denounced Greek physicians as the worst enemies of Rome and accused them of poisoning and murdering their clients. Indeed, some of the Greek practitioners were greedy quacks, incompetents, and adventurers who used their knowledge to mislead patients, manufacture poisons, and enter into conspiracies. Cato was fighting a losing battle, for Rome had been increasingly susceptible to Greek influences since the fourth century B.C.; the introduction of the cult of Asclepius and the coming of Greek physicians were indicative of this trend.

Traditionally, the head of the Roman household was expected to supervise the medical affairs of his family, slaves, and animals. The actual practice of medicine, however, was regarded as a menial craft suitable only for slaves and women. A Roman gentleman like Cato was aware of many traditional remedies, but his favorite was cabbage, which might even be superior to chicken soup because, in addition to being harmless, cabbage is a good source of vitamin C. In any case, Cato lived to the ripe old age of 84 during an era when the average life expectancy was about 25 years.

The writings of other Romans, almost by definition nonphysicians, reflect valuable insights into problems of hygiene, sanitation, water supplies, and public health, especially the importance of water supplies and sewage disposal. Rome obtained its water from a variety of supply systems, but the aqueducts that were bringing millions of gallons of water into Rome by the second century B.C. are generally thought of as the quintessentially Roman solution to one of the major problems faced by urban planners. Lower quality water was considered acceptable for the bathing establishments found in every Roman city and almost every town. Admission fees for the public baths were generally minimal, but the Romans should be credited with the establishment of the pay toilet. While public latrines were generally incorporated into the bathing establishments, independent public latrines were usually sited in the busiest sections of cities and towns. An admirable concern for the purity of water and the sanitary location of dwelling places is found in various well known texts from this period such as *On Architecture* (ca. 27 B.C.) by Vitruvius. Also of interest is the suggestion by Marcus Terentius Varro (116–27 B.C.) that swampy places might be inhabited by extremely minute animals that could enter the body through the mouth and nose and cause serious illnesses. While wealthy Romans could take advantage of the architectural and engineering skills for which Roman civilization is justly famous, and retreat to peaceful, quiet country villas, most people lived in crowded, unsanitary houses lacking proper kitchens and heating systems, piped water, private baths or latrines.

Most Romans relied on a combination of magic and folklore to fight disease. Each home had its special shrine and stock of herbal remedies. Appropriate rituals accompanied the administration of all drugs and the performance of any operation. It was an economical arrangement in which the same remedies, charms, and prayers served both man and beast.

Despite Cato's warnings, as Roman society became more complex and prosperous, or, as critics might say, less virtuous and self-sufficient, Roman citizens were soon eagerly consulting physicians who promoted a medical regimen more sophisticated than cabbages and incantations. The career of Asclepiades (ca. 124–50 B.C.) provides an instructive example of how Greek medicine was adapted to a Roman clientele. Asclepiades originally came to Rome as a rhetorician, but saw better prospects in medicine. Asclepiades offered treatments that worked "swiftly, safely, and sweetly." While his theoretical approach was mechanistic, in practice Asclepiades advised a sensible regimen, with individualized attention to diet, rest, and exercise, and simple remedies, such as wine, water, and cold baths, rather than bleeding and purging. Although Asclepiades provided a form of medical practice that could be successful in the framework of Roman expectations, suspicion and skepticism remained, as seen in the writings of Pliny the Elder (23–79 A.D.).

Like Cato before him, Pliny the Elder, exemplary Roman gentleman and author of one of the major encyclopedic works of antiquity, was suspicious of professional physicians. According to Pliny, physicians were incompetent, greedy, superfluous, and dangerous; Greek physicians had seduced Roman citizens away from their traditional herbal remedies and had contributed to the degeneration of Roman society. Pliny complained that physicians learned their craft by experimenting on patients and denounced them as the only men who could kill with impunity and then blame death on the victim for having failed to obey professional advice.

Pliny's *Natural History* provides an invaluable, far-ranging, if unsystematic survey of the science, medicine, agriculture, industries, and arts of the late republic and early empire. In lauding the virtues of Rome's traditional herbal remedies, Pliny claimed that everything had been created for the sake of man, making the whole world an apothecary shop for those who understood Nature's simple prescriptions, such as wound dressings made of wine, vinegar, eggs, honey, powdered earthworms, and pig dung. Among the remedies suggested by Pliny are some containing pharmacologically active compounds, such as ephedron (a valuable source of ephedrine) for asthma, cough, and hemorrhage.

In contrast, Dioscorides (ca. 40–80 A.D.), compiler of the text now known as *De materia medica* (*The Materials of Medicine*), one of the first Western herbals, exemplifies the generalization that Roman medicine was usually carried out by Greek physicians. Little is known about the life of Dioscorides, except that he may have studied at Alexandria before serving as *medicus* to Nero's armies. "Military physician" is probably too specialized a translation for this term, because it is unlikely that the Roman legions of this period were accompanied by an organized medical or surgical staff. Indeed the Roman army may have had more formal provisions for the care of sick horses than sick soldiers. Nevertheless, throughout the existence of the Roman Empire, the activities of its armies and its medical personnel diffused Greco-Roman medicine throughout Europe, North Africa, and the eastern Mediterranean world. Serving the Roman legions gave Dioscorides the opportunity to travel widely and study many novel plant species, hundreds of which were not known to Hippocrates. An acute observer and keen naturalist, Dioscorides provided valuable information about medically useful plants, their place of origin, habitat, growth characteristics, and proper uses. Remedies were also made from minerals and animals. Pharmacologists who have examined the text have found recipes for valuable therapeutic agents, including analgesics, antiseptics, emetics, laxatives, strong purgatives, and so forth.

Many of the herbal remedies identified and classified by Dioscorides can be found on the spice shelf of the average modern kitchen. However, the medical properties assigned to today's common spices would surprise the modern cooks. For example, cinnamon and cassia were said to be valuable in the treatment of internal inflammations, venomous bites, runny nose, and menstrual disorders. It is easy to single out bizarre recipes, such as the remedy for malarial fevers made of bed bugs mixed with meat and beans, but recent studies of the text suggest that Dioscorides classified his remedies according to subtle and sophisticated criteria. That is, Dioscorides appears to have based his classifications on a drug affinity system rather than on traditional methods such as plant morphology, or habitat. This required precise knowledge of the plants in the field, their preparation, and their effects on a significant number of patients.

In contrast to Dioscorides' widely used herbal, the writings of Celsus (ca. 14–37 A.D.) were essentially forgotten until the rediscovery of his *De re medicina* in 1426 presented Renaissance scholars with a source of pure classical Latin; it was one of the first medical texts to be turned out on the new printing press. Celsus had undertaken an ambitious encyclopedic work in four parts: agriculture, medicine, rhetoric, and warfare, but *On Medicine* is the only part to have survived. Almost

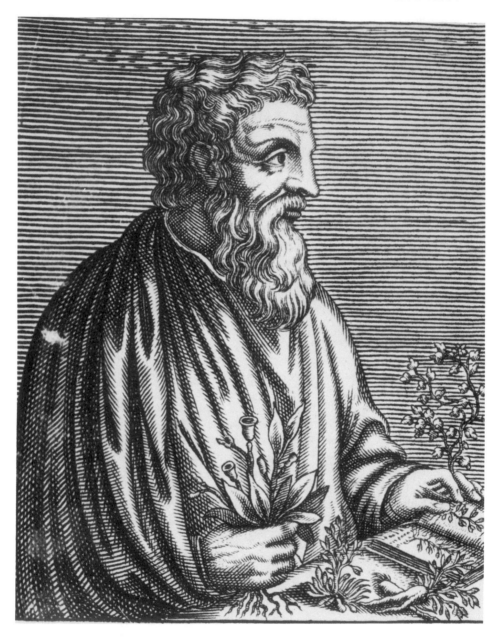

Dioscorides

nothing is known about the life of Celsus except for the fact that his contemporaries considered him a man of mediocre intellect. Although Celsus was clearly a master of organization, clarity, and style, the question of whether he composed, compiled, or plagiarized the text has been controversial.

In providing an historical context for his discussion of medicine, Celsus noted that the Greeks had cultivated the art of medicine more than any other people. The ancient Romans had enjoyed natural health, without medicine, because of their good habits. When they turned to lives of indolence and luxury, presumably under the malign influence of Greek culture, illness appeared and medicine became a necessity. After the death of Hippocrates, Greek medicine fragmented into various disputatious sects, some named after individuals and others, such as the Dogmatists, Empiricists, and Methodists, for their special approach to medical theory. Much about the origins, members, and practices of these sects remains obscure, but, thanks to Celsus, a fairly detailed account of the medical sects that flourished in his time can be reconstructed.

The Dogmatists emphasized the study of anatomy and claimed Erasistratus, Herophilus, and Hippocrates as their ancestors. Seeing medicine as practice, theory, and philosophy, the Dogmatists taught that physicians must study anatomy and physiology as well as the evident, immediate, and obscure causes of disease. Members of other sects might differ about many points, but they generally agreed that the Dogmatists were guilty of undue attention to speculative theories and a neglect of the practical goals of medicine.

Holding a more limited or more pragmatic view of the domain of medicine, the Empiricists believed it was necessary to understand evident or immediate causes, but that inquiry into obscure or ultimate causes was superfluous because nature was ultimately incomprehensible to human beings. In medicine, the physicians should be guided only by the test of experience as it answered the question: Does the patient get well? Some Empiricists claimed that the study of anatomy was totally useless for understanding living beings. They regarded human vivisection with horror and held it a crime to cause death in the name of the healing art. However, their emphasis on action was reflected in the excellent reputation of Empiric surgeons.

The Methodists believed that the body was composed of atoms and pores. Disease was the result of abnormal states of the pores due to excess tension or relaxation. Thus, knowledge of the three common conditions of the human body—the constricted, the lax, and the mixed—provided all the guidance the physician needed to treat his patients. Appropriate remedies relaxed or tightened the pores as needed. The Methodists claimed that their system was complete and that no further research into the causes of disease and therapeutics was necessary, but Juvenal, the satirist, said that the founder of the sect had killed more patients than he could count.

Wisely, Celsus concluded that no sect was wholly right or wrong. In seeking impartially for the truth it was necessary to recognize that some things which were not strictly pertinent to medical practice were valuable in stimulating and improving the mind of the practitioner. In dealing with cattle, horses, foreigners, and in the aftermath of disasters, it was sometimes necessary to look only at the simplest characteristics of disease. But a more sophisticated physician had to consider geography, climate, and the unique reactions of different patients.

Properly considered, the art of medicine could be divided into three parts: cure by diet (which in this case might better be translated by the term "lifestyle"); cure by medications; and cure by surgery. Experience taught the physician that standard medical practices were not equally appropriate to all patients. The art of medicine should be rational, Celsus concluded, and based on immediate causes, but ultimately medicine was an art that involved a great deal of guesswork. Anatomy was an important part of medical knowledge, but Celsus declared that vivisection was cruel and unnecessary. Students of medicine could learn about the positions and relations of the internal organs from dead bodies, but the practitioner should be alert to the possibility of gaining anatomical knowledge when "windows" of opportunity were presented to physicians engaged in treating the wounded.

While rejecting the Greek concept of the physician as necessary guide to proper regimen throughout life, Celsus considered it essential for every individual to acquire an understanding of the relationship between disease and the stages of life. Acute illnesses were the greatest threat to the young; chronic diseases threatened the old; the middle years were the safest, but disease could strike human beings at any age. Little could be added to Celsus' conclusion that the best prescription for a healthy life was one of variety and balance, proper rest and exercise, and avoidance of a self-indulgent obsession with medical advice.

Surgery, according to Celsus, should be the most satisfying field for the practitioner because it brought results that were more certain than treatment by drugs and diets. Physicians knew that some patients recovered without medicine, while some were not cured by the best medical treatment. In contrast, a cure effected by surgery was clearly the result of skill, not the result of supernatural forces or luck. After surgery, the physician must be ready to protect his patient from hemorrhage and the infections associated with the four cardinal signs of inflammation—*calor*, *rubor*, *dolor*, and *tumor* (heat, redness, pain, and swelling).

The Roman surgeon had mastered tools and techniques unknown to his Hippocratic predecessors, such as the use of the ligature for torn blood vessels and special spoons and dilators to remove barbed arrows from wounds. Roman surgeons could perform amputations and plastic surgery, as well as operations for bladder stones, goiter, hernia, cataract, and snake bites.

De re medicina provides a valuable survey of the medical and surgical practices of first-century Rome. However, during the European Middle Ages, Celsus and all the medical writers of antiquity, except Hippocrates, were eclipsed by the works of Galen of Pergamum (130–200 A.D.)

ON GALEN AND GALENISM

No other figure in the history of medicine has influenced concepts of anatomy, physiology, therapeutics, and philosophy as much as Galen, the physician known as

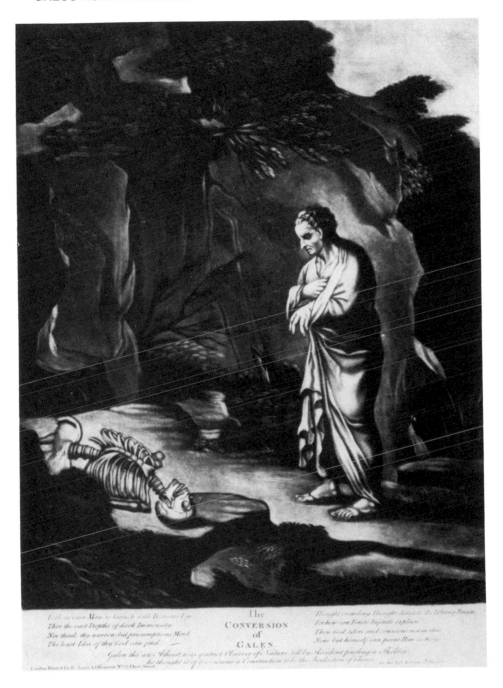

Galen

the Medical Pope of the Middle Ages and the mentor of Renaissance anatomists and physiologists. Galen left voluminous writings that touch on all the major medical, scientific, philosophical, ethical, and religious issues of his time. Contemporary admirers, including his patron the emperor Marcus Aurelius, called him the "First of Physicians and Philosophers." Other titles bestowed on Galen include "mulehead" and "windbag."

Galen was born in Pergamum, a city in Asia Minor, which saw itself as the cultural rival of Alexandria. In describing himself, Galen asserted that he had emulated the excellent character of his father, Nikon, a wealthy architect, known for his amiable and benevolent nature. Perhaps Galen could not totally dissociate himself from the example set by his mother, a bad-tempered woman, perpetually shouting at his father, provoking quarrels, and biting the servants. Galen had mastered mathematics and philosophy by the age of 14. Two years later, his father learned in a dream that his son was destined to become a physician. Galen began his medical studies at the age of 16 and composed at least three books while still a student at Pergamum. Later, in his advice to medical students and teachers Galen emphasized the importance of fostering a love of truth in the young that would inspire them to work day and night to learn all that had been written by the Ancients and to find ways of testing and proving such knowledge.

After the death of Nikon, Galen left Pergamum to continue his medical education with a series of teachers in Smyrna, Corinth, and Alexandria. On returning to Pergamum at the age of 28 after years of study and travel, Galen was appointed physician to the gladiators. Although he also worked at the Temple of Asclepius and established a flourishing private practice, within a few years Galen again became restless. In 161 he arrived in Rome where through good fortune, brilliant diagnoses, and miraculous cures he soon attracted many influential patients, patrons, and admirers. During this period, Galen engaged in public anatomical lectures, demonstrations, and disputes, and composed some of his major anatomical and physiological texts. Tired of the atmosphere in Rome, and aware of the danger of an epidemic that had entered the city along with soldiers returning from the Parthian War, Galen returned to Pergamum in 166. Not long afterwards, honoring a request from Emperor Marcus Aurelius, Galen returned to Rome and settled there permanently. Although strictly speaking Galen was not a "court physician," he did enjoy the friendship and protection of the emperors Marcus Aurelius, Commodus, and Septimius Severus and other prominent figures.

Late in life, stimulated by evidence that his writings were being corrupted by careless copyists, shameless impostors, and plagiarists, Galen composed a guide for the cautious reader called *On His Own Books,* which described the genuine works of Galen, as well as a reading program for physicians. Works for beginners were necessary, Galen complained, because many students lacked a good classical education and most "physicians" were pretenders who could barely read.

According to Galen, the best physician was also a philosopher. Thus, the true physician must master the three branches of philosophy: *logic*, the science of how to think; *physics*, the science of nature; and *ethics*, the science of what to do. With such knowledge, the physician could gain his patient's obedience and the admiration due to a god. Ideally, the physician would practice medicine for the love of mankind, not for profit, because the pursuit of science and money were mutually exclusive. In such passages, Galen portrayed himself as a scholar who realized that it was impossible to discover all that he passionately wished to know despite his persistent search for truth.

The essential features of Galen's system are a view of nature as purposeful and craftsmanlike and the principle of balance among the four qualities and the four humors. For Galen, anatomical research was the source of a "perfect theology" when approached as the study of form and function in terms of the "usefulness" of the parts. Instead of sacrificing bulls and incense, the anatomist demonstrated reverence for the Creator by discovering his wisdom, power, and goodness through anatomical investigations. The dissection of any animal revealed a little universe fashioned by the wisdom and skill of the Creator. Assuming that Nature acts with perfect wisdom and does nothing in vain, Galen argued that every structure was crafted for its proper function.

Dissection could be a religious experience for Galen, but most practitioners studied anatomy for guidance in surgical operations and the treatment of traumatic injuries. Systematic dissection was essential preparation for the surgeon, because a practitioner without anatomical knowledge could damage his patients. Where the surgeon could choose the site of incision, knowledge of anatomy would allow him to do the least damage possible. On the other hand, if the surgeon had to sever muscles to treat an abscess, his anatomical knowledge would allow him to predict subsequent damage and thus escape blame.

Anatomy could also be used to settle larger philosophical issues, such as the controversy about the seat of reason in the human body. Aristotelians placed reason in the heart, while others placed it in the head. One Aristotelian argument was that the voice, which is the instrument of reason, came from the chest. Thus, Galen's demonstration that the voice is controlled by the recurrent laryngeal nerves vindicated those who argued for control by the brain and also explained what happened when surgeons accidentally severed these nerves. Nevertheless, Galen believed that it was unnecessary to justify research by tenuous links to practical benefits. Interestingly, despite his own success in treating the gladiators of Pergamum, Galen seems to have harbored a deep antipathy for many aspects of surgery.

Because of his extensive writings, Galen was honored as the ultimate authority on anatomical and physiological questions without serious challenge until the sixteenth century, despite the fact that because of Roman prohibitions on human dissection, his "human anatomy" was based on dissection of other species. Often critical of his predecessors, especially Erasistratus and Herophilus, Galen obviously envied their resources and privileges. Certainly, Galen did not conceal the fact that his work was based on studies of other animals, including pigs and monkeys.

While Galen could not do systematic human anatomies, this does not mean that he never studied human cadavers. On one occasion a flood washed a corpse out of its grave and deposited the body on the bank of the river; the flesh rotted away, but the bones were still closely attached to each other. The enthusiasm with which Galen described such events suggests their rarity. As Celsus had suggested, a physician could learn a great deal about the form and functions of the internal organs by exploiting the wounds and injuries of his patients as "windows" into the body. Certainly, Galen would have taken full advantage of the opportunities he had enjoyed while binding up the gruesome wounds of the gladiators.

Never satisfied with pure anatomical description, Galen constantly struggled to find ways of proceeding from structure to function, from pure anatomy to experimental physiology. It is rare to encounter a problem in what might be called classical physiology that Galen did not attempt to cope with either by experiment or speculation. By extending medical research from anatomy to physiology, Galen established the foundations of a program that would transform the Hippocratic *art* of medicine into the *science* of medicine. In formulating his physiological principles, Galen was sometimes misled by preconceived and erroneous ideas and hindered by the technical difficulties inherent in such investigations. Given the magnitude of his self-imposed task, and the voluminous and prolix nature of his writings, the totality of his work has been more honored than understood. His errors, which ultimately stimulated revolutions in anatomy and physiology in the sixteenth and seventeenth centuries, tend to be overemphasized. It is important, therefore, to balance the merits and the defects in the powerful Galenic synthesis that was to satisfy the needs of scholars and physicians for hundreds of years.

Galen's system of physiology encompassed concepts of blood formation, respiration, the heartbeat, the arterial pulse, digestion, nerve function, embryology, growth, nutrition, and assimilation. Galenic physiology rests on the Platonic doctrine of a threefold division of the soul. This provided a means of dividing vital functions into processes governed by vegetative, animal, and rational "souls" or "spirits." Within the human body, *pneuma* (air), which was the breath of the cosmos, was subject to modifications brought about by the innate faculties of the three principle organs, the liver, heart, and brain, and distributed by three types of vessels: veins, arteries, and nerves. The system is complex and sometimes obscure. Moreover, it is difficult and perhaps counterproductive to attempt absolute distinctions between what Galen actually said and the way in which his doctrines were interpreted and handed down by later interpreters. In any event, Galen sometimes said different things in different texts and, since not all of his writings have survived, it is possible that interpretations made by commentators could have been based on manuscripts that have been lost.

In essence, according to Galen's system, pneuma was modified by the liver so that it became the nutritive soul or natural spirits which supported the vegetative functions of growth and nutrition; this nutritive soul was distributed by the veins. The heart and arteries were responsible for the maintenance and distribution of innate heat and pneuma or vital spirits to warm and vivify the parts of the body. The third adaptation, which occurred in the brain, produced the animal spirits required for sensation and muscular movement; the animal spirits were distributed through the nerves. Sometimes Galen's arguments concerning particular problems suggest reservations about the functions of the spirits, but he was certain that animal life is only possible because of the existence of pneuma within the body.

Because of the central role theories of the motion of the heart and blood have played in the history of medical science and therapeutics, Galen's views on these topics have been the subject of considerable attention and controversy. Part of the difficulty in recontructing a simplified version of Galen's concept of this problem resides in the fact that respiration and the movement of blood are so intimately linked in Galen's system that it is difficult to unravel the strands of each problem, or consider them apart from his doctrines concerning the elaboration and distribution of pneuma and spirits. Respiration, which was involved in cooling the excess heat of the heart, was obviously necessary for life. Therefore, vital spirit is necessarily associated with the organs of respiration, which in Galen's system included the heart and arteries as well as the lungs. *If* the natural spirit exists, Galen thought it would be contained in the liver and the veins. Attempting to simplify Galen's prolix arguments, his followers often transformed tentative "if there are" hypotheses into dogmatic "there are" certainties.

In Galen's physiological scheme, blood was continuously synthesized from ingested foods. The useful part of the food was transported as *chyle* from the intestines via the portal vein to the liver, where, by virtue of the innate faculty of the liver, it was transformed into dark venous blood. Tissues could then suck up the nutriments they need from the blood by virtue of their faculty for specific selection. The useless part of the food was converted into black bile by the spleen. Even Galen could not come to grips with the precise means by which such transformations—all the complex phenomena now subsumed by the term metabolism—might be effected.

Like Erasistratus, Galen assumed that there must be connections between the veins (which arose from the liver) and the arteries (which arose from the heart) because bleeding from any vessel could drain the whole system. But Galen ingeniously refuted the idea that, under normal conditions, the arteries contain only air. His arguments and experimental proof were set forth in a brief work entitled *Whether Blood Is Contained in the Arteries in Nature.* If the artery of a living animal is exposed and tied off at two points, the section of the vessel between the ligatures is full of blood. Moreover, when the chest of a living animal is opened, blood is found in the left ventricle of the heart. According to Galen's scheme, the arterial pulse was generated by the heart. During the diastole of the heart, the dilation of the arteries drew in air through the pores in the skin and blood from the veins. Thus, the arteries served the function of nourishing the innate heat throughout the body. This concept could be demonstrated by tying a ligature around a limb so that it was tight enough to cut off the arterial pulse. Below the ligature the limb would become cold and pale, because the arteries were no longer able to supply the innate heat.

Although Galen gave a good description of the heart, its chambers and valves, his preconceived concepts led to ambiguities, misinterpretations, and even misrepresentations of anatomical observations. For Galen's system to work, blood had to pass from the right ventricle to the left ventricle. Therefore, he assumed that blood in the right side of the heart could follow various paths; some of the blood carried impurities, or "sooty vapors," for discharge by the lungs via the artery-like vein (pulmonary artery). Blood could also pass from the right side to the left side of the heart by means of pores in the septum. The pores themselves were not visible, but Galen assumed that the pits found in the septum were the mouths of the pores.

After appropriate "digestion" in the lungs, inhaled air was brought to the heart by the pulmonary vein. The modified air was further acted on in the heart and transported to other parts of the body by the arteries. Arterial blood was especially fine and vaporous so that it could nourish the vital spirit. Further refinement was accomplished in the arteries that formed the *rete mirabile*—a network of vessels at the base of the brain of oxen and other animals, but not in humans. The transformation of arterial blood into animal spirits in the brain and their distribution via the nerves completed the threefold system of spirits. Clearly, the concept of blood circulation is incompatible with a scheme in which blood is constantly synthesized by the liver to be assimilated or used up as it ebbs and flows through the blood vessels. Of course, the nature of the Galenic system is so complex that "clearly" is hardly an appropriate word to use in a brief description of it; rather than throw any further obscurity on the subject, let us consider Galen's ideas about the treatment of diseases.

When writing about the nature of therapeutics, Galen argued that scientific knowledge of the causes of disease was essential for successful treatment. Like Hippocrates, Galen was an excellent clinician and a brilliant diagnostician who believed that the physician must explain disease in terms of natural causes. Indeed, an explanation for the genesis and essence of disease could always be found in humoral theory. According to Galen, the humors were formed when nutriments were altered by the *innate heat* which was produced by the slow combustion taking place in the heart. Foods of a warmer nature tend to produce bile, while those of a colder nature produce an excess of phlegm. An excess of bile produced "warm diseases" and an excess of phlegm resulted in "cold diseases." For prognosis, Galen relied on traditional tools, such as the examination of the pulse and the urine, and a rather rigid version of the Hippocratic doctrine of the "critical days."

Averting disease by rigid adherence to the principles of Galenic hygiene required continuous guidance by a competent physician, as set forth in his *On Hygiene*. The individualized health-promoting regimen prescribed by the physician required constant attention to the "six non-naturals," a confusing Galenic term for factors that, unlike geography, weather, season, and age, could be brought under the patient's control. Today's health and fitness experts would refer to the non-naturals as life-style choices, that is, food and drink, sleeping and waking, exercise and rest, "regularity," and "mental attitude." Eventually, in the hands of less gifted practitioners, Galen's program for a sophisticated individualized approach to the prevention and treatment of disease degenerated into a system of bleeding, purging, cupping, blistering, starvation diets, and large doses of complex mixtures of drugs.

Despite his reverence for Hippocrates, when confronted by disease, Galen was not willing to stand by passively, doing no harm, while waiting for Nature to heal the patient. A major work called *Method of Healing* and many other texts make this preference for action abundantly clear. Galen regarded bleeding as the appropriate treatment for almost every disorder, including hemorrhage and fatigue. Great skill was needed to determine how much blood should be taken, which vein should be cut, and the proper time for the operation. For certain conditions, Galen recommended two brisk bleedings per day. The first bleeding should be stopped just before the patient fainted, but the physician should not be afraid to provoke unconsciousness with the second bleeding, because patients who survived the first operation would not be harmed by the second. Galen was so enthusiastic about the benefits of venesection that he wrote three books about it.

As proof that nature prevented disease by discharging excess blood, Galen argued that women were spared many diseases that attacked men because their superfluous blood was eliminated by menstruation or lactation. Women with normal menstrual cycles supposedly enjoyed immunity from gout, arthritis, epilepsy, apoplexy, melancholy, and other diseases. Men who eliminated excess blood through hemorrhoids or nose bleeds could also expect to enjoy freedom from such diseases.

In terms of humoral doctrine, bleeding accomplished the therapeutic goals shared by patient and physician by apparently ridding the body of putrid, corrupt, and harmful materials. Moreover, some modern scientists suggest that venesection might have suppressed the clinical manifestations of certain diseases, such as malaria, by lowering the availability of iron in the blood; the availability of iron may determine the ability of certain pathogens to grow and multiply. Bleeding would also affect the body's response to disease by lowering the viscosity of the blood and increasing its ability to flow through the capillary bed. Bleeding to the point of fainting would also force the patient to rest. Given the importance of good nursing and a supportive environment, it should also be noted that when a feverish, delerious, and difficult patient is quieted to the point of fainting, the caretakers might enjoy a period of rest and recuperation.

Famous for his knowledge of drugs, Galen investigated the properties of simple medicines, complex concoctions, and exotics from distant places, such as "Balm of Gilead" from Palestine, copper from Cyprus, and the Lemnian Earths from the island of Lemnos. Lemnian Earths, or "Seals," were packets of specially prepared clay (much like Kaopectate) with the seal of the goddess stamped upon them. Galen brought back large supplies of these packets for use against poisons, bites of serpents, and putrid ulcers. Various kinds of ''earths'' have been used as medicines for hundreds of years; presumably adding the image of the goddess to Kaopectate would do no harm, but the consumption of unprocessed materials could be dangerous.

Complex drug mixtures were later called ''Galenicals'' and apothecary shops were often identified by the sign of ''Galen's Head'' above the door. Some Galenicals were pleasant enough to be used as beauty aids by wealthy Roman matrons. *Unguentum refrigerans*, an emulsion of water in almond oil, with white wax and scent of roses, is similar to modern ''cold cream.'' The Prince of Physicians also prescribed some rather nauseating remedies, such as bile from bulls, spiders' webs, skin shed by snakes, and a digestive oil compounded from cooked foxes and hyenas. As explained in one of Galen's minor works, the physician was often interested in detecting malingerers and may have used noxious remedies to test slaves who did not wish to work, or citizens and soldiers trying to escape political and military duties. However, Galen also developed elaborate speculative concepts about the way in which medical preparations worked and was able to provide rationalizations for the positive medical value of amulets and excrements. Anecdotes about the accidental discovery of the medical virtues of various noxious agents were also put to good use. For example, in *On Simples* Galen provided a lively account of the way in which a miserable old man suffering from a horrible skin disease was cured after drinking a jar of wine in which a poisonous snake had drowned.

Throughout the Roman Empire, the rich and powerful lived in fear of encountering poison at the banquet table, while poisonous plants and venomous creatures were constant threats to farmers, travelers, and soldiers. Galen was interested in the bites of apes, dogs, snakes, and, remembering his mother, human beings, all of which were presumed to be poisonous. Given the universal fear of poisons and venoms, the invention of bizarre antidotes was to be expected. Recipes for antidotes included herbs, minerals, and animal parts or products, such as dried locusts and viper's flesh. Roman recipes for theriacs, or antidotes, can be traced back to Mithridates, King of Pontus in Asia Minor. Mithridates (132–63 B.C.) was an investigator of medicinal herbs, poisons, antidotes, and an advocate of human experimentation. When exchanging recipes for antidotes with other researchers, Mithridates is said to have sent along a condemned prisoner to serve as a guinea pig. By taking a daily dose of his best antidotes, Mithridates made himself immune to all poisons. In 66 B.C., trapped in his fortress by the Roman army, Mithridates poisoned all his wives, concubines, and daughters, but no poison could kill Mithridates. According to Galen, Nero's physician Andromachus used Mithradates' poison lore to prepare the ultimate antidote, a formidable concoction containing some 64 ingredients, including opium and viper's flesh. Andromachus claimed that his theriac was a health tonic as well as a universal antidote.

Galen's skill and integrity were so highly regarded by his patrons that three Roman emperors entrusted the preparation of their theriac to him. Because others faced the danger of encountering inferior or counterfeit products, Galen suggested that they test the strength of theriacs by taking a drug that induced mild purging. If the alleged theriac prevented the normal effect of the drug, it might be genuine. Authentic theriac must be made with ingredients of the highest quality. Although the pounding, mixing, heating, and stirring of the final preparation could be accomplished in about 40 days, some authorities thought that a maturation period of 5–12 years was essential. During the Middle Ages, theriac became an important trade item for cities such as Venice, Milan, Genoa, Padua, Bologna, and Cairo. Theriac, viper's flesh and all, was still found in French and German pharmacopoeias at the end of the nineteenth century. In England, a degenerate form of the universal antidote became the candy known as "treacle."

Galen was apparently as skillful in the art of medicine as in the science. Aware of the bad repute brought to the profession by displays of ambition, contentiousness, and greed, Galen emphasized skill, dignity, and a disdainful attitude towards money. One important skill was the art of eliciting clues by casually questioning the messenger who called for the physician and the patient's friends and family. A secret examination of the contents of all basins removed from the sickroom on their way to the dung heap and the medicines already in use could provide further clues. The pulse, casually examined while observing the patient, was another valuable source of information. To escape blame for failures and to win universal admiration, the physician must cultivate the art of making his diagnoses and prognoses seem like acts of divination. A clever application of this tactic was to predict the worst possible outcome while reluctantly agreeing to accept the case. If the patient died, the physician's prediction was vindicated; if he recovered, the physician appeared to be a miracle worker.

In many ways Galen was truly a miracle worker; the remarkable quantity and quality of his work was acknowledged by his contemporaries. Even those who had engaged in bitter disputes with Galen respected his intelligence, productivity, and the passion with which he defended his doctrines. Yet, despite his brilliance in disputations, public lectures, and demonstrations, Galen seems to have had no students or disciples. Perhaps the personality traits that captivated Roman emperors and high government officials repelled colleagues and potential students. While some of his voluminous writings were lost in the centuries after his death and many were neglected, excerpts of his writings, commentaries, and translations were to form a major component of the medical curriculum and learned literature of late antiquity and the Middle Ages. In the transmuted and partially digested form known as Galenism, the Prince of Physicians dominated medical learning throughout the Middle Ages of Europe and the Golden Age of Islam. Galen's authority was not seriously challenged until the introduction of printing and a revival of interest in the true classics of antiquity made the genuine works of Galen and Hippocrates widely available. When Galen's anatomical and physiological doctrines were finally subjected to serious challenges in the sixteenth and seventeenth centuries, the physicians now remembered as reformers and revolutionaries began their work as Galenists. Perhaps their attacks on Galenism should be regarded as the triumph of the true spirit of Galen, physician, philosopher, and scientist.

SUGGESTED READINGS

Allbutt, Sir Thomas Clifford (1921). *Greek Medicine in Rome*. London: Macmillan.

Boswell, John (1984). *Expositio* and *oblatio*: The Abandonment of Children and the Ancient and Medieval Family. *American Historical Review* 89: 10–33.

Brain, Peter (1986). *Galen on Bloodletting*. New York: Cambridge University Press.

Celsus (1960–61). *De medicina*. 3 vols. (Trans. by W. G. Spencer). Loeb Classical Library. Cambridge, MA: Harvard University Press.

Dioscorides (1959). *The Greek Herbal of Dioscorides* (Illus. by a Byzantine in 512 A.D., trans. by John Goodyear, 1655 A.D.) Ed. by Robert T. Gunther. New York: Hafner.

Dodds, E. R. (1951). *The Greeks and the Irrational*. Berkeley: University of California Press.

Edelstein, Ludwig (1967). *Ancient Medicine*, Ed. by O. Temkin and C. L. Temkin. Baltimore, MD: Johns Hopkins University Press.

Edelstein, Emma, and Edelstein, Ludwig (1945). *Asclepius: A Collection and Interpretation of the Testimonies*. Baltimore, MD: Johns Hopkins University Press.

Galen (1951). *Galen's Hygiene* (Trans. Robert M. Green). Springfield, IL: Charles C. Thomas.

Galen (1968). *Galen's System of Physiology and Medicine* (Trans. by R. E. Siegel). Basel: Karger.

Galen (1962). *On Anatomical Procedures* (Trans. by W.L.H. Duckworth). Cambridge, England: Cambridge University Press.

Galen (1963). *On the Natural Faculties* (Trans. by A.J. Brock). Loeb Classical Library. Cambridge, MA: Harvard University Press.

Galen (1984). *On Respiration and the Arteries* (Ed. and trans. by D.J. Furley and J.S. Wilkie). Princeton, NJ: Princeton University Press.

Galen (1968). *On the Usefulness of the Parts of the Body* (Trans., intro., and commentary by Margaret Tallmadge May). Ithaca, NY: Cornell University Press.

Galen (1985). *Three Treatises on the Nature of Science* (Trans. by Richard Walzer and Michael Frede). Indianapolis, IN: Hackett Publishing Company.

Grmek, Mirko D. (1989). *Diseases in the Ancient Greek World*. Baltimore, MD: Johns Hopkins University Press.

Hanson, Ann Ellis (1975). Hippocrates: Diseases of Women. *SIGNS* 1: 567–584.

Hippocrates (1957–59). *Hippocrates*. 4 vols. (Trans. by W.H. S. Jones; vol. 3 by E.T. Withington). Loeb Classical Library. Cambridge, MA: Harvard University Press.

Hippocrates (1964). *The Theory and Practice of Medicine*. Trans. and intro. by E.C. Kelly. New York: Philosophical Library.

Hagg, Robin, ed. (1983). *The Greek Renaissance of the Eighth Century B.C.: Tradition and Innovation*. Stockholm: Paul Astroms Forlag.

Jackson, Ralph (1988). *Doctors and Disease in the Roman Empire*. Norman, OK: University of Oklahoma Press.

Jones, W. H. S. (1924). *The Doctor's Oath. An Essay in the History of Medicine*. Cambridge, England: Cambridge University Press.

Jones, W. H. S. (1909). *Malaria and Greek History*. London: Manchester University Press.

Kudlien, Fridolf, and Durling, Richard J., eds. (1990). *Galen's Method of Healing*. Proceedings of the 1982 Galen Symposium. New York: E. J. Brill.

Lain Entralgo, Pedro (1970). *The Therapy of the Word in Classical Antiquity*. New Haven, CT: Yale University Press.

Lloyd, G. E. R. (1987). *The Revolutions of Wisdom. Studies in the Claims and Practice of Ancient Greek Science*. Berkeley, CA: University of California Press.

Majno, G. (1975). *The Healing Hand: Man and Wound in the Ancient World*. Cambridge, MA: Harvard University Press.

Marek-Marsel, Mesulum, and Perry, Jon (1972). The Diagnosis of Love-Sickness: Experimental Psychology without the Polygraph. *Psychophysiology* 9: 546–551.

Milne, John Stewart (1907). *Surgical Instruments of Greek and Roman Times*. Oxford, England: Clarendon.

Nutton, Vivian, ed. (1981). *Galen: Problems and Prospects*. London: Wellcome Institute for the History of Medicine.

Onians, Richard Broxton (1951). *The Origins of European Thought About the Body, the Mind, the Soul, the World, Time, and Fate*. New York: Cambridge University Press.

Parsons, E. A. (1952). *The Alexandrian Library*. New York: Elsevier.

Pliny (1956-1966). *Natural History*. 10 vols. Trans. H. Rackham, W.H. S. Jones, and D.E. Eichholz. Loeb Classical Library. Cambridge, MA: Harvard University Press.

Rather, L. J. (1968). The 'Six Things Non-Natural': A Note on the Origins and Fate of a Doctrine and a Phrase. *Clio Medica* 3: 337–347.

Riddle, John M. (1985). *Dioscorides on Pharmacy and Medicine*. Austin, TX: University of Texas Press.

Sargent, Frederick (1982). *Hippocratic Heritage. A History of Ideas About Weather and Human Health*. New York: Pergamon Press.

Sarton, George (1954). *Galen of Pergamon*. Lawrence: University of Kansas Press.

Scarborough, John (1969). *Roman Medicine*. Ithaca, NY: Cornell Univeristy Press.

Smith, Wesley D. (1979). *The Hippocratic Tradition*. Ithaca, NY: Cornell University Press.

Staden, Heinrich von (1989). *Herophilus: The Art of Medicine in Early Alexandria*. New York: Cambridge University Press.

Steuer, Robert O., and Saunders, J. B. de C. M. (1959). *Ancient Egyptian and Cnidian Medicine. The Relationship of Their Aetiological Concepts of Disease*. Berkeley, CA: University of California Press.

Temkin, Owsei (1945). *The Falling Sickness: A History of Epilepsy from the Greeks to the Beginnings of Modern Neurology*. Baltimore, MD: Johns Hopkins Univeristy Press.

Temkin, Owsei (1973). *Galenism: Rise and Decline of a Medical Philosophy*. Ithaca, NY: Cornell University Press.

Watson, G. (1966). *Theriac and Mithradatium. A Study in Therapeutics*. London: The Wellcome Historical Medical Library.

Withington, E. T. (1909). *The History of Greek Therapeutics and the Malaria Theory*. Manchester, England: Manchester University Press.

5
THE MIDDLE AGES

No simple characterization can describe the state of medical theory and practice in the European Middle Ages, a period from about 500 to 1500 A.D. in which ideas about the nature of the physical universe, the nature of human beings and their proper place in the universe, and above all, their relationship to their Creator underwent such profound changes and dislocations. The Roman Empire, whose borders had encompassed the civilized Western world during the second century, had undergone its well-known ordeal of decline and fall after centuries of anarchy, turmoil, and warfare. Weakened by corruption, misgovernment, and insurrection, the city of Rome lost its role as undisputed political center of the crumbling Empire; in 330 Emperor Constantine established Byzantium (Constantinople) as his capital. By the end of the fourth century, the division of the empire between East and West had become permanent; the East was to become the Byzantine Empire and the West was to enter the era popularly known as the Dark Ages.

Medieval medicine has been described as everything from a pathological aberration to the dawn of a new chapter in the evolution of the medical profession. In recent years the literature on medieval medicine has become vastly richer and more sophisticated, particularly with respect to its relationship to religion, education, professional organization, alternative practitioners, patterns of morbidity and mortality, and the persistence of the classical tradition. The Middle Ages served as a stage for many remarkable scholars, doctors, and diseases, but rather than provide a catalogue of doctors and diseases, scholars and texts, we have selected only a small portion of all that made the Middle Ages both unique and instructive. In particular, we shall focus on leprosy and bubonic plague, diseases that are as inextricably, even if inappropriately, linked to the Middle Ages in the popular imagination as the term Dark Ages.

In facing AIDS, the disease that emerged in the 1980s to become the great modern pandemic, bubonic plague and leprosy are most often used as standards of comparative misery. If we can look into the Middle Ages as a "distant mirror," we may be able to think more clearly about the role of catastrophic diseases in society and in the human psyche. Plague and leprosy stand out among the myriad perils and adversities of the Middle Ages, much as AIDS has emerged as the pestilence emblematic of the last decades of the twentieth century. Many aspects of the origin, impact, and present and future threat of AIDS are unclear, just as there are many uncertainties about the historical meaning of leprosy and plague. But it is not unreasonable to hope that scientific knowledge concerning pathology and epidemiology, and historical research illuminating the social context in which particular diseases loomed so large, will eventually allow us to ask more meaningful questions about the ways in which people assess and respond to the threat of catastrophic disease.

The transition from Greco-Roman culture to medieval Christianity irrevocably transformed the status of the healing art. The Hippocratic tradition based on love of technique, intellectual curiosity, glorification of the healthy body, and the passionate pursuit of physical well-being were foreign to the spirit of the medieval Christian world. As a branch of learning, medicine, like all forms of secular learning, was considered inferior to and subordinate to theology. However, the actual state of medicine as the necessary healing art, rather than a branch of learning, is a more complex problem. If it were true that all sickness was the inexorable consequence of sin, or a test of faith, suffering through such trials and tribulations might well be the theoretically appropriate response.

The ancient Greeks regarded health as the highest good, but seeking health became problematic within Christian doctrine. Healing was good as an act of love; yet being healed, except by God and His servants, was not necessarily good. Disease could be punishment for sin or a test of faith. But the majority of people were not saints or ascetics; medicine continued to be part of normal life. With or without theological rationalizations, the quest for health and healing was never abandoned by the laity, nor did physicians and scholars wholly abandon the secular Hippocratic tradition. Hippocratic medicine won varying degrees of acceptance in Europe and Byzantium; while episodes of hostility and repression can be discovered, examples of accommodation and even respect can also be documented. Followers of Hippocratic medicine found ways to accommodate their art, with varying degrees of success, to the world of Christian beliefs. For their part, theologians found ways to justify the worthiness of healing and health, and the study of the authoritative texts that contined the ancient, secular knowledge that guided the physician. Setting aside major theologican concerns regarding body and soul, it could be argued that medicine was an art, like agriculture, architecture, and weaving, that God had granted to humankind. Moreover, the Hippocratic dietetic tradition could be rationalized as another means of the self-discipline essential to Christian life.

In the Middle Ages, as in all ages and cultures, religious healing and secular healing existed side by side, but the naturalistic basis of Hippocratic medicine gave it a non-Christian character that had not been a problem for cultures with more flexible and syncretic religious or ethical systems. The legendary Hippocrates as hard-working craftsman, motivated by love of humankind, could not be objectionable; he was anathema if portrayed as a healing god decended from Asclepius and Apollo, or a savior who could perform miracles of healing independent of God and His representatives. The physician could maintain some degree of medical autonomy and continue to honor the traditional wisdom of Hippocrates, but would have to learn to award ultimate credit for any cures to God.

The Greeks had venerated health and regarded the healthy human body as beautiful and essentially god-like; Christians were taught to despise the flesh and its desires, especially sexual desire. But, since the body housed the soul, or was a temple of God, it deserved some measure of care and respect, even if we ignore the complex theological debate about the physiological possibility of the resurrection of the body. Theologians could divide medicine into two parts: religious medicine concerned with "heavenly things" and human medicine concerned with "earthly things." Human medicine relied on empirical methods such as dietary management, drugs, bleeding, and simple surgical operations. Religious medicine involved prayers, penitence, exorcism, holy relics, charms, and magical incantations. The two parts of medicine differed in origin and efficacy: experience had taught physicians about the power of herbs, but Christ, "the author of heavenly medicine," could cure the sick by his word alone and even raise the dead from the grave. Thus, the Church, which acted for Christ, could heal without earthly medicine.

Some of the early Church Fathers taught that it was sinful to try to cure bodily ills by earthly medicines and that the spirit of God was not found in healthy bodies. Disease served as a test of faith by forcing a choice between secular medicine and the Church. But it was also possible to argue that the body should be kept strong because those who were sick and weak might more easily succumb to the Devil. Moreover, if disease was punishment for sin, and forgiveness was the province of the Church, healing must be part of the Church's mission of mercy and charity. In any case, except for those who deliberately chose mortification of the flesh, there is ample evidence that popes, priests, and peasants sought remedies for their pain and disease. As the cynic says, everyone wants to go to heaven, but no one wants to die.

Theologians recorded many miracle tales in which pious men and martyred saints cured the sick after human medicine proved useless. Medieval scholars believed that the universe was governed by general laws which had been assigned by God, but theologicans established an important role for miracles. Priests and physicians might care for the sick with kindness and recognize the medical virtues of drugs, but every cure was ultimately a miracle. Healing miracles were often ascribed to the direct action of saints or their relics. Strictly speaking, ''relic'' refers to the mortal remains of a saint, but the term was also used to describe objects that had been in contact with these holy persons.

By the fourth century the remains of certain saints were the objects of public cults, despite the doubts expressed by some theologians as to the propriety of honoring such objects. Those who argued for the veneration of relics triumphed and the increasing popularity of this form of worship encouraged the discovery, multiplication, and theft of relics. The display of such obvious frauds as hairs from Noah's beard, drops of the Virgin's milk, and other wonders was enough to provoke the skepticism of a saint.

In spite of the veritable flood of relics that washed over Europe during the Crusades, the insatiable demand posed the threat of a relic shortfall. One solution was to make a little bit of relic go a long way: saints and martyrs were dismembered so that the parts could be shared by several shrines. ''Contact relics''—water, cloths, or earth that had been in contact with the remains—could also be venerated. When the need was acute, some relics were invested with the power of self-reproduction.

Miraculous cures were not uncommon incidents in the lives of martyrs and saintly kings. For example, when Edward the Confessor washed the neck of a scrofulous, infertile woman, her scrofula disappeared and within a year she gave birth to twins. The diluted blood of St. Thomas of Canterbury cured blindness, insanity, leprosy, and deafness, but, like their Egyptian and Roman counterparts, most saints tended to specialize. The martyred brothers Cosmas and Damian, famous for their skill in medicine and their refusal to take payment for their services, became the patron saints of physicians and pharmacists. Unlike many of the other texts of this genre, the stories dealing with Cosmas and Damian often advised the sick to seek the aid of both physicians and healing saints. One of their more spectacular cures involved grafting the leg of a dead pagan onto one of their converts. In another episode, the saints appeared to a physician in a dream and told him how to perform a surgical operation and apply healing drugs to a woman with breast cancer. When the doctor went to the church where the woman had gone to pray to Cosmas and Damian, he found that the operation had been miraculously performed. The saints left the final phase of treatment, application of healing ointments, to the physician.

Some saints became associated with particular diseases or parts of the body through the manner of their death. St. Apollonia became patron saint of toothache because all her teeth had been knocked out during her martyrdom. Pestilential disease became the specialty of St. Sebastian, who had been wounded but not killed by Diocletian's archers. Sebastian's recovery suggested that he was immune to the arrows of death. In portraits of the saint, arrows pierce his body at the sites where plague buboes usually appear. An arrow in the heart symbolized sudden death.

Just as the pagan gods were replaced by Christian saints, the rituals of Asclepius were absorbed into Christian practice. Temples were transformed into churches where the worship of Christ the Healer, or his healing saints, provided a familiar setting for medical miracles. In contrast to the Asclepiads who excluded the incurable from the sanctuary, the Church took on the nursing of hopeless cases and promised relief in the next world if faith failed to effect an immediate cure.

In the writings of theologians, secular physicians are generally mentioned only to show how relics and prayers were effective after earthly medicine failed. Given the bias of these authors, such stories can be looked upon as proof that the sick often turned to lay healers. Medieval writings contain many complaints about the physician's love of "filthy lucre" and the high cost of medical aid. On the other hand, biographies of medieval kings, nobles, and clergymen also refer to dedicated physicians who won the respect and friendship of their patrons.

In making his diagnosis, the medieval physician relied primarily on the patient's narrative of symptoms, but many healers were regarded as masters of the ancient art of uroscopy (urine inspection). Using a specially marked flask, the physician studied the color of the urine and the distribution of clouds, precipitates, and particles at various levels of the flask in order to determine the nature of the illness and the condition of the patient. A story about the Duke of Bavaria indicates that even in the tenth century some patients were skeptics. To test his physician, the Duke substituted the urine of a pregnant woman for his own. After making his inspection, the physician solemnly announced that God was about to bring about a great event: the Duke would soon give birth to a child.

The influence of Christianity on medical thought is only one aspect of the way in which the Church attained a virtual monopoly on all forms of learning during the Middle Ages. The task of translating Greek medical texts into Latin had begun by the fifth century. For the most part, the study of ancient texts and the preparation of extracts and compilations reflect interest in logic and philology rather than science, but there is evidence that medical manuscripts were consulted for practical purposes. Indeed, the marginal comments found on medical manuscripts provide evidence of interest in medicine and even experimentation with drugs.

The writings of certain medieval theologians, such as Isidore, Bishop of Seville (ca. 560–636), provide a good example of informed interest in medical matters. Isidore believed that it was possible to prepare useful encyclopedic texts that would conform to Christian faith and morals through the study of both pagan and Christian writings. Such studies supported the idea that medicine embraced all the other liberal disciplines of study. Medicine was the art of protecting, preserving, and restoring health to the body by means of diet, hygiene, and the treatment of wounds and diseases. But medicine was also a "second philosophy" which cured the body, just as the first philosophy cured the soul. Thus, the physician had to be well grounded in literature, grammar, rhetoric, and dialectic, in order to understand and explain difficult texts and study the causes and cures of disease in the light of reason. Many medical manuscripts were written in the form of a dialogue, the format used in medieval teaching. The dialogues usually began with a standard question, such as:

''What is medicine?'' Students were expected to memorize standard answers and the teacher's exposition of the text.

By the ninth century medieval scholars had established the concept that medical studies were an integral part of Christian wisdom. If all learning, including the science of health, came from God, the religious need not fear a conflict between the study of the medical literature and religion. Medical knowledge could be enjoyed as an intellectual ornament, an area of serious study, and a potentially useful technique.

One of the major innovations of the Middle Ages was the formal establishment of university education in medicine during the twelfth and thirteenth centuries. However, only a tiny fraction of all medical practitioners between the thirteenth century and the fifteenth century had any university training. The influence of the faculties of medicine was more closely related to the establishment of a regular curriculum, authoritative texts, technical knowledge and information, and a medical elite enjoying high intellectual and social status and prestige than to the absolute number of university trained physicians.

The establishment of universities and faculties of medicine throughout Europe was very uneven; students often had to undertake long journeys in search of suitable mentors. Moreover, the universities of the Middle Ages were very different from both the ancient centers of learning and their modern counterparts, especially in terms of the relationships among students, faculty, and administrators. The exact origins of some of the major universities are obscure. The term ''university'' was a rather vague term which originally referred to any corporate status or association of persons; eventually it came to be used for institutions of higher learning. Large numbers of students, all of whom shared Latin as the language of learning, were drawn to universities to study with teachers known for particular areas of excellence. Many students entered the universities at the age of 14 or 15 after securing the rudiments of the seven liberal arts: grammar, rhetoric, logic, arithmetic, geometry, astronomy, and music.

The medical texts available for use by the time medical faculties were established included many translations from Greek and Arabic manuscripts, as well as new Latin commentaries and compendia. But before the fifteenth century students and professors had access to only a portion of the writings of Hippocrates, Galen, and other ancient writers. Some of Galen's most important texts, including *On Anatomical Procedures*, were not translated into Latin until the sixteenth century. Some manuscripts were extremely rare and could not have served many scholars and teachers. Moreover, many of the Latin texts attributed to Hippocrates and Galen were spurious.

While the rise of the university as a center for training physicians is an important aspect of the history of medieval medicine, for much of this period learned medicine was still firmly associated with the church and the monastery. With its library, infirmary, hospital, and herbal gardens, the monastery was a natural center for medical study and practice. On the other hand, charitable impulses towards the sick were sometimes obliterated by an all-consuming concern for the soul, coupled with contempt for the flesh. Some ascetics refused to make allowances for the "indulgence" of the flesh, even for sick flesh. St. Bernard of Clairvaux (1091–1153), a mystic who engaged in harsh, self-imposed penances, expected his monks to live and die simply. Building infirmaries, taking medicines, or visiting a physician were forbidden. The lives of saints and ascetics contained many exemplary cases suggesting that a regimen of self-imposed privations that Galen would have found abhorrent led to health, longevity, and peace of mind. Ascetics might fast several days a week, eat nothing but bread, salt, and water, stay awake all night in prayer, and give up bathing and exercise (some saints were famous for sitting on pillars for years at a time). But the reaction of saints and ascetics to diseases and accidents that were not self-inflicted might be quite different. Here the stories vary widely. Some ascetics accepted medical or surgical treatment for disorders such as cancer and dropsy, while others categorically refused to accept drugs or doctors. Some were fortunate enough to be cured in a rather Asclepian fashion by ministering angels who appeared in dreams to wash their wounds and anoint their bruises.

A more temperate view of the needs of the sick was taken by the founders of other religious orders, and infirmaries and hospitals were established as adjuncts to many monasteries in order to provide charity and care for the sick. In such cases, the rules of St. Benedict (ca. 480–547) provided reasonable guidelines for care of the sick. Although the monastic routine called for hard work, special allowances were to be made for the sick, infirm, and aged. The rules of St. Benedict called for the establishment of an infirmary as a Christian duty. The care of the sick was such an important duty that those caring for them were enjoined to act as if they served Christ directly. There is suggestive evidence that monks with some medical knowledge were chosen to care for the sick.

By the eleventh century, some monasteries were training their own physicians. Ideally, such physicians would uphold the Christianized ideal of the healer who offered mercy and charity towards all patients, whatever their status and prognosis. The gap between ideal and reality is suggested by evidence of numerous complaints about the pursuit of "filthy lucre" by priest-physicians. When such physicians gained permission to practice outside the monastery and offered their services to wealthy nobles, accusations of luxurious living and the decline of monastic discipline were raised.

The apparently simple question of whether medieval clergymen were or were not forbidden to practice medicine and surgery has been the subject of considerable controversy. Only excessive naiveté would lead us to expect that official records and documents are a realistic reflection of the status of forbidden practices. The official Church position was made explicit in numerous declarations and complaints about the study and practice of medicine and surgery by clergymen. Several twelfth-century papal decisions expressed a desire to restrict the practice of medicine by monks. The declarations of the Council of Clermont (1130), the Council of Rheims (1131), and the Second Lateran Council (1139) all contain the statement: "Monks and canons regular are not to study jurisprudence and medicine for the sake of temporal gain." This decision referred specifically to the pursuit of money, not to the study and practice of medicine or law. It was clearly the pursuit of money that was disreputable, not the practice of medicine or law. Obviously, the need for so many official prohibitions indicates how difficult it was to make practice accord with policy.

Another myth about medieval medicine is the assumption that the Church's opposition to "shedding human blood" prohibited surgery. However, this prohibition was based on opposition to shedding blood because of hatred and war, not to surgery in general, and certainly not to venesection. The idea that this position had any medical significance was essentially an eighteenth-century hoax.

The processes that led to the establishment of medicine as a profession based upon a formal education, standardized curriculum, licensing, and legal regulation were set in motion in the Middle Ages. Of course, laws differed from place to place, as did enforcement and the balance of power between unofficial practice and legally sanctioned practice. Law codes might specify the nature of the contract between patient and doctor and the penalties and fines for particular errors. Physicians could be fined for public criticism of other doctors, failure to consult other physicians in cases of serious illness, or for treating a female patient in the absence of proper witnesses. The law might even require giving more weight to the patient's spiritual welfare than physical well-being. The law could compel the doctor to advise the patient to seek confession, even though the fear inspired by this custom might be dangerous in itself.

Despite some unwelcome constraints, the doctor achieved the benefits of a legally defined status. As a consequence, healers who practiced without a state-approved license became subject to criminal prosecution and fines. Professional physicians argued that standards of practice would be raised by eradicating unfit practitioners, identified as "empirics, fools, and women." However, formal requirements also excluded many skilled healers. Another unfortunate consequence of medieval legal codes was the tendency to separate medicine from surgery and diminish the status of the surgeon.

Not all medical practitioners were either highly educated priests or scholars or illiterate empirics. For example, the Anglo-Saxon leechbooks of early medieval England provide some insights into the concerns of practitioners and patients separated from the "high medical culture" of the learned centers of Europe. Little is known about the education and practice of the typical medieval English healer, but both monastic physicians and secular physicians appear in illustrations and paintings. Early medieval English medical books were generally compilations of ancient texts, unique only in that many were written in Old English, rather than Latin. Presumably most English doctors, known as "leeches," were literate, at least in the vernacular. By the fourteenth century, monastic centers of learning were producing scholars with little tolerance for the Anglo-Saxon leechbooks. Considering the fact that parchment was a valuable and reusable resource, it is surprising that any of the early English medical texts did in fact survive.

The nineteenth-century revival of interest in folklore inspired the Rev. Thomas Oswald Cockayne to rescue surviving Anglo-Saxon medical texts and prepare a three-volume collection called *Leechdoms, Wortcunning and Starcraft of Early England, Illustrating the History of Science in This Country Before the Norman Conquest.* The leechbooks provided instructions for surgical techniques, herbal remedies, rites, and charms to prevent all kinds of diseases including sudden illness caused by "flying venom" and "elf-shot." Chronic diseases were attributed to "the worm," a term applied to all manner of worms, insects, snakes, and dragons. Some rather colorful descriptions of "worms" were probably inspired by observations of the very real creatures that live on human beings and domestic animals. Bits of tissue and mucus in excretions, vomit, or blood, or maggots in putrid wounds could also provide evidence of "worms."

Anglo-Saxon leechbooks reflect the mingling of Greek, Roman, Teutonic, Celtic, and Christian concepts of medicine and magic. Disease could be cured by invoking the names of the saints, exorcism, or by transferring it to plants, animals, earth, or running water. The preparation of almost every remedy required the recitation of some prayer or charm, along with the number magic of the pagan "nines" and the Christian "threes." Despite condemnation of amulets as magical objects, Christianized versions of these protective devices were widely used.

The prescriptions in the leechbooks suggest the common disorders endured by medieval people, such as arthritis, eye disorders, burns and scalds, unwanted pregnancies, impotence, and infertility. A wealth of recipes testify to the universal presence of the louse. Iatrogenic disorders (caused by medical treatment), such as complications resulting from phlebotomy, were not unknown; in retrospect, it would not be surprising to find infection or tetanus among patients whose venesection wounds were dressed with "horses tords." Remedies and charms to regulate the menses, prevent miscarriage, ensure male offspring, and ease the pains of childbirth were discussed at great length. Patients had to follow instructions carefully, or the results could be disastrous. For example, a son would be born if both man and wife drank a charm prepared from a hare's uterus, but if only the wife drank this preparation she would give birth to a hermaphrodite.

Given the importance of domestic animals to the medieval economy, the use of many of the same remedies for man and beast is not surprising, but the religious aspects of medieval veterinary medicine are another matter. Whatever beneficial effects holy water and prayers might have on humans, it is difficult to imagine that religious rites would greatly impress sheep, pigs, and bees. The use of pagan and magical rituals to protect domestic animals was as much condemned as their use in treating humans, with much the same results. Some of the "cures" must have tormented the animals more than the disease. For example, one ritual for horses required cutting crosses on the forehead and limbs with a knife whose haft had been made from the horn of a fallow ox. After pricking a hole in the horse's left ear and inscribing a Latin charm on the haft of the knife, the healer declared the beast cured.

Another interesting example of somewhat later English medicine is found in the life and work of John of Gaddesden (1280–1361), physician to Edward II. Author of *The Rose of England, the Practice of Medicine from the Head to the Feet*, John might have been the model for Chaucer's Doctor of Physic. According to Chaucer, the *Rosa Anglica* was an inevitable part of a typical physician's library. John modestly claimed that his treatise was so well organized and detailed that surgeons and physicians would need no other book. Remedies are suggested for both wealthy and poor patients. Thus, the treatment of dropsy could be managed with expensive diuretic remedies if the patient were rich, but a poor patient should be advised to drink his own urine every morning. One of the most famous recommendations in the *Rosa Anglica* was the "red therapy" for smallpox, which involved surrounding a victim of smallpox with red things to expedite healing and prevent the formation of scars.

With a few rare exceptions, women as practitioners and patients are largely invisible in the older literature concerning the history of medicine in general and the Middle Ages in particular. Although women presumably suffered from most of the diseases and disasters that afflicted men, "women's complaints" were generally discussed only in terms of pregnancy, childbirth, lactation, and menstrual disorders. Women practitioners were generally thought to be subsumed by the term "midwife." Recent scholarship has helped to correct this picture and enrich our knowledge of women's medical practice and medical care during the Middle Ages. Just as women practitioners were not restricted to the role of midwife, women patients did not restrict their choice of medical advisor to members of their sex, even if their "complaint" involved sensitive issues such as infertility.

Before discussing what might be considered the problems of the "rank and file" of women practitioners and patients, it is of interest to look at the life and work of Hildegard of Bingen (1098–1179), one of the twelfth century's most remarkable writers on cosmological and medical questions. Known and respected as an apocalyptic prophet, writer, composer, and healer, from England to Byzantium during her lifetime, she was soon all but forgotten, except in her native Germany. St. Hildegard has been called a mystic, a visionary, and a prophet; nevertheless, her writings suggest practical experience and boundless curiosity about the wonders of nature. A revival of interest in St. Hildegard during the twentieth century has brought her to the attention of scholars, feminists, musicians, poets, herbalists, and homeopathic practitioners.

As the tenth and last child of a noble family, Hildegard was offered to God as a tithe and entered a life of religious seclusion at the age of 8; she took monastic vows in her teens and was chosen abbess of her Benedictine nunnery in 1136. At about 15 years of age, Hildegard, who had experienced certain forms of visions since early childhood, began receiving revelations about the nature of the cosmos and humankind. The visions were explained to her in Latin by a voice from heaven. In

1141 a divine call commanded her to write down and explain her visions. When she began writing at the age of 43, Hildegard thought that she was the first woman to embark on such a mission. The names of other women writers were unknown to her. After a papal inquiry into the nature of her revelations, Hildegard became a veritable celebrity and was officially encouraged to continue her work. Her advice was sought by popes, kings, and scholars. Hildegard's *Physica, The Book of Simple Medicine,* or *Nine Books on the Subtleties of Different Kinds of Creatures* is probably the first book by a female author to discuss the elements and the therapeutic virtues of plants, animals, and metals. The text includes much traditional medical lore concerning the medical uses or toxic properties of many herbs, trees, mammals, reptiles, fishes, birds, minerals, gems, and metals. It was also the first book on natural history composed in Germany. Hildegard's other major work, the *Book of Compound Medicine,* or *Causes and Cures,* included material on the nature, forms, causes, and treatments of disease, human physiology and sexuality discussed in terms of Adam and Eve, astrology, and so forth. The two books on medicine made no claims to divine inspiration. At the age of 60, Hildegard began another difficult mission as public preacher for monastic and clerical reform.

Relying primarily on traditional humoral theory, Hildegard usually suggested treatments based on the principle of opposites. Foods, drugs, and precious stones were prescribed to prevent and cure disease. For example, sapphire was good for the eyes and served as an anti-aphrodisiac, which made it an appropriate gem to have in a convent or monastery. Remedies calling for parts of exotic animals, such as unicorn liver and lion heart, were recommended for dreaded diseases like leprosy.

In exploring mental as well as physical diseases, Hildegard discussed frenzy, insanity, obsession, and idiocy. According to Hildegard, even the most bizarre mental states could have natural causes. Thus, people might think a man was possessed by a demon when the real problem might be a simultaneous attack of headache, migraine, and vertigo. Hildegard probably had a special interest in these disorders; modern medical detectives have diagnosed her visions as classic examples of migraine.

Most of the women healers who practiced medicine and midwifery during the Middle Ages left no traces of their activities in the written records. Indeed, coming to the attention of the authorities and directly competing with licensed practitioners was dangerous for those forced to live at the margins of society. Thus, although few women were able to attain the learning and influence reached by St. Hildegard in her safely cloistered position, many other medieval women served as nurses, herbalists, and healers in hospitals and infirmaries in Europe and the Holy Land. For example, St. Walpurga (d. 779) was an English princess who studied medicine and founded a monastery in Germany. She is often depicted holding a flask of urine in one hand and bandages in the other. From the twelfth century to the fourteenth century, some Italian universities allowed women to study and teach medicine. At the University of Salerno, where Trotula (or Trota), author of the *Practica secundum Trotam*, taught and practiced medicine in the twelfth century, the subject of "women's diseases" fell within the province of women professors. But the exclusion of women from formal medical education, and thus from the legal and lucrative professional practice of the art, was far more common. Nevertheless, it is possible to find women practitioners among all the ranks of the medieval medical community—physicians, surgeons, barber-surgeons, apothecaries, leeches, healers, and assorted empirics. As in the modern university or corporation, their distribution would tend to include larger numbers at the bottom of the hierarchy than at the top. While medieval practitioners battled fiercely for control over the paid practice of medicine, there is little doubt that much of the routine, unpaid care of the sick took place in the home and was carried out by women.

During the Middle Ages, women could practice medicine or surgery in some French towns if they passed an examination. However, the medical faculty of Paris often complained about quacks of both sexes in the city. As medical faculties and professional organizations gained prestige and power, laws governing medical practice became increasingly restrictive throughout Europe. Unlicensed practitioners were prosecuted, fined, or excommunicated for disregarding these laws. As indicated by the case of Jacoba Felicie in Paris in 1322, the lack of a formal education did not necessarily mean a lack of skill and experience. The Dean and Faculty of Medicine of the University of Paris charged Jacoba with illegally visiting the sick of both sexes, examining their pulse, urine, bodies, and limbs, prescribing drugs, collecting fees, and, worse yet, curing her patients.

Not only did Jacoba feel competent to practice medicine, she also thought herself capable of pleading her own case. Patients called to testify praised her skill; some noted that she had cured them after regular physicians had failed. Jacoba argued that the intent of the law was to forbid the practice of medicine by idiots and incompetents. Because she was both knowledgeable and skillful, the statute of 1271 did not apply to her. Moreover, natural modesty about the "secret nature" of female infirmities created a need for women doctors. The Dean and Masters of Medicine who prosecuted Jacoba did not deny her skill, but they argued that medicine was a science transmitted by texts, not a craft to be learned empirically. The Court agreed with the Masters of Medicine. Licensed women physicians essentially vanished by the sixteenth century, but hordes of quacks were busily peddling herbs, amulets, and charms. This army of empirics included barber-surgeons, herbalists, nurses, and midwives. As the fear of witchcraft increased during the waning years of the Middle Ages, the position of women healers became even more precarious.

Whatever the relative merits of scholars, physicians, and empirics might have been, probably the best physicians of the Middle Ages were those recommended in the popular health handbook known as the *Regimen of Salerno*: Doctors Quiet, Rest, Diet, and Merryman. Unfortunately, these doctors were unlikely to be on the staff of the typical hospital or to make housecalls at the hovels of the poor.

Hospitals have been called the greatest medical innovation of the Middle Ages, but because the modern hospital is so closely associated with advances in research, medical education, and surgery, the term "hospital" conjures up images that are inappropriate to previous time periods. Certainly, medieval hospitals played an important social role, but their primary goals were religious, not scientific. Medieval hospitals provided comfort, nursing, and medical care as well as charity.

Confusion about the origins and development of the medieval hospital reflects the paradoxes and tensions of this complex era. Many hospitals were no more than cottages, but in the major towns relatively large institutions served as infirmaries, almshouses, hostels, and leper houses. Of course the number and nature of these charitable enterprises changed throughout the Middle Ages. During the fourteenth century some hospitals were trying to discharge the sick poor and replace them with paying clients, while others became so intolerable that the inmates rebelled and demolished them.

One problem exacerbated during the Middle Ages was the separation between surgery and medicine. Although the leech of the early medieval period was both physician and surgeon, his "surgery" was generally limited to routine procedures, such as phlebotomy, cupping, and cauterization, and simple emergency measures for coping with the usual run of burns, bruises, wounds, ulcers, sprains, dislocations, toothaches, and broken bones. A few more daring practitioners had the special skills needed for couching cataracts, tooth extraction, and lithotomy (the surgical removal of stones in the urinary bladder). Modern specialists might be surprised to find their medieval counterparts among the lowly oculists, bone-setters, tooth extractors, cutters of the stone, and other empirics, rather than in the company of learned physicians. Nevertheless, during the Middle Ages, ambitious surgeons were trying to win a more respectable professional status for surgery as a branch of knowledge with its own body of technical writings and an eminently useful occupation. A special technical literature of surgery was growing by the thirteenth century, but some clues to earlier, less learned traditions can be glimpsed in the epic poetry of earlier centuries.

Since the need for surgeons is a common by-product of warfare, semi-legendary stories of great heroes and battles often reflect actual practice with more immediacy than learned texts. According to Scandinavian epic poets, if professional doctors were not available, the men with the softest hands were assigned to care for the wounded. Many famous physicians were said to have descended from warriors with gentle hands. Truly heroic warriors bound up their own wounds and returned to the battle. Sometimes women cared for the wounded in a special tent or house near the battlefield. One saga describes a woman who cleaned wounds with warm water and extracted arrows with tongs. When she could not find the arrow, she made the patient eat boiled leeks. Then the hidden wound could be located because it smelled of leeks.

Although epic heroes emerged from crude battlefield surgery completely healed and eager to fight, the subjects of more mundane operations often succumbed to bleeding, shock, and infection. Despite their familiarity with the soporific effects of poppy, henbane, and mandrake, surgeons did not routinely use these drugs before an operation. Potions made of wine, eggs, honey, and beer were used to wash and

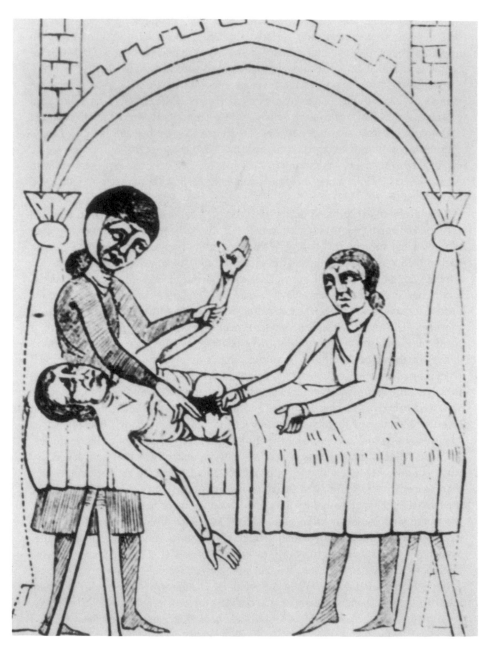

Medieval depiction of an operation on the liver

dress external and internal wounds. A dressing for burns might be as gentle as a mixture of egg whites, fats, and herbs, or it might be strengthened by the addition of goat droppings.

Medieval medicine is also notable for the appearance of some outstanding practitioners who deplored the separation between medicine and surgery. The learned doctors of Salerno, the most famous Western medical school of the Middle Ages, maintained high standards of surgery and taught anatomy and surgical techniques by dissections of animals. Medieval authors created simplified new Latin texts based on the work of Salerno and the Arabic literature. A treatise on surgery, based on the lectures of Roger Frugard, who taught and practiced surgery at Parma in northern Italy, was prepared about 1180 by his colleague Guido Arezzo the Younger. Roger's highly influential and often copied *Surgery* described methods of wound closure, trephination, and lithotomy, recommended mercury for skin diseases and seaweed for goiter. In the mid-thirteenth century, Roland of Parma produced an important new edition of Roger's surgical treatise which became known as the *Rolandina*. Roland, who taught at the new medical center in Bologna, based his teaching and practice on Roger's methods. Even as late as the sixteenth century, after newer Latin texts and translations of Galen and Arabic authors became available, Roger's treatise was respectfully studied. By the beginning of the fourteenth century, texts for surgeons who were literate but had not mastered Latin were appearing in vernacular languages. These texts provided practical information on medicine and surgery and collections of recipes.

Hugh of Lucca (ca. 1160–1257), town surgeon of Bologna, and his son Theodoric, Bishop of Cervia (1210–1298) may have been the most ingenious of medieval surgeons. Theodoric is said to have attacked the two great enemies of surgery, *infection* and *pain*, and rejected the idea that the formation of pus was a natural and necessary stage in the healing of wounds. Indeed, Theodoric realized that the generation of pus, sometimes deliberately provoked by surgeons, obstructed wound healing. He also objected to the use of complex and noxious wound dressings. To overcome the pain caused by surgery, Theodoric attempted to induce narcosis by the use of a "soporific sponge" containing drugs known to produce a sleep-like state. Just how effective his methods were in practice is unclear. Sponges were prepared by soaking them in a mixture of extracts from mandrake, poppy, henbane, and other herbs. Before surgery began, the dried sponges were soaked in hot water and the patient was allowed to chew on the sponge and inhale the vapors.

Sometime in the early fourteenth century, Henri de Mondeville, surgeon to Philip the Fair of France, composed a major treatise on surgery. The text was still unfinished when Henri died about 1320. In addition to being unfinished, Henri's text was polemical and argumentative in style and tone and hostile to the medical authorities. Proud of his skills and accomplishments as a surgeon, Henri struggled vainly against the separation of surgery from medicine. By the end of the century the gentlemen of the Faculty of Medicine in Paris were demanding that graduate physicians take an oath that they would not perform any surgical practices. Henri's work was gradually forgotten and his text was not printed until 1892. The title "father of French surgery" was bestowed on Guy de Chauliac (ca. 1298–1368), eminent physician and surgeon and author of a treatise on surgery which remained a standard work into the eighteenth century. Until the sixteenth century, most of the Latin and vernacular texts on surgery produced in Europe were essentially derivatives of the work of Roger Frugard and Guy de Chauliac.

EPIDEMIC DISEASES OF THE MIDDLE AGES

Many of the afflictions described in medieval texts are still common today, but the most feared of all pestilential diseases, leprosy and bubonic plague, still color our perceptions of this era. Indeed, the most devastating pandemics the world has ever experienced—the Plague of Justinian and the Black Death—provide an appropriate frame for the medical history of the Middle Ages. It might be said that plague and leprosy should not be discussed as "medieval diseases." Indeed, epidemics of bubonic plague continued into the nineteenth century and both plague and leprosy continue to claim victims in the twentieth century.

Medieval astrologers blamed the Black Death on a malign conjunction of Saturn, Jupiter, and Mars; epidemiologists now trace the cause of epidemic plague to an unfortunate conjunction of *Yersinia pestis*, fleas, and rats. A brief overview of the complex ecological relationships of microbes, fleas, rodents, and human beings will help us understand the medieval pandemics, the waves of plague that continued well into the seventeenth century, and the status of plague today. It is worth discussing the components of this web of relationships in order to dispel the notion that discovering the "cause" of epidemic disease is a simple matter of naming the microbe involved and as a reminder that rodents, fleas, mosquitoes, ticks, and microbes are still part of the web of life. Moreover, the magnitude of the pandemics caused by bubonic plague is an instructive lesson about how powerful a force disease can be in human history. Such reminders are essential now that molecular biologists are able to identify, isolate, and manipulate the genetic factors responsible for the awesome virulence of the microbes that cause bubonic plague and other epidemic diseases.

Plague provides an interesting example of the way in which a specific microbe can cause different clinical patterns. In this case, the major forms of illness are known as *bubonic* and *pneumonic* plague. In the absence of appropriate antibiotics, the mortality rate from bubonic plague may exceed 50%; the deadly pneumonic form probably kills 100% of its victims. Even today, despite streptomycin, tetracycline, and chloramphenicol, many plague victims succumb to the disease.

If the plague bacillus enters the body via the bite of an infected flea, the disease follows the pattern known as bubonic. After an incubation period of about 6 days, victims suddenly experience pains in the chest, coughing, difficulty in breathing,

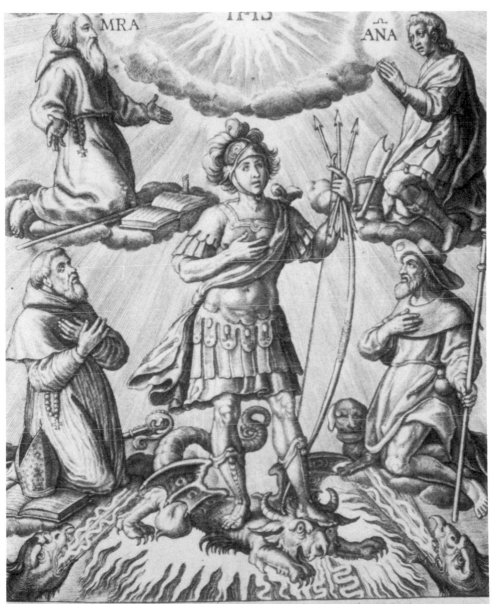

Plague

vomiting of blood, high fever, and dark splotches on the skin. The most characteristic signs of bubonic plague are the hard, painful swellings called "buboes" that appear in the lymph nodes, usually in the groin, armpit, neck, and behind the ears. Restlessness, anxiety, headaches, mental confusion, hallucinations, and finally coma and death may follow. In some cases, referred to as *septicemic* plague, the patient may rapidly weaken, become delirious or comatose, and die in 1–3 days without the appearance of buboes.

Spread directly from person to person by droplets of saliva, pneumonic plague is highly contagious and exceptionally lethal. Just what circumstances lead to the transformation of bubonic plague to the pneumonic form is uncertain. However, if victims of bubonic plague develop pulmonary abscesses, their fits of coughing will release hordes of bacteria. When inhaled, the bacteria make their way through the mucous membranes to spread and multiply in their new hosts, who are classified as victims of primary pneumonic plague. The incubation period for pneumonic plague is usually only 1–3 days and the onset of symptoms is very abrupt. Pain in the chest is accompanied by violent coughing which brings up bloody sputum. Neurological disorders progress rapidly and incapacitate the victim. Hemorrhages under the skin produce dark purple blotches. Coughing and choking, the patient finally suffocates and dies.

As if to provide unequivocal proof that plague was not a medieval disease, bubonic plague swept across Asia in the 1890s, from Canton to Hong Kong to Bombay, killing about one million people in India in 1903, while invading Java, Japan, Asia Minor, South Africa, the shores of North and South America, Portugal, Austria, and parts of Russia. Alexandre Yersin (1863–1943) discovered the plague bacillus during an outbreak in Hong Kong in 1894. Shibasaburo Kitasato (1852–1931), studying the same outbreak for the Japanese government, also contributed to early studies of the bacterium. Originally called *Pasteurella pestis*, the plague bacillus was renamed *Yersinia pestis* in honor of Yersin.

At least three naturally occurring varieties of *Yersinia pestis* are known today. All three varieties cause virulent infections in humans and most mammals. The microbe can remain viable for many months in the congenial microclimate of rodent warrens. Its life span in putrefying corpses is limited to a few days, but it may survive for years in frozen cadavers. Thus, local outbreaks depend on the state of rodent communities and the means used to dispose of the bodies of plague victims.

Although *Yersinia pestis* can easily penetrate the mucous membranes, it cannot enter the body through healthy, unbroken skin. Therefore, the microbe is generally dependent on the flea to reach new hosts. In the 1890s, scientists began to present evidence that the flea was involved in the transmission of plague, but the "flea theory" was greeted with such skepticism that members of the British Plague Commission in Bombay carried out experiments to prove that fleas did not transmit plague. They "proved" their hypothesis because they assumed that "a flea is a flea is a flea." Further progress in "fleology" revealed that all fleas are not created equal.

Out of some 2000 different kinds of fleas, the black rat's flea, *Xenophylla cheopsis*, has been awarded first prize as the most efficient vector of plague, but at least eight species of fleas can transmit the microbe to humans. The flea itself becomes a victim of the plague bacillus, as its stomach becomes blocked by a plug of bacteria. When the flea bites a new victim, the ingested blood comes in contact with this plug and mixes with the bacteria. Part of the ingested material, containing a huge number of bacteria, is regurgitated into the wound.

Fleas are usually fairly loyal to their host species. Unfortunately, *X. cheopsis* finds human beings an acceptable substitute for the rat. *Pulex irritans*, the human flea, cannot approach the infective power of the rat flea, but under appropriate conditions quantity could make up for quality. Despite the flea's role as ubiquitous nuisance and vector of disease, Thomas Moffet (1553–1604), father of Little Miss Moffet, noted that, in contrast to being lousy, it was not a disgrace to have fleas.

Once the connection between rats and plague was elucidated, many authorities believed that the black rat, *Rattus rattus*, was the only source of plague epidemics. However, almost 200 species of rodents have been identified as possible reservoirs of plague. The concept of "sylvatic plague" acknowledges the ecological significance of *Yersinia pestis* among various species of wild rodents.

There is some controversy about the status of the black rat in Europe during the early Middle Ages. Adding to the confusion is the fact that ancient chroniclers did not distinguish between rats and mice when they spoke of "vermin" and the strange behaviors that were considered omens of disaster. Medieval physicians and peasants rightly feared that when rats, mice, moles, and other animals that normally lived underground came to the surface, acted as if drunk, and died in great multitudes, pestilential disease would follow. However, these strange portents were easily reconciled with the idea that noxious vapors generated deep within the earth could escape into the atmosphere where they produced deadly *miasmata* (poisonous vapors).

Sometime during the Middle Ages, the black rat made its way to Europe and, finding excellent accommodations in its towns and villages, took up permanent residence. The medieval town may seem picturesque through the misty lens of nostalgia, but it was a filthy, unhealthy place of narrow, winding alleys, not unlike rodent warrens, surrounded by haphazard accumulations of garden plots, pig pens, dungheaps, shops, houses, and hovels shared by humans and animals. Perhaps it is not just a coincidence that a marked decline in the incidence of European plague occurred at about the same time that the black rat was being driven out by a newcomer, the large brown rat, *Rattus norvegicus*.

Although epidemic bubonic plague may have occurred in very ancient periods, early descriptions of "plagues and pestilences" are too vague to provide specific diagnoses. Thus, the Plague of Justinian in 540 is generally regarded as the first definitive bubonic plague epidemic in Europe. Further waves of plague can be charted over the next several centuries. However, the disease seems to have died out in the West only to be periodically reintroduced from Mediterranean ports.

According to our best eyewitness, the historian Procopius (ca. 500–560), the plague began in Egypt in 540 and soon spread over the entire earth, killing men, women, and children in every nation. Although the disease always seemed to spread inland from coastal regions, no human habitation, no matter how remote, was spared. Many people saw phantoms before they were struck by the disease, some people collapsed in the streets as if struck by lightning, others locked themselves into their houses for safety, but phantoms appeared in their dreams and they too succumbed. Panic and terror mounted with the death toll as civil life ceased; only the corpse-bearers made their way through streets littered with rotting bodies. As the daily toll reached into the thousands, graves and gravediggers became so scarce that ships were filled with corpses and abandoned at sea. Those who survived were not attacked again, but depravity and licentiousness seemed to consume those who had witnessed and survived the horrors of the plague.

The sick were objects of great fear, but Procopius noted that the disease was not necessarily contagious, because nurses, gravediggers, and even physicians who examined the bodies of the dead and opened plague buboes at post-mortems might be spared. Physicians could not predict which cases would be mild and which would be fatal, but they came to believe that survival was most common in cases where the plague bubo grew large, ripened, and suppurated.

There are many gaps in our knowledge of the early waves of plague; however, there is no lack of speculation. Some argue that the death and disorder caused by the plague led to the decline of the Byzantine Empire. A shift of power in Europe from south to north, Mediterranean to North Sea, may have been the consequence of the failure of plague to penetrate the British Isles, northern Gaul, and Germania. Establishing the death toll is virtually impossible. Overwhelmed by panic and fear, witnesses resorted to symbolic or exaggerated figures to convey the enormity of the disaster. Many accounts of medieval pestilence state that mortality was so great that there were not enough of the living to bury the dead.

Surviving records are essentially silent about the status of plague between the ninth century and its catastrophic return in the fourteenth. Of course, the absence of specific references to plague does not prove that the disease did not occur during that period. For the medieval chroniclers, the causes of all great "perils and adversities"—earthquakes, floods, famines, pestilential diseases—were beyond human comprehension or control, and so common that only the most dramatic were worth recording.

During the twelfth and thirteenth centuries, Europe attained a level of prosperity unknown since the fall of Rome. Population growth began to accelerate in the eleventh century and reached its peak by the fourteenth. Europe remained a largely agricultural society, but the growth of towns and cities reflected a demographic and economic revolution. Nevertheless, even before the outbreak of plague, conditions seem to have been deteriorating. By about 1300, Europe could no longer bring more land into use or significantly improve the yield of land already under cultivation. The harvests from 1315 to 1317 were disastrous; food prices soared and malnutrition apparently became more prevalent. Contemporary observers said that clergymen and nobles prayed for a pestilence to reduce the lower class population so that others could live in more comfort. If this is true, the fourteenth-century pandemic is an awesome testimonial to the power of prayer. The pandemic that has come to be called the Black Death surpassed all previous pestilences as a remedy for overpopulation, while creating more havoc, misery, and fear than any protagonist on the stage of history before the twentieth century.

Although we do not know exactly where or how the Black Death began, it is clear that many plague outbreaks originated in the urban centers of the Near and Middle East. From these foci of infection, plague spread by ship and caravan trade routes. There are many uncertainties about the route taken by the plague and the rapidity of its progress, but the outlines of its journey by ship via the major ports of the Mediterranean and along the overland trade routes have been charted. The ships of the Italian city states probably served as the vehicles that brought the plague to western Europe in 1347 via the Crimean ports on the Black Sea. Within 2 years the Great Plague had spread throughout Europe, reaching even Greenland.

Survivors of the plague years predicted that those who had not experienced the great pestilence would never be able to comprehend the magnitude of the disaster. Indeed, the dispassionate analytical accounts of modern historians attempting to confirm or disconfirm some hypothesis about cause and effect relationships between the plague and subsequent events make a grim contrast to eyewitness accounts of the pandemic. Some historians see the Black Death as the event that ended the Middle Ages and destroyed medieval social, economic, and political arrangements. Others warn against confusing sequential relationships with cause and effect. Even the mortality caused by the plague remains a matter of controversy. In some areas the death rate may have been about 12%, whereas in others it apparently exceeded 50%. Estimates of the numbers killed in Europe alone range from 20 to 25 million; throughout the world more than 42 million people may have died.

The plague years provided a significant turning point for the medical profession. Many contemporary accounts speak of the lack of physicians, but it is not always clear whether this was due to their death from pestilence or because they had hidden themselves away for fear of contagion. The effect of the plague on the Church was also undeniably profound. Mortality among the clergy seems to have reached 50% between 1348 and 1349. Estimates of mortality in the higher orders of the Church are about 30%. Mortality in the Pope's court at Avignon was about 25%. In some areas, monasteries, churches, and whole villages were abandoned. Many writers complained that deaths among clergymen led to the ordination of men of lower qualifications and demoralization within the ranks. On the other hand, fear of death among the general populace increased the level of bequests to the Church.

With many physicians convinced that a catastrophic new disease had appeared, hundreds of plague tractates (treatises devoted to explanations of the disease and suggestions for its prevention and treatment) were written. But perhaps the most compelling account of the ravages of the plague is Giovanni Boccaccio's (1313–1375) introduction to the *Decameron*, a collection of stories supposedly told by 10 young men and women who left Florence in an attempt to escape the plague. According to Boccaccio, who had survived an attack of plague, Florence had become a city of corpses as half of Italy succumbed to the disease. Very few of the sick recovered, with or without medical aid, and most died within 3 days.

Many died not from the severity of their disease, but from want of care and nursing. The poor were the most pitiable; unable to escape to the countryside, they died by the thousands and the stench of rotting corpses overwhelmed the city. Every morning the streets were filled with bodies beyond number. Customary funeral rites were abandoned; corpses were dumped into trenches and covered with a little dirt. Famine followed plague, because peasants were too demoralized by fear to care for their crops or their animals. Worse than the disease itself, according to Boccaccio, was the barbarous behavior it unleashed; the healthy refused to aid friends, relatives, or even their own children. A few believed that asceticism would avert the plague, but others took the threat of death as an excuse for satisfying every base appetite. Criminal and immoral acts could be carried out with impunity for there was no one left to enforce the laws of man or God.

A surprisingly cheerful and optimistic view of the great pestilence was recorded by French cleric and master of theology Jean de Venette. According to de Venette, during the epidemic, no matter how suddenly people were stricken by the plague God saw to it that they died "joyfully" after confessing their sins. Moreover, the survivors hastened to marry and women commonly produced twins and triplets. Pope Clement VI graciously granted absolution to all plague victims who left their worldly goods to the Church. The Pope sought to win God's mercy and end the plague with an Easter pilgrimage to Rome in 1348. The power of faith proved to be no match for the power of pestilence. Prayers, processions, and appeals to all the patron saints were as useless as medicines.

Guy de Chauliac confessed that doctors felt useless and ashamed because the plague was unresponsive to medical treatment. Physicians, knowing the futility of medical intervention, were afraid to visit the sick for fear of becoming infected themselves. Worse yet, if they did take care of plague victims they could not expect to be paid because patients died and escaped their debts. Guy did not join the physicians who fled from Avignon; he contracted the disease, but recovered. Pope Clement VI was more fortunate than his physician. The Pope remained shut up in his innermost chambers, between two great protective fires, and refused to see anyone.

Physicians could not cure the plague, but they could offer advice, much of it contradictory, on how to avoid contracting the disease. Abandoning the affected area was often advised, but opinions varied about the relative safety of potential retreats. If flight was impossible, another option was to turn one's home into a medieval version of a fallout shelter. To reduce contact with tainted air, doctors suggested moving about slowly while inhaling through aromatic sponges or "smelling apples" containing exotic and expensive ingredients such as amber and sandalwood, strong-smelling herbs, or garlic, the traditional theriac of the poor. Bathing was regarded as a dangerous procedure because baths opened the pores and allowed corrupt air to penetrate the outer defenses. Physicians eventually developed elaborate protective costumes with long robes, gloves, boots, and "bird-beaked" masks which held a sponge steeped in protective aromatic substances. Those fortunate enough to secure medical attention were fortified by theriacs and dietary regimens designed to remove impurities and bad humors. Once symptoms of the disease appeared, physicians prescribed bleeding and purging, and attempted to hasten the maturation of buboes by scarification, cupping, cauterization, poultices, and plasters.

During later outbreaks of plague, secular and clerical authorities attempted to limit the spread of the disease with prayers and quarantine regulations. Of course, infected rats had no respect for either approach. By the fifteenth century, Venice, Florence, and other Italian cities had developed detailed public health measures. Less advanced states throughout Europe used the Italian system as a model for dealing with epidemic disease. Unfortunately, the well-meaning officials who formulated quarantine rules were ignorant of the natural history of plague. Some measures, such as the massacre of dogs and cats, were clearly counterproductive. Long periods of quarantine for those suspected of carrying the contagion caused unnecessary hardships and promoted willful disobedience (today a quarantine of 7 days is considered adequate).

Perhaps the combination of faith and quarantine regulations, along with more subtle changes in plague ecology, eventually mitigated the effects of further waves of plague, at least in the countryside. During the fifteenth century the rich could expect to escape the plague by fleeing from the city. Eventually, patterns of mortality were established which convinced the elite that plague was a contagious disease of the poor. However, the situation is complicated by diagnostic confusion between true bubonic plague and other infectious diseases. The public health authorities preferred to err on the side of caution and were likely to suspect plague given the slightest provocation. Much "plague legislation" after the Black Death was actually more concerned with protecting the personal safety and property of the elite than with control of plague itself. But the concept of granting authority to secular public health officials was established. Epidemic plague essentially disappeared from the western Mediterranean by the eighteenth century; it remained a threat in the eastern Mediterranean area well into the nineteenth century, but later outbreaks never achieved the prevalence or virulence of the Black Death.

Plague is still enzootic among wild rodents throughout the world, leading to sporadic human cases in Africa, Asia, Latin America, and the United States. Thus, unforeseen changes in the ecology of a plague area could release a wave of plague among animals and humans. For example, the massive disruption of sanitary and medical organizations that would follow a nuclear war could provide a fertile killing field for plague.

In the first decade of the twentieth century, while California politicians and merchants acted as if bad publicity was more dangerous than plague, bubonic plague escaped from San Francisco and established itself as an endemic disease among the rodents of the western United States. Prairie dog colonies in Colorado provide a large reservoir of plague threatening cities and tourists, but New Mexico has had the largest number of human cases. Because human plague is now rare and unexpected, sporadic cases are often misdiagnosed. If appropriate treatment is not begun soon enough, the proper diagnosis may be made at the autopsy. Between 1949 and 1980, 97 cases of human plague were diagnosed in the United States; 17 were fatal. Moreover, whereas only 5% of the cases identified between 1949 and 1974 were of the pneumonic form, between 1975 and 1980 this highly virulent form accounted for about 25% of New Mexico's plague cases. The extent of plague transmission between rural and urban animals is unknown, but the danger is not negligible. People have been infected by domestic cats, bobcats, coyotes, and cottontail rabbits.

Perhaps the most dangerous characteristic of *Yersinia pestis* today is its ability to camouflage itself in popular historical memory as a "medieval plague" of no possible significance to modern societies. Much about the disappearance of plague from the ranks of major epidemic diseases is obscure, but we can say with a fair degree of certainty that medical breakthroughs had nothing to do with it. In its animal reservoirs, the plague is very much alive and presumably quite capable of taking advantage of any disaster that would significantly alter the ecological relationships among rodents, fleas, and humans.

FROM LEPROSY TO HANSEN'S DISEASE

More than any other disease, leprosy demonstrates the difference between the biological nature of illness and the attributes ascribed to the sick. Indeed, it is fair to say that leprosy and Hansen's disease (the modern name for true leprosy) stand for different *ideas* more than different *diseases*. The word *leper* is still commonly used to mean one who is hated and shunned by society. Medieval attitudes towards the leper were based on biblical passages pertaining to "leprosy," a vague term applied to various chronic, progressive skin afflictions, from leprosy and vitiligo to psoriasis and skin cancer. The leper, according to medieval interpretations of the Bible, was "unclean" and, therefore, a dangerous source of physical and moral pollution.

According to the biblical rules governing leprosy, persons and things with suspicious signs were brought to the priests for examination. Leprosy dwelled not only in human beings, but also in garments of wool or linen, objects made of skins, and even in houses. Diagnostic signs included a scaly eruption, boil, scab, or bright

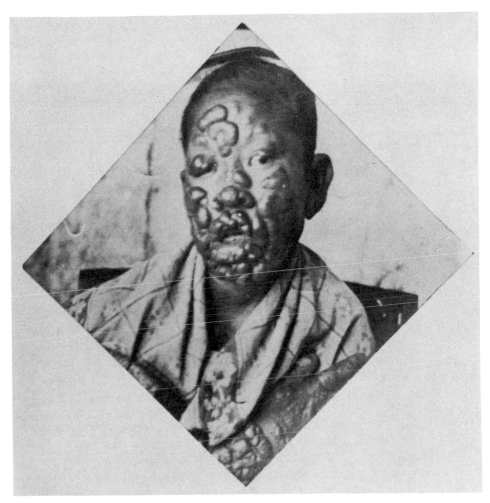

Leprosy (photographed in Manila in 1899)

spot. When the signs were ambiguous, the priest shut the suspect away for as long as 2 weeks for further observations. When a final judgment had been reached, the leper was instructed to dwell in isolation and call out as a warning to those who might approach him, ''unclean, unclean.''

Islamic teachings also reflected fear of leprosy. ''Fly from the leper,'' warned the Prophet Muhammad, ''as you would fly from a lion.'' According to Islamic law and custom, people suffering from leprosy were not allowed to visit the baths. It was said that foods touched by a leper could transmit the disease, and that no plants would grow in soil touched by the bare feet of a leper.

A brief survey of modern findings about this disease may help us understand the ambiguities and complexity of the medieval literature concerning leprosy. *Mycobacterium leprae*, the bacillus that causes leprosy, was discovered in 1874 by the Norwegian physician Gerhard Hansen (1841–1912). Hansen had observed leprosy bacilli as early as 1871, but it was very difficult to prove that the bacteria found in skin scrapings of patients actually caused the disease. No animal model was available and the putative leprosy bacillus refused to grow in artificial media. It took almost 100 years for scientists to overcome these obstacles. To honor Gerhard Hansen and avoid the stigma associated with the term leper, the disease was renamed Hansen's disease.

What is most surprising about Hansen's disease is the fact that it is only slightly contagious. Many people having extended and intimate contact with lepers, such as spouses, nurses, and doctors, do not contract the disease, while others with little contact become infected. Evidence of the limited degree of contagiousness of leprosy today does not, of course, prove that the disease was not more contagious in the past. Nevertheless, leprosy could not have been as contagious as medieval writers assumed; religious and medical authorities argued that leprosy could be spread by the glance of a leper or an unseen leper standing upwind of healthy people.

Various indeterminate patterns exist between the two polar forms of Hansen's disease, known as tuberculoid and lepromatous. The more severe form, lepromatous leprosy, which accounts for about 20% of all cases, is characterized by skin lesions consisting of raised blotches, nodules, and lumps. Eventually, the thickening of the skin of the forehead and face, exaggeration of natural lines, and loss of facial hair produce the so-called "lion face." As the disease progresses, ulcerating skin lesions lead to destruction of cartilage and bone.

The early symptoms of tuberculoid leprosy include skin lesions and loss of sensation in the affected areas. Patients with the tuberculoid form mount a partially effective cell-mediated immune response; unfortunately this weak response may lead to damage to tissues rather than elimination of the bacteria. About 30% of all victims of Hansen's disease eventually develop crippling deformities due to damaged joints, paralysis of muscles, and loss of soft tissue and bone, especially the fingers and toes. Loss of sensitivity due to nerve damage results in repeated injuries and infections.

Leprosy seems to have been rare in Europe before the fall of Rome. Although the disease was creeping into the Mediterranean arena by the sixth century, the Crusades of the eleventh and twelfth centuries created ideal conditions for a major invasion. Indeed, there are estimates that by the end of the twelfth century one out of every 200 Europeans was infected with leprosy. The high incidence of leprosy among pious persons, especially Crusaders and pilgrims returning from the Holy Land, was a source of embarrassment to the Church. The Crusades were part of massive movements of human populations that broke down ancient barriers and carried

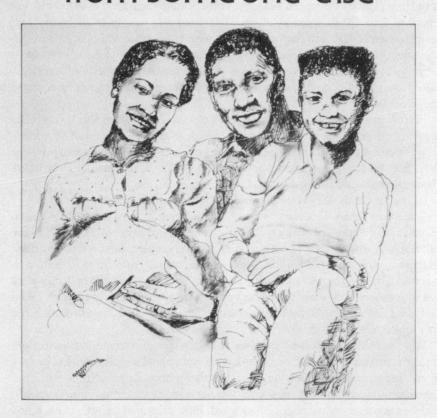

Hansen's Disease

infectious diseases to new populations. However, after reaching its peak in the thirteenth century, leprosy all but disappeared from Europe.

Priests, doctors, and lepers were involved in the examination of alleged medieval lepers. If incriminating signs of leprosy were found—bright spots, depigmented patches, sores, thickened skin, hoarse voice, and "lion face" —the accused was found guilty; a funeral service, rather than an execution, followed the verdict. Although the rites of exclusion could be held in a church, performing them in a cemetery with the leper standing in a grave made the symbolic death and burial more dramatic. Sprinkling earth on the leper's head, the priest declared him dead to the world, but reborn to God. While hated by all men, the leper was said to be loved by God; compensation for the sufferings of the leper were to be expected in the next world. The rules concerning lepers and marriage reflect the ambiguity of the leper's status. Leprosy was not necessarily accepted as a cause for the dissolution of marriage. Indeed, the Church decreed that a male leper could require a healthy wife to continue sexual relations.

Feared by all and condemned to live in isolation, lepers were also conspicuous targets of religious charity. Thousands of leper houses were established by various religious orders throughout Europe. Where lepers were granted the special privilege of begging for alms, other impoverished people seem to have pretended to be lepers in order to receive alms or be admitted to leper houses. Miserable as these places might be by our standards, they were presumably better than the alternatives.

Sometimes lepers were the objects of "heroic charity," such as that of Queen Mathilda, who expressed her piety by bringing lepers into her own rooms where she fed them and washed their feet. On finding her so occupied, her brother was filled with revulsion and warned her that King Henry might not enjoy being intimate with a woman who spent her days caressing the feet of lepers. However, Mathilda's piety was so contagious that she soon had her brother kissing the lepers. In contrast, Philip the Fair of France thought that lepers should be buried alive or burned to death rather than subjected to symbolic rites of isolation and burial.

When in public, lepers were supposed to wear a special costume and warn others of their approach with a bell, or rattle. Lepers were not allowed to speak to healthy people, but could point with a long stick to indicate items they wished to purchase. (Presumably money taken from a leper was not a source of contagion.) As always, justice or injustice was not equally distributed. Enforcement of the rules of exclusion varied from laxity to extreme brutality. The role forced upon the leper was not that of a sick person, but that of a scapegoat.

Given the ambiguity of the early signs of leprosy, how was it possible to "discover" medieval lepers? Theoretically, lepers were supposed to report their disease to the authorities, but "closet lepers" were probably detected and exposed by suspicious neighbors. Medieval descriptions of all diseases contain highly stylized and speculative material expressed in terms of humoral pathology. However, the divergence between modern and medieval "observations" is more striking in the case of leprosy than for other diseases. In the absence of microbiological tests even the most skillful modern diagnostician may find it difficult to distinguish leprosy from other diseases that produce chronic, progressive skin lesions. Although some change in clinical patterns may occur over time, it seems likely that medieval authors, whether physicians or priests, described what they expected to see rather than what they actually saw.

Many medical authorities assumed that leprosy was caused or transmitted by improper sexual acts, such as intercourse with a menstruating woman, or by contact with a healthy woman who had previously had intercourse with a leper. The presumption of a link between leprosy and "moral defilement," specifically lechery, persisted into the twentieth century. But sex and sin were not the only causes of leprosy recognized by medieval physicians. The disease could be inherited from a leprous ancestor or acquired from the bite of a poisonous worm, rotten meat, unclean wine, infected air, and corrupt milk from a leprous wet nurse. Various diets were commonly recommended to prevent or cure leprosy; almost every food fell under suspicion at one time or other. Indeed, many years of research convinced Sir Jonathan Hutchinson (1828–1913) that rotten fish caused leprosy.

Although the only useful medieval response to leprosy was isolation of the afflicted, physicians, quacks, the Bible offered hope of miraculous cures. According to Matthew, Jesus healed a leper simply by touching him and saying "be thou clean." In contrast to this instantaneous cure, Naaman, who was cured by the prophet Elisha, had to wash himself in the Jordan River seven times. Bartolomeus Anglicus (fl. 1250) admitted that leprosy was difficult to cure, except of course by the help of God, but he did suggest a remedy made from the flesh of a black snake cooked in an earthen pot with pepper, salt, vinegar, oil, water, and a special "bouquet garni." Because this powerful snake soup would make the patient dizzy and cause his body to swell, theriac was needed to counteract undesirable side effects. Eventually, the patient's flesh would peel and his hair fall out, but these problems would subside. An equally promising remedy from a fifteenth-century leechbook combined a bushel of barley and half a bushel of toads in a lead cauldron. The mixture was simmered until the flesh of the toads fell from the bones. The barley brew was dried in the sun and then fed to newly hatched chicks. The chicks were roasted or boiled and fed to the leper.

Driven by fear and hope, desperate lepers might attempt even the most gruesome of cures, be it eating human gall bladder or bathing in blood. Because many transient skin lesions were probably mistaken for Hansen's disease, appeals to saints, baths, bizarre recipes, and strange diets were sometimes followed by miraculous cures of the *post hoc ergo propter hoc* variety (the logical fallacy in which sequence is confused with cause).

Perhaps the most surprising aspect of medieval European leprosy is the virtual disappearance of the disease by the fourteenth century. Obviously, this change was not the result of any medical breakthrough. Even the cruel measures taken to isolate lepers were of dubious efficacy in breaking the chain of transmission because the disease has a long latent period during which susceptible individuals are exposed to infection. Changing patterns of commerce, warfare, and pilgrimages may have broken the chain of contagion by which leprosy reached Europe from areas where the disease remained, and still remains, endemic.

If leprosy all but vanished from Europe with minimal medical or public health advances, could it not be totally eradicated today through deliberate efforts? There are good reasons to consider Hansen's disease a logical candidate for a global eradication campaign. Unlike bubonic plague, leprosy does not seem to have a natural animal reservoir. Therefore, breaking the chain of person-to-person transmission should eventually eliminate the disease. Leprosy was one of six infectious tropical diseases that the World Health Organization slated as targets of a worldwide public health campaign launched in 1975. However, malaria, schistosomiasis, filariasis, leishmaniasis, trypanosomiasis, and leprosy do not present a major threat to wealthy nations or individuals. Thus, they do not receive the attention that has been awarded to smallpox, poliomyelitis, measles, and other incurable, but preventable infectious diseases.

Because the early symptoms of Hansen's disease are similar to many other ailments, its victims may be misdiagnosed and subjected to inappropriate treatments for long periods of time. The drugs most frequently used to treat leprosy are dapsone, rifampicin, and clofazimine. Despite the appearance of strains of *M. leprae* resistant to each of these drugs, public health authorities argue that if a partial course of therapy were instituted for all lepers, the disease could be eradicated. Even if the afflicted individual is not completely cured, drug treatment renders the patient noninfectious and breaks the chain of transmission. Unless resources are allocated for a major assult on leprosy the worldwide incidence of the disease will inevitably increase and Hansen's disease will become more difficult to treat.

Politics and poverty account for much of the difficulty in mounting a global campaign against leprosy, but research on Hansen's disease has also been hindered by the reluctance of *M. leprae* to multiply and be fruitful in laboratory animals and artificial media. Research has been facilitated by the discovery that the bacilli will multiply in the footpads of mice, the nine-banded armadillo, and several nonhuman primates.

The World Health Organization estimates that more than 100 years after the discovery of the causative agent for leprosy, about 15 million people still suffer from the disease. The number could actually be much higher, because Hansen's disease is often misdiagnosed or unreported. Many patients still think of the diagnosis as an ineluctable curse rather than a curable disease.

SUGGESTED READINGS

Amundsen, Darrel W. (1978). Medieval Canon Law on Medical and Surgical Practice by the Clergy. *Bulletin of the History of Medicine* 52:22-44.

Anderson, Frank J. (1977). *An Illustrated History of the Herbals*. New York: Columbia University Press.

Andrews, Michael (1977). *The Life That Lives on Man*. New York: Taplinger.

Arano, Luisa Cogliato (1976). *The Medieval Health Handbook; Tacuinum Sanitatis*. Trans. and adapted by Oscar Ratti and Adele Westbrook. New York: Braziller.

Artz, Frederick B. (1980). *The Mind of the Middle Ages. An Historical Survey, A.D. 200-1500*. Chicago: University of Chicago Press.

Bell, Walter George (1924). *The Great Plague in London in 1665*. London: John Lane.

Benton, John (1985). Trotula, Women's Problems, and the Professionalization of Medicine in Medieval Europe. *Bulletin of the History of Medicine* 59: 30-53.

Biraben, J.-N., and Le Goff, Jacques (1975). The Plague in the Early Middle Ages. In Robert Forster and Orest Ranum, eds. *Biology of Man in History*. Baltimore: Johns Hopkins University Press, pp. 48-80.

Bonser, Wilfrid (1963). *The Medical Background of Anglo-Saxon England: A Study in History, Psychology, and Folklore*. London: The Wellcome Historical Medical Library.

Bowsky, William M., ed. (1971). *The Black Death. A Turning Point in History?* New York: Holt, Rinehart and Winston.

Brody, Saul Nathaniel (1974). *The Disease of the Soul; Leprosy in Medieval Literature*. Ithaca, NY: Cornell University Press.

Brown, Peter (1980). *The Cult of the Saints. Its Rise and Function in Latin Christianity*. Chicago: University of Chicago Press.

Campbell, Anna Montgomery (1931). *The Black Death and Men of Learning*. New York: Columbia University Press.

Carmichael, Ann G. (1986). *Plague and the Poor in Renaissance Florence*. New York: Cambridge University Press.

Cholmeley, H. P. (1912). *John of Gaddesden and the Rosa Medicinae*. Oxford, England: Clarendon Press.

Cipolla, Carlo M. (1973). *Cristofano and the Plague*. Berkeley, CA: University of California Press.

Cipolla, Carlo M. (1979). *Faith, Reason, and the Plague in Seventeenth-Century Tuscany*. Ithaca, NY: Cornell University Press.

Clay, Rotha Mary (1909). *The Medieval Hospitals of England*. New York: Barnes & Noble.

Cobban, Alan B. (1988). *The Medieval English Universities. Oxford and Cambridge to c.1500*. Berkeley, CA: University California Press.

Cockayne, Rev. Thomas Oswald (1864-66). *Leechdoms, Wortcunning and Starcraft of Early England*. Illustrating the history of science in this country before the Norman conquest. Collected and edited by Rev. T. O. Cockayne. New intro. by Charles Singer (1961). London: The Holland Press.

Contreni, John (1981). Masters and Medicine in Northern France During the Reign of Charles the Bald. In Margaret Gibson and Janet Nelson, eds. *Charles the Bald: Court and Kingdom*. Oxford, England: BAR International Series 101, pp. 333-350.

Crawford, Sir Raymond Henry Payne (1914). *Plague and Pestilence in Literature and Art*. Oxford, England: Clarendon Press.

Dawson, Warren R. (1935). *The Bridle of Pagasus: Studies in Magic, Mythology and Folklore*. London: Methuen.

Dols, Michael W. (1977). *The Black Death in the Middle East.* Princeton, NJ: Princeton University Press.

Dronke, Peter (1984). *Women Writers of the Middle Ages.* New York: Cambridge University Press.

Evans, J. A. S. (1972). *Procopius.* New York: Twayne Publishers.

Flanagan, Sabina (1989). *Hildegard of Bingen, 1098-1179: A Visionary Life.* New York: Routledge.

Forster, Robert, and Ranum, O. (1975). *Biology of Man in History.* Baltimore, MD: Johns Hopkins Press.

Gottfried, Robert S. (1983). *The Black Death: Natural and Human Disaster in Medieval Europe.* New York: The Free Press.

Gottfried, Robert S. (1986). *Doctors and Medicine in Medieval England, 1340-1530.* Princeton, NJ: Princeton University Press.

Green, Monica (1989). Women's Medical Practice and Medical Care in Medieval Europe. *SIGNS* 14: 434–473.

Gussow, Zachary (1989). *Leprosy, Racism, and Public Health: Social Policy in Chronic Disease Control.* Boulder, CO: Westview Press.

Hansen, G. Armauer, and Looft, Carl (1895). *Leprosy.* London: Simpkin, Marshall, Hamilton, Kent and Co., Ltd.

Haskins, C. H. (1927). *The Renaissance of the Twelfth Century.* Cambridge, MA: Harvard University Press.

Hinton, M. A. C. (1931). *Rats and Mice as Enemies of Mankind.* 3rd ed. London: British Museum of Natural History. Economic Series, No. 8.

Hirst, Leonard Fabian (1953). *Conquest of Plague. A Study of the Evolution of Epidemiology.* Oxford, England: Clarendon Press.

Howard-Jones, N. (1975). Kitasato, Yersin and the Plague Bacillus. *Clio Med.* 10(1):23–27.

Hughes, Muriel Joy (1943). *Women Healers in Medieval Life and Literature.* New York: King's Crown Press.

Isidore, Bishop of Seville (1954). *Isidore of Seville: The Medical Writings.* Intro., trans. and commentary by W. D. Sharpe. Philadelphia: American Philosophical Society.

Jackson, Robert (1982). Hutchinson on Leprosy. *International Journal of Dermatology* 21: 614-619.

Jacquart, Danielle, and Thomasset, Claude (1988). *Sexuality and Medicine in the Middle Ages.* Trans. by Matthew Adamson. Princeton, NJ: Princeton University Press.

Kealey, Edward J. (1981). *Medieval Medicus: A Social History of Anglo-Norman Medicine.* Baltimore, MD: Johns Hopkins Press.

Kibre, Pearl (1984). *Studies in Medieval Science: Alchemy, Astrology, Mathematics and Medicine.* London: Hambledon Press.

Lawn, Brian (1963). *The Salernitan Questions: An Introduction to the History of Medieval and Renaissance Problem Literature.* Oxford, England: Oxford University Press.

MacKinney, Loren C. (1937). *Early Medieval Medicine.* Baltimore, MD: Johns Hopkins Press.

Mason-Hohl, Elizabeth (1940). *The Diseases of Women: A Translation of Passionibus mulierum curandorum.* Los Angeles: Ward Ritchie Press.

Martin, Betty (1950). *Miracle at Carville.* Ed. by Evelyn Wells. Garden City, NY: Doubleday.

Maugh, Thomas M (1982). Leprosy Vaccine Trials to Begin Soon. *Science* 215: 1083–1086.

McEvedy, Colin, and Jones, Richard (1978). *Atlas of World Population History*. New York: Penguin Books.

Newman, Barbara (1987). *Sister of Wisdom: St. Hildegard's Theology of the Feminine*. Berkeley: University of California Press.

Obermann, Julian, ed. (1954). *The Code of Maimonides: Book Ten, the Book of Cleanness*. Trans. H. Danby. New Haven, CT: Yale University Press.

Pouchelle, Marie-Christine (1990). *The Body and Surgery in the Middle Ages*. New Brunswick, NJ: Rutgers University Press.

Preuss, Julius (1923). *Biblical and Talmudic Medicine*. Trans. by Fred Rosner. New York: Sanhedrin Press.

Procopius (1954). *Procopius*. With an English Translation by H. B. Dewing. In Seven Volumes. Cambridge, MA: Harvard University Press.

Richards, Peter (1977). *The Medieval Leper and His Northern Heirs*. Cambridge, England: D.S. Brewer Ltd.

Rosner, Fred (1984). *Medicine in the Mishneh Torah of Maimonides*. New York: KTAV.

Rothenberg, Gunther E. (1973). The Austrian Sanitary Cordon and the Control of Bubonic Plague: 1710-1874. *JHMAS* 28:15-23.

Rowland, Beryl, ed. and trans. (1981). *Medieval Woman's Guide to Health*. London, England: Croom Helm.

Rubin, Stanley (1974). *Medieval English Medicine*. New York: Barnes & Noble.

Sacks, Oliver (1985). *Migraine. Understanding a Common Disorder*. Berkeley, CA: University of California Press.

Siraisi, Nancy G. (1990). *Medieval and Early Renaissance Medicine*. Chicago: University of Chicago Press.

Stuart, S. M. (1975). Dame Trot. *SIGNS* 1:537-542.

Talbot, Charles H. (1967). *Medicine in Medieval England*. London: Oldbourne.

Temkin, Owsei (1973). *Galenism: Rise and Decline of a Medical Philosophy*. Ithaca, NY: Cornell University Press.

Temkin, Oswei (1990). *Hippocrates in a World of Pagans and Christians*. Baltimore, MD: Johns Hopkins University Press.

Thompson, James Westfall, ed. (1939). *The Medieval Library*. Chicago: University of Chicago Press.

Tuchman, Barbara W. (1978). *A Distant Mirror. The Calamitous 14th Century*. New York: Alfred A. Knopf.

Twigg, G. (1984). *The Black Death: A Biological Reappraisal*. New York: Schocken.

Voigts, Linda E. (1979). Anglo-Saxon Plant Remedies and the Anglo-Saxons. *ISIS* 70: 250-268.

Wu Lien-teh (1959). *Plague Fighter: The Autobiography of a Modern Chinese Physician*. Cambridge, England: Heffer.

Wu, Lien-teh (1926). *A Treatise on Pneumonic Plague*. Strasburg, France: Berger-Levrault. League of Nations.

Ziegler, Philip (1969). *The Black Death*. New York: Harper Torchbooks.

6

ISLAMIC MEDICINE

T he Middle Ages of European history roughly correspond to the Golden Age of Islam. Contacts between the Islamic and the Western world began with conflict and misunderstanding and have generally persisted in this pattern ever since. Ignorance concerning Islamic culture is obviously a perpetual source of danger in a world where by the 1980s about one in every five human beings was a Muslim, that is, a follower of Islam. Islam, the religion founded by Muhammad (570–632), literally means "to submit to God's will or law." When Muhammad was about 40 years old, he received the call to prophethood and a series of visions in which the *Qur'an* (Koran) was revealed to him. By the time of his death, practically all of Arabia had accepted Islam and a century later his followers had conquered half of Byzantine Asia, all of Persia, Egypt, North Africa, and Spain.

Early Western accounts of "Arabian medicine" reflect the legacy of conflict rather than an analysis of Islamic medicine as a component of a system of faith and a means of dealing with the universal problem of illness. For many European scholars, Arabian medicine was significant only in terms of the role it played in preserving Greek philosophy during the European Dark Ages. Arabian medicine was understood as synonymous with Arabic medicine—Arabic being the language of learning throughout areas of the world under Islamic influence. Thus, Arabic texts need not have Arab authors; Persians, Jews, and Christians took part in the development of the Arabic medical literature. Indeed, the literary sources for the study of classical Islamic medicine come from a geographic area stretching from Spain to India and a time span of some 900 years. Just as the term "Chinese medicine" is broadly used with respect to medical practice in the countries that came within the sphere of China's influence, the term "Islamic medicine" is used to designate the system of ideas and practices which was widely transmitted with the Arab conquests. Like Chinese medicine and Ayurvedic medicine, Islamic medicine is a living system still respectfully studied and practiced by traditional healers.

Discussions of Arab achievements in science, medicine, and philosophy once focused on a single question: Were the Arabs merely the transmitters of Greek achievements or did they make any original contributions? Such a question is inappropriate when applied to a period in which the quest for empirical scientific knowledge was unknown. Physicians, philosophers, and other scholars accepted the writings of the ancients as truth, example, and authority, to be analyzed, developed, and preserved. Having no attachment to the doctrine of the primacy of originality and progress, scholars saw tradition as a treasure chest, not as a burden or obstacle. Like their counterparts in the Christian West, scholars in the Islamic world had to find a means of peaceful coexistence with powerful religious leaders who took the position that knowledge could come only through the prophet Muhammad and his immediate followers.

Human well-being can be seen as central to the fundamental Islamic view of life. The *Qur'an* itself was given to believers as "a guide and a medicine" and the restorer of both spiritual and physical health. In a literal sense, the *Qur'an* could be taken as a medicine by writing a passage from the sacred book on a cloth, washing out the ink, and drinking the wash water. Fragments concerning medical lore culled from the *Qur'an* and the "sayings and doings" (*Hadith*) of the Prophet were gathered together as the "Medicine of the Prophet." These sayings reflect the Prophet's general approval of traditional Arab medicine, but later commentators apparently supplied many additional sayings. Some of the medical *Hadiths* encourage medical care of the sick and suggest broad principles of health, others refer to particular diseases and health problems and medical or spiritual treatments.

One of the most widely quoted sayings of the Prophet is: "God has sent down a treatment for every ailment." The Prophet was also quoted as saying that valid knowledge was of only two kinds, "knowledge of faith and knowledge of the body." The idea that "stress" induces diseases seems to be inherent in the saying that "Excessive worry makes for physical illness in a person." The sayings of the Prophet provided guidance on medical ethics and tradition, consolation of the sick, the evil eye, magic, amulets, and protective prayers. Some orthodox Muslims considered the Medicine of the Prophet superior to secular medicine in providing care for the soul and the body.

Many of the Prophet's "medical sayings" dealt with sensible eating and drinking to prevent disease. Others were complex or subtle statements about the relationship between suffering and sin. "A believer will suffer no sickness nor even a thorn to pierce his skin," Muhammad declared, "without expiating one of his sins." But there was also the promise that sickness and suffering could confer religious merit, because Muhammad promised that ''He who dies on a sickbed, dies the death of a martyr.'' Another saying promised that a woman who died in childbirth gained the rank of a martyr.

The Prophet generally recognized natural causes of illness and the natural effects of medical treatments. Of course, other passages in the *Qur'an* and the sayings of the Prophet refer to divine or supernatural aspects of illness. When God tested a person by sending misfortune or disease, the faithful could gain religious merit by bearing the trial patiently. Several passages suggest that the sick should bear their suffering and call for a doctor only when the situation became unbearable. Thus, while many factors in the evolution of Islamic culture favored the development of science and medicine, as in the Christian world certain forms of orthodoxy were hostile and intolerant of secular studies in general and medicine in particular. Traditionalists who wanted to preserve indigenous customs fought the infiltration of Greek ideas by attempting to sanctify Bedouin medical lore by attributing traditional beliefs to the Prophet. While Arab medicine during Muhammad's life time was essentially Bedouin folk medicine, a few scholar-physicians of that period were already familiar with the principles of Greek and Indian medicine and may have successfully prescribed such remedies for Muhammad.

Some theologians justified the acceptance of Greek medicine by reminding the faithful that the Prophet had come to teach only the Sacred Law and not medicine or other practical matters. His allusions to medicine, therefore, were not part of divine revelation, but spontaneous comments on folk-medicines, such as henna for gout, camel urine for stomach disorders, and antimony for eye disorders. Such folklore predated Islam and was neither religious nor scientific. On the other hand, if Muslims used a traditional remedy like honey, it could have a positive effect through the power of faith because Muhammad called honey a health-restoring food.

Although the Prophet unquestionably recommended cupping and the use of honey in treating certain illnesses, his position on cauterization was ambiguous. After

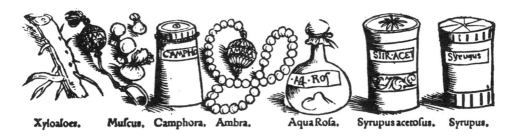

Xyloaloes.   Muſcus, Camphora, Ambra.   AquaRoſa.   Syrupus aceroſus.   Syrupus.

Pharmaceuticals

admitting that cauterization could restore health, the Prophet reportedly prohibited its use. But other passages indicate that on some occasions Muhammad ordered the use of cautery and even treated some of his wounded followers by cauterization. To rationalize use of the cautery, commentators argued that the prohibition was only intended to stop practitioners from boasting that the cautery was a totally effective measure. *All* remedies worked only by God's will. The Prophet's position on the use of amulets and faith healing represents an interesting compromise not unlike that reached by the Christian Church. Some of his followers reported that the Prophet originally forbade the use of all amulets because they might contradict strict monotheism by invoking supernatural agents. Eventually, he accepted the use of amulets whose contents were in keeping with the teachings of the *Qur'an*. Faith healing was apparently allowed in the treatment of venomous bites and the evil eye. Muslims were strictly forbidden to resort to star-cults, the reading of omens, and "black" or "white" magic.

Over the years, scores of books of "Prophetic Medicine" were compiled by traditionalists who hoped to counter the growing influence of Greek medicine by providing simple and safe Islamized medical handbooks for ordinary people. The authors were usually theologians and religious leaders, not medical practitioners. But all of these books failed to resolve the basic question: Is it more meritorious to trust completely in God, or to seek medical treatment? Nevertheless, despite the competing claims of traditionalists, theologians, and skeptics, Greek philosophy, science, and medicine eventually captivated Arab physicians and scholars, resulting in the formation of the modified Greco-Arabic medical system that continues to flourish today as *unani medicine*.

Finding a means of justifying a scientific or secular approach to medicine was a challenge to Muslim scholars, much as it had been to Christians. While the value of medicine was generally accepted, some theologians accused doctors of confusing the priorities of the common people by encouraging them to place physical health before religious values. However, Prophetic Medicine, whatever the uncertainties of interpretation, clearly taught that "after faith, the art and practice of medicine is the most meritorious service in God's sight." Medical writers justified the study and practice of medicine as a form of religious service which was pleasing to God, so long as it relieved human suffering while acknowledging the primacy of faith.

By the end of the seventh century, under the leadership of the first four *caliphs* (successors to the Prophet), the Arabs had completed the conquest of Syria, Persia, and Egypt, and the process of assimilating Greek philosophy, science, and medicine into Islamic culture began. Muhammad had said: "Seek knowledge, even in China," but it was originally the Persian city of Jundi Shapur that served as a intellectual magnet for Muslim scholars. Located in southwestern Iran not far from the city of Susa, the ancient city of Jundi Shapur provided a uniquely tolerant and peaceful meeting point for the study of the philosophical and medical traditions of Persians,

Greeks, Indians, Zoroastrians, Jews, and Nestorians. The hospital at Jundi Shapur seems to have functioned as a medical school. The scholars of Jundi Shapur carried out the monumental task of assembling and translating Greek texts, including those of Hippocrates and Galen, into Syriac, which was then the language of the university. Many of the Greek texts were eventually translated into Arabic from these Syrian editions. The Arabs captured the city in 636, but treated the university with respect. Two of the prophet's physicians were said to have studied at Jundi Shapur. Ten years later Alexandria was also conquered.

After the triumph of the Abbasid caliphs in 750 and the establishment of Baghdad as the capital of the Islamic Empire, the Hellenization of Islamic culture accelerated rapidly. By the end of the tenth century, Baghdad and Cairo had developed into independent centers of scholarship. The library established in Cairo in 988 was said to house well over 100,000 volumes. The city had 36 public libraries by 1258. In 1258 the Mongols conquered Baghdad and its great libraries were destroyed. So many manuscripts were thrown into the river that, according to one observer, the Tigris ran black, red, and green with ink for 3 days. Another chronicler said that the river was so thick with manuscripts that one could walk across it.

Assimilating the intellectual treasures of antiquity into Islamic culture began in the "Age of Translations" (ca. 750–900) with prodigious efforts to translate philosophical and scientific classics into more accessible forms. At the school for translation established during the reign of the Caliph Al-Ma'mun (813–33), many of Galen's medical and philosophical works were translated into Arabic versions. One of the most important translators was Hunayn Ibn Ishaq (809–875), a scholar who was often heard reciting Homer in Greek as he walked the streets of Baghdad. Hunayn's work was a major factor in creating the great Galenic synthesis, but he and his disciples translated other texts, including some of the works of Hippocrates and the *Materia medica* of Dioscorides. A major task for a scholar taking on such an unprecedented challenge was to create an appropriate nomenclature for concepts never before expressed in Arabic. Hunayn composed influential summaries, commentaries, and study guides for medical students, including the *Questions on Medicine for Scholars*. This ancient version of the ever-popular student "cram book" was a popular genre among Arab scholars; hundreds have survived. In therapeutics, Hunayn followed Galen's preference for complex remedies, rather than the simple remedies of Prophetic Medicine.

Certain elements in Islamic theology, especially the call for total resignation to the will of God, might have inhibited the faithful from actively pursuing practical private and public health initiatives. On the other hand, the Prophet himself made it a point to visit those who had been confined to their homes by sickness to bring comfort, hope, and advice. Thus, some strands of Islamic doctrine encouraged passivity and fatalism, but others emphasizing action and good deeds provided the inspiration for the establishment of charitable institutions to promote the general welfare.

One of the most significant achievements of the Golden Age of Islamic medicine was the development of hospitals and hospital-based clinical training of medical practitioners. Hospitals did not exist during the time of Muhammad, but eventually charitable services, such as hospitals, hospices, religious centers, and educational institutions, were established as part of Islamic culture. Financial support was encouraged, or demanded, by the religious law of charitable endowments. Records concerning the first Islamic hospitals are fragmentary, but there is general agreement that such institutions were founded in the early eighth century. Some were apparently modeled on the hospital and school of Jundi Shapur, but others served more specific roles such as caring for the blind and disabled and the isolation of lepers. More than 30 hospitals were distributed throughout the Islamic world by the end of the ninth century. Records of such institutions provide information concerning administration, finances, budget, salaries of medical personnel, arrangements of wards, dispensaries, libraries, and teaching arrangements. Other charitable enterprises included the organization of teams of physicians and female medical personnel to visit the sick in prisons and mobile dispensaries which served rural areas.

Hospitals were founded in Baghdad, Damascus, and other major cities. The largest and most famous hospital in the Muslim world was established in Cairo in 1286 by al-Mansur Qalawun, who dedicated it to serve all who needed care, rich and poor, old and young, male and female. Formerly a palace, the hospital was said to have a capacity of 8000. The hospital had special wards for various physical and mental diseases, a surgery, pharmacy, dispensary, library, lecture rooms, a chapel for Christians, and a mosque for Muslims. Although orthodox Muslims objected to musical diversions, some hospitals had musicians and singers to comfort and cheer up the patients through music therapy. Despite the inspiration afforded by Jundi Shapur, the hospital movement does not seem to have been established in Persia until the fifteenth century. In the later medieval period, the status of many formerly great hospitals deteriorated as Islamic medicine and science experienced a period of decline.

Admirably detailed records were compiled and edited by clinicians at many of these hospitals in the form that became known as "treatments based on repeated experience." Such resources were important in allowing the larger Islamic hospitals to assume much of the task of medical education and clinical research. It was the reputation of individual sages and masters of medicine rather than that of the hospital per se that attracted students. It was the master, not the institution, who granted a student a certificate indicating achievements in medical theory and clinical experience which allowed the student to teach and practice the subjects indicated. A truly dedicated student might travel to several different cities to study special areas of medicine with famous masters. Women were trained separately by private tutors as nurses, midwives, and gynecologists.

A scandal concerning the death of a patient in a Baghdad hospital in 931 is said to have been the stimulus for the initiation of a more formal system of testing doctors. Reports on the impact of testing say that 160 out of 860 medical practitioners in

Baghdad failed the examination. Official testing of pharmacists had begun in the ninth century. Rules and regulations appear to have varied considerably with time and place throughout the Muslim world. In response to the lack of "quality control" for practitioners, an interesting new medical genre developed in the form of handbooks for laymen on "How to Test a Doctor." Such stories about how patients tested their doctors seem to be of universal appeal. One famous example involved a man who presented his physician with the urine of a mule and claimed it was that of a favorite slave girl. The physician responded that the girl must have been bewitched, because only a mule would pass such urine. When the doctor recommended a good feed of barley as the appropriate remedy, he was appointed chief personal physician to the caliph.

As institutions of religious learning known as "madrasas" developed, the medical sciences became an optional part of the curriculum. By the thirteenth century, students at some of these institutions could specialize in either religion or natural sciences. Many physicians complained that standards of medical education and practice deteriorated as teaching hospitals lost their role to the religious educational institutions where theology and religious law overshadowed medicine and science. Some doctors acquired huge fortunes and a few are remembered for establishing hospitals and charitable clinics. It is notable that wealth accumulated by politicians and generals was sometimes considered so tainted that it was subject to confiscation by Muslim governments, but doctors were exempt from such actions. Most experts in medical ethics argued that it was appropriate to charge fees for treating the sick. The physician needed to earn enough to marry and educate his children, without having to engage in work that would interfere with the study of science. Thus, it was important for the rich to pay large fees so that the doctor could care for the poor without charge.

Dressed in his white shirt and cloak, distinctive doctor's turban, carrying a silver-headed stick, perfumed with rose-water, camphor, and sandalwood, the physician was an impressive figure. But, despite the honors accorded to scholar-physicians, skepticism about medical practice remained strong. Just as Cato and Pliny had decried the insidious growth of Greek medicine in Rome, Islamic traditionalists warned that the medical art was foreign to Arab culture and doubted that the physician could really do anything to cure disease or ward off death. In many Persian stories the Devil appears disguised as a physician, or the physician kills his patient through ignorance or treachery. In one such story, a physician murdered his patient by poisoning the lancet used for venesection. Months later the physician himself needed bleeding; by accident, he used the poisoned lancet. Another eminent physician proved he had a fool for a patient when he treated himself for elephantiasis by allowing starving vipers to bite him. This treatment is reminiscent of a story told by Galen, but in this case when the poison drove out the elephantiasis it induced leprosy, deafness, and loss of vision.

The persistence of this attitude towards medicine is apparent in the autobiography of the seventeenth-century emperor Jehangir, son of the great Mogul emperor Akbar

(1542–1605). After describing how medical treatment of the aged Akbar had turned diarrhea into dysentery and dysentery into constipation and constipation into diarrhea and death, Jehangir said that, except for God's decree and doctors' mistakes, no one would ever die.

THE GREAT SAGES OF ISLAMIC MEDICINE

Although medieval physicians, whether Muslims, Jews, or Christians, generally assumed that Galenism was a complete and perfect system, the great sages of Islamic medicine are worth studying in their own right, not just in terms of their role in preserving classical medicine. Latin translations of the works of a few authors, including Rhazes, Avicenna, and Albucasis, were most influential in Europe, but the Arabic works of many other scholars held a place in the Muslim world which had no parallel in the West. Western scholars were most interested in recovering Greek medical knowledge and had less interest in practical aspects of Islamic medicine, such as the development of hospitals and clinical training. Some Muslim physicians became well known in the West as philosophers and alchemists.

Rhazes (ca. 850–ca. 923; al-Rāzī; Abū-Bakr Muhammad 'ibn Zakariy-yā-Razi) has been revered as the greatest physician of the Islamic world, one of most scientifically minded physicians of the Middle Ages, and one of the great physicians of all time. The indefatigable Rhazes was the author of at least 200 medical and philosophical treatises, including his massive unfinished masterpiece the *Continens*, or *Comprehensive Book of Medicine*. The *Continens* was translated into Latin by the Jewish physician Faraj Ibn Salim (known in Latin as Farragut) for King Charles of Anjou. The work was completed in 1279 and finally printed in 1486. The two printed volumes weighed more than 20 pounds. Rhazes' manual of the healing art, *Kitab al-Mansuri (Almansor)*, was very influential in the West into the sixteenth century. Rhazes was chosen as director of one of the first great hospitals in Baghdad in competition with 100 other candidates. He is said to have selected the most healthful location for the hospital by hanging pieces of meat at likely sites and finding the one where there was the least putrefaction.

Insights into the tension between orthodoxy and philosophy in the Muslim world can be found in *The Conduct of a Philosopher*, a book Rhazes wrote to rebut attacks on his personal conduct. In answer to charges that he had overindulged in life's pleasures, Rhazes answered that he had always been moderate in everything except acquiring knowledge and writing books. By his own reckoning, he had written more than 20,000 pages in one year and had damaged his eyes and hands by working day and night for more than 15 years. Although Rhazes taught that a middle road between extreme asceticism and overindulgence was the most healthful, he offered his own conduct as an appropriate model for those willing to commit themselves to the life of the mind. All biographical accounts agree that Rhazes became blind near the end of his life and that he refused treatment because he was weary of seeing the world and unwilling to undergo the ordeal of surgery to see any more. Eventually, biographers adopted the spurious but irresistible story that Rhazes lost his vision when his patron al-Mansur had the physician beaten on the head with one of his own books for failing to produce evidence in support of his alchemical theories. Presumably the text used in the beating was a treatise on alchemy.

The case histories compiled by Rhazes provide insight into the relationship between patient and physician, the range of complaints for which his contemporaries consulted physicians, which signs and symptoms the physician thought significant, the kinds of treatment used, and even the occupations and family background of his patients. Just as physicians had ethical obligations to patients, patients had an ethical duty to trust and cooperate with their physician. It was most important, according to Rhazes, for people to follow the doctor's advice. "With a learned physician and an obedient patient," Rhazes promised, "sickness soon disappears." Unfortunately, not all patients were obedient and not all physicians were learned or even competent. Rhazes had seen impostors who claimed to cure epilepsy by making a cut at the back of the head and then pretending to remove stones or blood clots. Other quacks pretended to draw snakes through the patient's nose, worms from the ears or teeth, frogs from under the tongue, and bones from wounds and ulcers.

In dealing with his wealthy and powerful patients, Rhazes' was generally ingenious and sometimes daring. One story concerns Rhazes treatment of al-Mansur, who was suffering from an apparently incurable crippling ailment. Before beginning treatment, Rhazes asked al-Mansur for his best horse and mule. The next day he had his patient take a hot bath and administered various remedies. Suddenly Rhazes threatened the amir with a knife and shouted insults at him. In a frenzy, al-Mansur scrambled from the bath, but the physician ran outside where his servant waited with the horse and mule. Later Rhazes sent his patient a letter explaining that he had provoked him in order to use fear and anger as a means of increasing his innate heat and obtaining an instantaneous cure. Having recovered from both his ill health and his anger, the amir showered his physician with gifts.

One of Rhazes' case histories appears to be the first written description of "rose-fever," to use the term adopted in the nineteenth century. Rhazes noticed that one of his patients seemed to suffer from a kind of catarrh (runny nose) or cold every spring. Convinced that the problem was caused by the scent of roses, Rhazes advised his patient to avoid aromatic things such as roses, herbs, onions, and garlic. If the symptoms became particularly troublesome, he recommended cupping on the neck and bleeding from arteries of the temples.

Rhazes' book *On Smallpox and Measles* provides further evidence of his clinical acuteness as well as valuable information about diagnosis, therapy, and concepts of diseases. Among the ancients, diseases were generally defined in terms of symptoms, e.g., fevers, diarrheas, skin lesions, and so forth. Therefore, Rhazes' treatise on smallpox and measles has been called a major landmark in establishing the concept of specific disease entities. According to Rhazes, smallpox was caused by impurities in the blood derived from bad menstrual blood that had been present during gestation. During puberty, these impurities tended to boil up in a manner analogous to the fermentation of wine. The problem was essentially universal, and children rarely escaped the disease. Measles, which Rhazes recognized as a separate disease, was caused by very bilious blood. However, even an experienced physician might have trouble distinguishing smallpox from measles. To protect his reputation, the physician should wait until the nature of the illness was obvious before giving his diagnosis.

Proper management before the onset of smallpox might lessen its virulence, but when the disease was inevitable the physician should encourage eruption of the pox by wrapping, rubbing, steaming, purging, and bleeding and take special precautions to prevent blindness. According to Rhazes, pustules that became hard and warty instead of ripening properly indicated that the patient would die. Various recipes were supposed to remove pockmarks, but the nearly universal presence of smallpox scars suggests that these remedies—which included sheep dung, vinegar, sesame oil, and the liquid found in the hoof of a roasted ram—were about as useful as modern wrinkle creams. In reality, once smallpox appeared medicine could do little to alter the course of the disease, except to make it worse, but an elaborate regimen gave the physician and patient a sense of control, comfort, and hope.

Islam's "Prince of Physicians," Avicenna (980–1037; Abu Ali Hysayn ibn Abdullah ibn Sina), was the first scholar to create a complete philosophical system in the Arabic language. In medicine and philosophy Avicenna's erudition and influence cannot be underestimated. Indeed, critics contended that his influence inhibited further developments in medicine, because no physician was willing to challenge the reasoning of the master of philosophy, natural science, and medicine. Thanks to Avicenna's autobiography and the devotion of his students, we have a fairly complete account of the prodigy who amazed his father and teachers by mastering the *Qur'an* by the age of 10. After surpassing his teachers in jurisprudence and philosophy, the young scholar turned to the natural sciences and was soon teaching medicine to established physicians. But when Avicenna began to study clinical medicine, he realized that some things could be learned only from experience and not from books. Thereafter, Avicenna spent his days catering to his wealthy patrons and devoted his nights to lecturing to his students, dictating notes for his books, and drinking wine. Temperance was certainly not one of Avicenna's virtues. Eventually, wine, women, and work affected his constitution. Unwilling to wait for a gradual improvement, he prescribed medicated enemas 8 times per day; these treatments caused ulcers, seizures, colic, and extreme weakness. When his strength was all but gone, he abandoned further treatment and died. His enemies exulted that his medicine could not save his life and his metaphysics could not save his soul.

Avicenna's great medical treatise, the *Canon*, was written for general practitioners, but an abridgment called the *Poem on Medicine* provided laymen with an accessible summation of medical theory. Because the information in the *Canon* was essential for medical practice, Avicenna suggested that doctors should memorize the entire book. With Avicenna's *Canon* as their guide, traditional healers still diagnose illness by feeling the pulse and inspecting urine, cure diseases that Western medicine cannot name, comfort their patients with satisfying explanations of their conditions, and care for patients who do not accept and cannot afford modern psychiatric methods. Followers of Avicenna learned to find diagnostic clues in the size, strength, speed, elasticity, fullness, regularity, and rhythm of the pulse and the color, density, transparency, turbidity, sediments, quantity, odor, and froth of urine samples.

Having made his diagnosis, the physician could find much practical advice in the works of Avicenna for treating illness and maintaining the health of his patients under different conditions. For example, to provide partial relief from lice, the traveler should rub his body with a woolen ribbon that had been dipped in mercury and wear the ribbon around his neck until a thorough attack on the pests was possible. Practical medicine required management of the healthy body to preserve well-being and management of the sick body to restore health through diet, simple and compound drugs, and surgical procedures. Establishing an appropriate regimen in infancy provided the foundations of a life-long plan for the preservation of health. Much of Avicenna's advice on infant care seems quite sensible, but his remedies for deficient lactation include a daily dose of white ants or dried earthworms in barley water. Elderly patients required a regimen emphasizing moistening and warming measures, such as soothing olive oil baths. Boiling a fox or lizard in the oil made it more effective when treating severe joint pain. Avicenna expected the physician to be able to assess the quality of water because bad water caused a host of disorders, including enlargement of the spleen, constipation, hemorrhoids, diarrhea, and insanity. Avicenna's advice concerning water quality implies a remarkably fine balance. Water samples should be weighed; the water which was lighter per similar volume was of the best quality. Waters containing metallic substances and those infested with leeches were dangerous, but Avicenna noted that water containing iron strengthened the internal organs, stopped diarrhea, and stimulated the sexual organs.

Elegant expositions of the philosophical principles of medicine and the relationship between mind and body are woven into Avicenna's case histories. For example, his use of the pulse as a "lie-detector" demonstrated how physiological phenomena betray our hidden thoughts. In treating a case of "love-sickness," Avicenna unobtrusively kept his finger on the patient's wrist and detected the irregularity of the pulse that corresponded to mention of the lover's name. Another challenging case involved a young man who suffered from melancholy and the delusion that he was a cow. The man mooed loudly, refused to eat, and begged to be killed and made into stew. The patient cheered up immediately when Avicenna sent word that the butcher would soon come to slaughter him. Finally, Avicenna came to the sickroom with a butcher's knife and asked for the cow. Mooing happily, the young man was bound hand and foot, but after a thorough examination, Avicenna declared that the cow was too thin to be butchered. The patient ate so eagerly that he soon recovered his strength and was cured of his delusion.

Avicenna also expected the physician to master surgical techniques for treating a wide variety of wounds and injuries. Although the doctor might prescribe drugs to relieve pain before the operation, the patient still had to be bound and restrained by the surgeon's assistants. After the operation, warm water, vinegar, or wine was sponged over the site. Nevertheless, postsurgical infection was so common that the same Persian word meant both wound and pus.

A more specialized guide to Arab surgery was provided by Albucasis (Abu 'l-Qasim Khalaf ibn-'Abbas al-Zahrawi, d. 1013), an extremely ascetic man who devoted much of his time to working among the poor. His *On Surgery and Instruments* is one of the first comprehensive illustrated treatises on this important subject. Of course, bleeding, cupping, and cauterization are extensively discussed because they represented the mainstays of surgical practice. In discussing the uses of cauterization from ''head to heel,'' Albucasis praised the cautery as an instrument with ''universal application'' for almost every disorder, organic or functional. Despite his piety, he was obviously not inhibited by the uncertainties surrounding the Prophet's position on its use. Recommendations for the use of the cautery to arrest hemorrhage, prevent the spread of destructive lesions, strengthen organs that became cold in temperament, and remove putrefactive matter are also found in the works of Avicenna. By counteracting excessive humidity and coldness of the brain, cauterization cured a host of disorders from headache and epilepsy to lethargy and apoplexy. To perform the operation on the patient's shaved head, the surgeon placed his hand on the root of the nose between the eyes and applied the cautery to the spot marked by his middle finger. If the bone was exposed when the sizzling stopped, the operation was complete; if not, cauterization should be repeated. Some surgeons believed in keeping the wound open, but Albucasis advised readers that it was safer to avoid further interventions. If the cautery failed to cure chronic migraine or acute catarrh, Albucasis suggested bleeding from arteries.

Both Albucasis and Avicenna provided detailed discussions of the theory and practice of bloodletting. In all but the very old and very young, venesection was valuable for both the preservation of health and the treatment of disease. Drugs assisted the body in the elimination of noxious humors through purging, vomiting, and diuresis, but venesection was the most effective method because it removed excess humors in the same proportion as they were present in the blood vessels. As stipulated by Galen, venesection was even useful in the treatment of hemorrhages, because it diverted blood to the opposite side of the body. Doctors commonly used about 30 blood vessels for venesection; 16 of these were in the head, 5 in the arms and hands, and 3 in the legs and feet. Despite the danger of damage to nerves, the elbow veins were frequently used for disorders of the chest, abdomen, and eyes.

The patient's strength and the color of the blood determined the amount to be taken. If the blood was initially black, the doctor should continue bleeding until it became red; if the blood was thick, he should bleed until it became thin. Bleeding could be carried out in several small installments for a weak patient, but a person with hot, sharp, abundant blood and fever should be bled until he fainted. Albucasis warned the doctor to keep his finger on the pulse during bleeding to avoid the possibility that the patient might die rather than faint. For some conditions leeches, cupping, and cauterization were preferable to venesection. Cupping, with or without scarification, was considered less debilitating than venesection, but leeches were sometimes more appropriate because the creatures could be applied to parts of the body unreachable with cupping vessels. Leeches were excellent for drawing blood from deep tissues, but they had to be carefully selected; large-headed leeches that were black, gray, or green, or had hairy bodies with blue stripes were said to cause inflammation, hemorrhage, fever, fainting, and paralysis. Albucasis described methods of removing a leech stuck in the throat, but did not explain how the leech got there.

Female patients presented special difficulties, because a chaste woman would not expose her body to a male doctor. If a woman required surgery, Albucasis suggested calling for a competent woman doctor, a eunuch doctor, or an experienced midwife. The midwife should know the signs and manner of normal delivery, have wisdom and dexterity, and be skillful in dealing with abnormal presentation, prolonged labor, and the extraction of a dead fetus. It is interesting that Albucasis said that women doctors were "uncommon," rather than nonexistent. The reference to eunuchs is also notable because castration was forbidden by Moslem law. Nevertheless, after apologizing for mentioning this operation, Albucasis described it in some detail. Albucasis' surgical text and Rhazes' treatise on smallpox were among the earliest classical Arabic texts to be printed in England. Both were edited and translated into Latin by an apothecary named John Channing (d. 1775) in the eighteenth century.

Other areas of great interest to Arab scientists were pharmacology, alchemy, and optics. Arabic treatises on drugs, drug products and their nomenclature, and aromatic medicinal plants, such as musk, ambergris, aloe, camphor, and saffron, were composed in the eighth and ninth centuries. Many treatises on specialized aspects of pharmacy were written. These texts can be divided into four main types: formularies and compendiums, herbals and books on medicinal materials, toxicology, diet and drug therapy. In large measure, the Arabic literary tradition served as a force in shaping the development of pharmacy as an independent profession.

The medical formulary of al-Kindi (Yaqub ibn-Ishaq al-Kindi, ca. 800–870) served as a model for Arabic treatises on pharmacology, botany, zoology, and mineralogy. Persian and Indian drugs that were unknown to Hippocrates and Galen appear in such formularies, as did new kinds of drug preparations. Linguistic analysis of the medical materials discussed by al-Kindi indicates that 33% of the drugs came from Mesopotamian and Semitic traditions, 23% from Greek sources, 18% Persian, 13% Indian, 5% Arabic, and 3% from ancient Egyptian sources. Unfortunately, many of al-Kindi's other writings—some 270 treatises in logic, philosophy, physics, mathematics, music, astrology, natural history, and medicine—were lost. Many Arabic works deal specifically with the anatomy of the eye, its role in vision, and the treatment of eye diseases. Presumably, the high frequency of eye diseases in the Near

East stimulated a special interest in theories of vision and practical ophthalmology. Although the theory of vision may seem a rather esoteric branch of knowledge, al-Kindi argued that it would prove to be the key to the discovery of nature's most fundamental secrets. The Latin version of his work on optics, *De aspectibus*, was very influential among Western scientists and philosophers.

THE STRANGE CASE OF IBN AN-NAFIS

Western scholars long maintained that the major historical contribution of Arabian medicine was the preservation of ancient Greek wisdom and that nothing original was produced by medieval Arabic writers. Because the Arabic manuscripts thought worthy of translation were those which most closely followed the Greek originals (all others being dismissed as corruptions), the original premise—lack of originality—was confirmed. The strange story of Ibn an-Nafis (Al-Qurashi, d. 1288) and the pulmonary circulation demonstrates the unsoundness of previous assumptions about the Arabic literature. The writings of Ibn an-Nafis were essentially ignored until 1924 when Dr. Muhyi ad-Din at-Tatawi, an Egyptian physician, presented his doctoral thesis to the Medical Faculty of Freiburg, Germany. If a copy of Dr. Tatawi's thesis had not been brought to the attention of Prof. Max Meyerhof, Ibn an-Nafis' discovery of the pulmonary circulation might have been forgotten.

Honored by his contemporaries as a learned physician and ingenious investigator, Ibn an-Nafis was described as a tireless writer and a pious man. His medical writings included the *Comprehensive Book of Medical Science*, the *Well Arranged Book on Ophthalmology*, and the *Commentary on the Canon of Ibn Sina*. He also wrote on logic, law, ethics, language, rhetoric, and tradition. Unfortunately, only a few of his books have survived. While serving as Chief of Physicians in Egypt, Ibn an-Nafis became seriously ill. His colleagues advised him to take wine as a medicine, but he refused because he did not wish to meet his Creator with alcohol in his blood.

It is not clear how Ibn an-Nafis reached his ingenious conclusions as to the pulmonary circulation, however, he was known to have been critical of Galen's style and theories. While anatomical research was conducted on various animals, such as monkeys and sheep, human dissection was generally prohibited by Islamic law and custom. While some physicians might have been tempted by clandestine opportunities to violate this rule, in the *Commentary*, an-Nafis specifically explained that the prohibitions of religious law and his own "natural charity" prevented him from performing dissections. It is quite unlikely that the physician who refused to take wine to save his life would have acted against religious law and his own conscience to satisfy scientific curiosity. Human dissection was not acceptable in the Muslim world, because the mutilation of a cadaver was considered an insult to human dignity. This revulsion concerning the mutilation of dead bodies might have been a reaction to memories of the pre-Islamic Arab wars in which victors sometimes deliberately

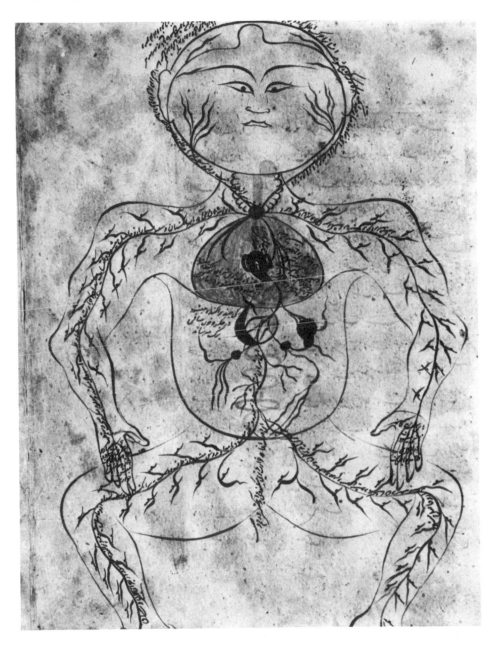

Human anatomy

mutilated the bodies of their enemies. Islamic law prohibited this ritualistic mutilation and orthodox legal experts argued that scientific dissection was essentially the same violation of the dignity of the human body. These prohibitions were invoked in modern times in response to progress in organ transplantation. The general population seemed eager to accept such medical progress, but some religious authorities tried to forbid it.

In the midst of a fairly conventional discussion of the structure and function of the heart, an-Nafis departed from the accepted explanation of the movement of the blood. His description of the two ventricles of the heart accepts the Galenic doctrine that the right ventricle is filled with blood and the left ventricle with vital spirit. His next statement, however, boldly contradicted Galen's teachings on the pores in the septum. An-Nafis insisted that there were no visible or invisible passages between the two ventricles and argued that the septum between the ventricles was thicker than other parts of the heart in order to prevent the harmful and inappropriate passage of blood or spirit between them. Thus, to explain the path taken by the blood, he reasoned that after the blood had been refined in the right ventricle, it was transmitted to the lung where it was rarefied and mixed with air. The finest part of this blood was then clarified and transmitted from the lung to the left ventricle. That is, the blood can only get into the left ventricle by way of the lungs.

Perhaps some still obscure Arabic, Persian, or Hebrew manuscript contains a commentary on the curious doctrines of Ibn an-Nafis, but there is as yet no evidence that later Arab authors or European anatomists were interested in these anti-Galenic speculations. Thus, although Ibn an-Nafis did not influence later writers, the fact that his concept was so boldly stated in the thirteenth century should lead us to question our assumptions about progress and originality in the history of science. Since only a small percentage of the pertinent manuscripts have been studied, edited, translated, and printed, the question may go unanswered for quite some time.

THE SURVIVAL OF YUNANI MEDICINE (UNANI TIBB OR GRECO-ISLAMIC MEDICINE)

Islamic medicine did not disappear at the end of the Middle Ages, but continued to develop and spread to other areas. During the nineteenth century, traditional practitioners came under increasing pressure from competing Western-style doctors and government officials. In 1838 the Ottoman sultan Mahmud II established the first Western-style medical school and hospital in Istanbul and staffed it with French doctors. The Sultan claimed that traditional Islamic medicine had become stagnant and sterile and he expected to see a strong trend towards secularization. Many other Muslim countries eventually followed this example and tried to ban the practice of traditional medicine.

Even where twentieth-century laws regulating medical practice drove traditional practitioners underground, diligent explorers could still find them. For example, in French-ruled Algeria, traditional healers and their patients were reluctant to talk to outsiders because it was illegal for people without the proper French qualifications to perform surgery. Nevertheless, traditional healers performed eye surgery, tooth extractions, cupping, cautery, bloodletting, and assisted in difficult births. Although anesthetic drugs were available, most practitioners did not use them before surgery. Some healers claimed that their methods were so gentle that the patient did not suffer, but assistants were invariably needed to restrain the patient. Many people treated themselves with yunani drugs and cauterization in order to avoid the costs of seeing a doctor and because of their faith in such remedies.

Under British rule in the Indian subcontinent both Muslim and Hindu traditional systems survived. In the 1960s, the Pakistani government ordered the registration, licensing, and utilization of *hakims* (traditional scholar-physicians), because modern medicine was too expensive or totally unavailable to the rural population. Western-style doctors strenuously objected to this official recognition of their rivals.

With official recognition by the Governments of Pakistan and India and regulations administered through the Ministries of Health, male and female yunani practitioners, known as *tabibs* and *tabibas*, respectively, now flourish in urban as well as rural settings. Many practitioners learn the art as apprentices, but others become academically qualified through a 4-year course of study at recognized yunani medical colleges where the curriculum includes the *Canon* of Avicenna as well as the standard components of modern medicine. The tabib still diagnoses illness by the inspection of the pulse, urine, stools, and tongue, and prescribes traditional drugs and diets. Scientific analyses of yunani remedies have confirmed the value of many medicinal plants, but hundreds of traditional drugs have not been investigated. In general, however, modern Muslim societies have not succeeded in establishing the complete acculturation of modern medicine into Islam, despite the fact that medieval Islam successfully assimilated Greek, Persian, and Indian medical traditions. Despite the explosive revival of Islamic fundamentalism in the 1980s, India and Pakistan appear to be the only nations where a serious effort is being made to incorporate valuable features of the surviving medical system of the Islamic Golden Age into health-care planning.

SUGGESTED READINGS

Albucasis (1973). *Albucasis on Surgery and Instruments*. Translation and Commentary by
    M. S. Spink and G. L. Lewis. Berkeley: University of California Press.
Arberry, A. J. (1985). *The Koran Interpreted*. New York: Macmillan.
Arberry, Arthur J. (1950). *The Spiritual Physick of Rhazes*. London: John Murray.
Avicenna (1974). *The Life of Ibn Sina*. A Critical Edition and Annotated Translation by
    Wiliam E. Gohlman. Albany, NY: New York: State University of New York Press.
Avicenna (1930). *A Treatise on the Canon of Medicine of Avicenna Incorporating a
    Translation of the First Book*. Trans. by O.C. Gruner. London: Luzac.
Bannerman, Robert H., Burton, Johns, Che'en Wen-Chieh, eds. (1983). *Traditional*

Medicine and Health Care Coverage. A Reader for Health Administrators and Practitioners. Geneva: WHO.

Baquai, F. U. (1977). *Traditional Medicine in Pakistan.* Karachi, Pakistan: Hamdard Foundation.

Browne, Edward Granville (1921). *Arabian Medicine.* London: Cambridge University Press. Westport, CT: Hyperion Press, repr., 1983.

Campbell, Donald (1926). *Arabian Medicine and Its Influence on the Middle Ages.* 2 vols. London: Kegan, Paul.

Dols, Michael W., and Gamal Adil S., ed. and trans. (1984). *Medieval Islamic Medicine: Ibn Ridwan's Treatise "On the Prevention of Bodily Ills in Egypt."* Berkeley, CA: University of California Press.

Dols, Michael W. (1987). The Origins of the Islamic Hospital: Myth and Reality. *Bulletin of the History of Medicine* 62: 367-390.

Eastwood, Bruce S. (1982). *The Elements of Vision: The Micro-Cosmology of Visual Theory According to Hunayn Ibn Ishaq.* Philadelphia, PA: American Philosophical Society.

Elgood, Cyril (1951). *A Medical History of Persia and the Eastern Caliphate from the Earliest Times to the Year A.D. 1932.* London: Cambridge University Press. Reprinted, with additions and corrections, ed. by G. van Heusden. Amsterdam: APA-Philo Press, 1979.

Goichon, A. M. (1969). *The Philosophy of Avicenna and Its Influence on Medieval Europe.* Trans. from the French, with notes, annotations and a preface by M.S. Khan. Delhi, India: Motilal Banarsidass.

Gruner, O. Cameron (1967). *Commentary on the Canon of Avicenna.* Karachi, Pakistan: Hamdard Foundation.

Hamarneh, Sami Khalaf (1983-4). *Health Sciences in Early Islam: Collected Papers.* Ed. by Munawar A. Anees. 2 vols. Blanco, TX: Zahra Publications.

Hameed, A., ed. (1983). *Avicenna's Tract on Cardiac Drugs and Essays on Arab Cardiotherapy.* Karachi, Pakistan: Institute of History of Medicine and Medical Research, and New Delhi, India: Institute of Health and Tibbi (Medical) Research.

Hays, John R., ed. (1978). *The Genius of Arab Civilization: Source of Renaissance.* Cambridge, MA: MIT Press.

(Hunayn) Humain ibn Ishaq (1980). *Questions on Medicine for Scholars.* Trans., preface, historical note by Paul Ghalioungui. Cairo, Egypt: al-Ahram Center for Scientific Translations.

Hilton-Simpson, M. W. (1922). *Arab Medicine and Surgery. A Study of the Healing Art in Algeria.* London: Oxford Univeristy Press.

Khan, M. S. (1986). *Islamic Medicine.* London: Routledge & Kegan Paul.

Kreuger, Haven C. (1963). *Avicenna's Poem on Medicine.* Springfield, IL: Charles C. Thomas.

Leslie, Charles, ed. (1976). *Asian Medical Systems: A Comparative Study.* Berkeley, CA: University of California Press.

Levey, Martin (1973). *Early Arabic Pharmacology. An Introduction Based on Ancient and Medieval Sources.* Leiden: E. J. Brill.

Levey, Martin (1966). *The Medical Formulary of Al-Kindi.* Madison, WI: University of Wisconsin Press.

Lindberg, David C. (1976). *Theories of Vision from Al-Kindi to Kepler*. Chicago: University of Chicago Press.

Meyerhof, Max (1984). *Studies in Medieval Arabic Medicine: Theory and Practice*. London: Variorum Reprints.

Nasr, S. H. (1968). *Science and Civilization in Islam*. Cambridge, MA: Harvard University Press.

Padover, S. K. (1939). Muslim Libraries. In J. W. Thompson, ed. (1939). *The Medieval Library*. Chicago: University of Chicago Press.

Rahman, F. (1952). *Avicenna's Psychology*. London: Oxford University Press.

Rahman, Fazlur (1987). *Health and Medicine in the Islamic Tradition: Change and Identity*. New York: Crossroad.

Rhazes (1948). *A Treatise on the Smallpox and Measles*. Trans. from the original Arabic by W. A. Greenhill (1848). London: Sydenham Society.

Said, H. M. (1979). *Traditional Greco-Arab and Modern Western Medicine: Conflict or Symbiosis*. Karachi, Pakistan: Hamdard Foundation.

Savage-Smith, Emilie (1988). Gleanings from an Arabist's Workshop: Current Trends in the Study of Medieval Islamic Science and Medicine. *Isis* 79: 246-272.

Savage-Smith, Emilie (1988). John Channing: Eighteenth-Century Apothecary and Arabist. *Pharmacy in History* 30: 63-80.

Shah, M. H. (1958). *Avicenna: His Life and Works*. Karachi, Pakistan: Hamdard Medical Digest.

Shah, M. H. (1966). *The General Principles of Avicenna's Canon of Medicine*. Karachi, Pakistan: Naveed Clinic.

Shah, M. H. (1966). *Canon of Avicenna* (English translation). Karachim, Pakistan: Interservices Press.

Siraisi, Nancy, G. (1987). *Avicenna in Renaissance Italy. The Canon and Medical Teaching in Italian Universities After 1500*. Princeton, NJ: Princeton University Press.

Sonnedecker, Glenn (1976). *Kremers and Urdang's History of Pharmacy*. Philadelphia: J.B. Lippincott Company.

Temkin, Owsei (1977). Was Servetus Influenced by Ibn an Nafis? In *The Double Face of Janus and Other Essays in the History of Medicine*. Baltimore, MD: The Johns Hopkins University Press, pp. 284–286.

Ullman, M. (1978). *Islamic Medicine*. Edinburgh University Press.

Vohora, S. B. and Khan, S. Y. (1979). *Animal Origin Drugs Used in Unani Medicine*. New Delhi, India: Vikas Publishing House.

Watt, W. M. (1973). *The Influence of Islam upon Medieval Europe*. Edinburgh University Press.

Wickens, G. M., ed. (1952). *Avicenna: Scientist and Philosopher*. A Millenary Symposium. London: Luzac.

7

MEDICINE AND THE RENAISSANCE

T he term Renaissance designates the rebirth of the arts and sciences that accompanied the complex and often painful economic, social, political, and intellectual
transformations taking place in Europe between about 1300 and 1650. The
Renaissance was a new age of exploration of the word, the world, the mind, and the
human body. During this period, Europe experienced the disintegration of medieval
economic and social patterns, the expansion of commerce, cities, and trade, and the
growth of the modern state. While such a profound transformation might seem to
imply a sharp break with the past, in many ways the Renaissance was the natural
culmination of the Middle Ages. As an area of scientific and philosophical interest,
if not therapeutic advances, the Renaissance is a time of special importance for
medicine. However, the exact relationship between the Renaissance and the
renaissance of medicine is extremely complicated. It is possible to speak of a long
medical renaissance which began in the twelfth century, a distinct medical renaissance
of the sixteenth century, and a medical revolution of the seventeenth century.
    A witness from the era known as the Scientific Revolution (1450–1630), Francis
Bacon (1561–1639), England's premier philosopher of science and Lord High
Chancellor, said that if we considered the "force, effect, and consequences" of all
the products of human ingenuity, the three most important inventions were printing,
gunpowder, and the compass. Moreover, Bacon noted, the three inventions that had
changed the appearance and the state of the whole world were unknown to the
ancients. The establishment of printing presses throughout Europe in the 1460s

launched a communications revolution which might, in part, account for the permanence of the Renaissance. The "print revolution" accelerated the trend towards literacy, the diffusion of ideas, the establishment of a vernacular literature, and transformed a "scribal" and "image culture" into a "print culture." Interest in educational problems was not limited to higher learning and university curricula, but included reform programs for elementary education. Despite the inevitable grumbling about the vulgarity of printed books as compared to manuscripts and the fear that an excess of literacy might be subversive, scholars were generally more concerned with acquiring the new treasures than in complaining about the end of scribal culture. In print, a text could speak to students directly, rather than through the professor or keeper of manuscripts. The mass-produced book made it possible for the young to study, and perhaps even learn, by reading on their own. Gunpowder weapons have an important place in the history of medicine because they forced surgeons to deal with problems unknown to Hippocrates and Galen. The Chinese are thought to have invented gunpowder, which was first reported in Europe in the thirteenth century, but others have claimed prior or independent invention. As Europeans followed the compass around the world, they brought back new plants, animals, and remedies that would transform agricultural and medical practice and left in their wake a series of ecological and demographic catastrophes.

THE MEDICAL HUMANISTS

Just as the Renaissance transformed the arts, the Scientific Revolution transformed ideas about the nature of the universe and the nature of man. During the period from about 1450 to 1700, the Greco-Islamic tradition was replaced by modern science. Applying this new mode of thought to anatomy, physiology, and medical education would have been impossible without the work of the humanist scholars. Like the scholastics of the Middle Ages, the humanists were devoted to words and books and the difficult task of integrating experience and practice with classical learning, but their interests had turned from heaven to earth. While the humanist scholars were generally more concerned with art and literature than science, their new perspective served the needs of the medical sciences as well. As staunch supporters of the newly purified Galenic texts, humanist scholars rejected corrupt medieval translations. Nevertheless, their reverence for ancient authorities made them skeptical of attempts to create a new medical science that would be independent of the ancient authorities. The work of Thomas Linacre (1460?–1524) and John Caius (1510–1573), outstanding English medical humanists, illustrates the nature of scholarship and medical education in this period.

Thomas Linacre studied Greek in Florence and Rome before receiving the degree of Doctor of Medicine from the University of Padua in 1496. In addition to his scholarly work, Linacre maintained a lucrative private medical practice, taught

Greek, and served as physician to King Henry VII. As founder and guiding light of the College of Physicians, Linacre helped to mold the character of the English medical profession. Under the leadership of Linacre's devoted disciple John Caius, the College of Physicians grew in power and prestige, taking control of medical licensing away from religious authorities and using strict regulations to enhance the status of approved physicians. Nevertheless, Caius was troubled by his perception of a decline in English medical humanism. Indeed, in terms of the development of scholarship, universities, and the learned professions, England lagged behind the intellectual centers of the continent. Thus, like other English scholars, Caius had to pursue his studies abroad. After abandoning his theological studies, Caius became a medical student at the University of Padua where he met the anatomist Andreas Vesalius. Both men were involved in editing and publishing new Latin versions of Galenic texts, but their reactions to discrepancies between Galenic anatomy and the human cadaver were quite different. While Vesalius insisted on returning to the "true book of the human body," Caius was confident that once all the writings of Galen were critically edited medical knowledge would be virtually complete. In 1546 Caius was appointed anatomical demonstrator to the United Company of Barbers and Surgeons. Since 1540, the Company of Barbers and Surgeons had been allotted the bodies of four convicted felons per year for anatomical demonstrations. After considerable lobbying by Caius and other elite physicians, the College of Physicians received a similar bequest in 1565.

Whereas other presidents of the College of Physicians had generally ignored unqualified practitioners, especially outside London, Caius wanted to control medical licensing for all of England. Although his goal of raising standards for medical education and practice was laudable, efforts to limit the number of practitioners by dictating their credentials had adverse effects, especially for women and the poor. Obviously, the needs of the common people could not be met by the small number of physicians who belonged to the medical aristocracy, which was not necessarily a meritocracy. Because women were not admitted to the universities, female practitioners were easy targets for licensing reforms. In addition to his campaigns against unlicensed practitioners, quackery, witchcraft, and superstition, Caius zealously challenged those who publicly criticized Galen.

Respect for the ancients did not blunt Caius' ability to observe and describe new phenomena, as shown in his account of the "English sweating sickness." The *Boke or Counseill Against the Disease Called the Sweate* (1552) was the first original description of disease to be written in England in English. In all probability, Caius would be distressed to know that his vernacular description of the "sweats" is now regarded as his most important medical work. Outbreaks of the "English Sweats" or "Sudor Britanica" struck in 1485, 1506, 1517, 1528, and 1551. The disease was characterized by copious sweat, fever, nausea, headache, cramps, pain in the back and extremities, delirium, hallucinations, and a profound stupor. Within about 24 hours the disease reached a critical stage when either the disease or the patient came to an abrupt end. Even among strong, healthy men the mortality rate was extremely high. According to Caius, a stricken town was fortunate if only half of all souls were claimed by the disease. After carefully evaluating the clinical pattern and natural history of the disease, he concluded that the sweate was a new disease. Both the exact nature of these epidemics and the reason for their apparent localization are still obscure.

AUTOPSIES, ART, AND ANATOMY

While the artists and anatomists of the Renaissance are inextricably associated with the reform of anatomy, the study of human anatomy—from bodies, as well as from books—had not been entirely neglected since the death of Galen. During the Middle Ages, human dissection was not pursued with the freedom and intensity so briefly enjoyed by Herophilus and Erasistratus, but it had not been absolutely forbidden or abandoned. There are various examples of medieval post-mortems and dismember-ments. Sometimes autopsies were conducted to investigate suspicious deaths, outbreaks of plague, or even to search for special signs inside the body of purported saints. Human dissection was practiced to a limited extent during the thirteenth and fourteenth centuries in those universities in southern Europe having medical faculties. Bologna University statutes dated 1405 recognized the practice of dissection; in 1442 the city of Bologna was authorized to provide two cadavers each year to the university for dissection. During the fifteenth century similar provisions were made for most of the major European universities. Thus, students were able to observe a limited number of human dissections. However, they knew that examinations and disserta-tions required knowledge of accepted texts, not the ability to perform practical demonstrations; they primarily attended dissections to confirm their readings of the ancient authorities and prepare for examinations. Medieval and Renaissance students were probably not too different from students running a typical "cookbook" experiment today. Such experiments are performed to teach a standard technique or confirm some accepted fact, not to make novel observations. By about 1400, human dissection was part of the curriculum of most medical schools. However, well into the sixteenth century medical students were in little danger of being forced to confront radically new ideas about the nature of the human body.

For teachers as well as students, the purpose of dissection was to supplement the study of Galenic texts, but simplified guides were needed. One of the best known of the early dissection manuals was the *Anatomy* (1316) by Mondino de Luzzi (ca. 1275–1326), who served as public lecturer at the University of Bologna from 1314–1324. Mondino's *Anatomy* was practical and succinct. The first printed edition of Mondino's popular text appeared in 1478 and was followed by at least 40 editions. But medical humanists rejected Mondino's text and turned to newly restored anatomical works by Galen, especially *On the Use of the Parts* and *On Anatomical*

Procedures. A major problem with the early texts was the lack of anatomical illustrations as opposed to simple diagrams and images that had nothing to do with the explication of anatomical materials. Mastery of the principles of artistic perspective in the fifteenth century made the new art of anatomical illustration possible.

The development of a special relationship with the sciences, especially anatomy, mathematics, and optics, gave Renaissance art much of its distinctive character. Both artists and physicians sought accurate anatomical knowledge. Artists placed a new emphasis on accurately representing animals and plants, scientific use of perspective, and above all the idea that the human body was beautiful and worthy of study. To make their art true to life and death, artists attended public anatomies and executions and studied intact and flayed bodies in order to see how the muscles and bones worked. While many Renaissance painters and sculptors turned to dissection, none exceeded Leonardo da Vinci (1452–1519)—painter, architect, anatomist, engineer, and inventor—in terms of artistic and scientific imagination. Leonardo's notebooks present a man of formidable genius and insatiable intellectual curiosity; they also reveal the problem of Leonardo as an historical figure. His notebooks are full of brilliant projects, observations, and hypotheses about human beings, animals, light, mechanics, and more. But the projects were never completed, and thousands of pages of notes and sketches went unpublished. The left-handed artist kept his notebooks in code, a kind of mirror writing. It is tempting to speculate that if Leonardo had systematically completed his ambitious projects and conscientiously published and publicized his work, he might have revolutionized several scientific disciplines. Instead, Leonardo's legacy has been assessed as "the epitome of greatness in failure," because that which is incomplete, disorganized, and unknown cannot be considered a contribution. To regard Leonardo as typical of his era is of course unrealistic, although he had many brilliant contemporaries. Nevertheless, Leonardo's work indicates the scope of the ideas and work that a person of genius might achieve with the materials available in the fifteenth century.

At 14 years of age, Leonardo was apprenticed to Andrea del Verrochio (1435–1488), painter, sculptor, and the foremost teacher of art in Florence. Verrochio insisted that all his pupils learn anatomy. Within 10 years Leonardo was recognized as a distinguished artist and had acquired wealthy and powerful patrons. Despite these advantages, Leonardo led a restless and adventurous life, serving various patrons, prosecuted on charges of homosexuality, beginning and discarding numerous projects for machines, statues, and books. It was art that first led Leonardo to dissection, but he pursued anatomical studies of animals and humans with almost morbid fascination for nearly 50 years, dissecting pigs, oxen, horses, monkeys, insects, etc. Leonardo was granted permission to study cadavers at a hospital in Florence. Thus, while planning a revolutionary treatise on the anatomy of "natural man," the artist spent many sleepless nights surrounded by corpses. Convinced that all problems could be reduced to mechanics and mathematics, Leonardo was contemptuous of astrology and alchemy and distrustful of medicine. Indeed, he believed that preserving one's health was most easily accomplished by avoiding physicians and their drugs. Like Cato and Pliny, he denounced physicians as "the destroyers of life," who lusted after wealth despite their inability to make an informed diagnosis.

ANDREAS VESALIUS ON THE FABRIC OF THE HUMAN BODY

Just as Copernicus and Galileo revolutionized ideas about the motions of the earth and the heavens, Andreas Vesalius (1514–1564) transformed Western concepts of the structure of the human body. Vesalius's great treatise on the microscosm, *The Fabric of the Human Body* (*De humani corporis fabrica libri septum*), appeared in 1543, the year in which Copernicus published the revolutionary text that placed the sun, rather than the earth, at the center of the universe. Vesalius was heir to the humanist medical tradition that had rediscovered the original writings of Hippocrates and Galen; he was a member of the first generation of scholars to enjoy access to the complete works of Galen. Given the scope of his work, Vesalius can be considered a classical scholar and humanist, as well as a physician, anatomist, and artist. Unlike Linacre and Caius, however, Vesalius was able to renounce the errors of the ancients clearly and publicly. Through his scholarship and his own observations he came to realize that human anatomy must be read from the "book of the human body," not from the pages of Galen. Vesalius regarded his work as the first real advance in anatomical knowledge since the time of Galen. It is not unreasonable to say that Vesalius took up the study of human anatomy at the point it had reached when Galen died.

A horoscope cast by Girolamo Cardano, a Milanese physician, fixes the birth of Andreas Vesalius in Brussels, Belgium, on December 31, 1514, at 5:45 a.m. Vesalius was born into a world of physicians, pharmacists, and royal patronage. His father was imperial pharmacist to Charles V and often accompanied the Emperor on his travels. As a youth, Vesalius began to teach himself anatomy by dissecting mice and other small animals. Although he studied at both the University of Paris and Louvain, institutions notable for their extreme conservatism, his innate curiosity was not destroyed by the benefits of education.

While a student at the University of Paris, Vesalius served as assistant to Jacobus Sylvius (1478–1555), an arch-conservative who saw human dissection only as a means of pursuing Galenic studies. Unfortunately, the atmosphere in Paris became so threatening that Vesalius found it necessary to leave without a degree. In the fall of 1537, Vesalius enrolled in the medical school of the University of Padua, a venerable, but relatively enlightened institution. He was awarded the M.D. in December 1537, and appointed lecturer-demonstrator in anatomy and surgery. Vesalian dissection-lectures occupied the anatomist and his audience from morning to night for 3 weeks at a time. To minimize the problem of putrefaction, anatomies were scheduled for the winter term. Several bodies were used simultaneously so that different parts could be clearly demonstrated. Anatomies began with a study of the

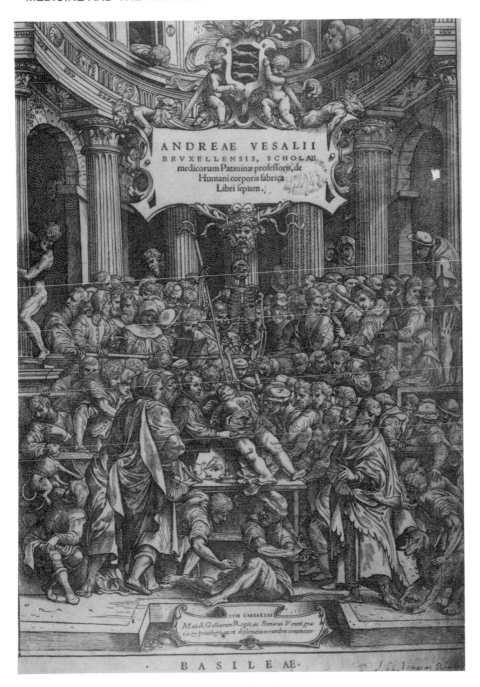

Andreas Vesalius

skeleton, and then proceeded to the muscles, blood vessels, nerves, organs of the abdomen, chest, and brain.

By 1538 Vesalius was beginning to recognize differences between Galenic anatomy and his own observations, but when the young anatomist publicly challenged Galen, Sylvius denounced his former student as "Vesanus" (madman), purveyor of filth and sewage, pimp, liar, and various epithets unprintable even in our own permissive era. Vesalius in turn told his students that they could learn more at a butcher shop than at the lectures of certain blockhead professors. Referring to the dissection skills of his former teacher, Vesalius said that Sylvius and his knife were more at home at the banquet table than the dissecting room. In 1539 Marcantonio Contarini, a judge in Padua's criminal court, became so interested in Vesalius's work that he awarded the bodies of executed criminals to the university and obligingly set the time of execution to suit the anatomist's convenience.

Finally, to mark his independence from Galen, Vesalius arranged a public dissection lecture in which he demonstrated over 200 differences between the skeletons of apes and humans, while reminding his audience that Galen's work was based on the dissection of apes. Hostile reactions from outraged Galenists were inevitable; Vesalian anatomists were villified as the "Lutherans of Physic" on the grounds that the heresy of such medical innovators was as dangerous as Martin Luther's (1483–1546) effect on religion. Tired of the controversy, Vesalius took a position as court physician to Charles V, Holy Roman Emperor and King of Spain, to whom he dedicated the *Fabrica*. Soon Vesalius discovered that imperial service was almost as unpleasant as the stormy academic world.

The patronage of a king, pope, or wealthy nobleman might allow a scientist to continue his research, but such patrons were often difficult and demanding patients. Charles V suffered from gout, asthma, and a variety of vague complaints exacerbated by his predilection for quack remedies. Moreover, kings often loaned their physicians to other royal courts. Thus, when Henry II of France was injured while jousting, Vesalius and the French surgeon Ambroise Paré were among the physicians in attendance. Using the heads of four recently decapitated criminals, Paré and Vesalius carried out experiments to ascertain the nature of the injuries and correctly predicted that the wound would be fatal. According to a doubtful, but persistent tradition, Vesalius went on a pilgrimage to the Holy Land to extricate himself from the Emperor's service, or as a penance for initiating a premature autopsy. Vesalius may have used the excuse of a pilgrimage to explore the possibility of returning to a professorship at Padua. Unfortunately, he died on the return voyage.

What led Vesalius, a man steeped in conservative academic scholarship, to reject Galen's authority and demand that anatomists study only the "completely trustworthy book of man"? Vesalius attributed his own disillusionment with Galen to his "discovery" that Galen had never dissected the human body. However, a minor work, known as the "Bloodletting Letter," suggests that practical problems concerning venesection forced Vesalius to question Galenic dogma. Venesection was the subject of violent controversies among sixteenth-century physicians. No one suggested abandoning bloodletting; rather, the medical humanists attacked what they called corrupt Arabist methods and called for a return to the pure teachings of Hippocrates and Galen.

Unfortunately, even after "purification," Galen's teachings on the venous system remained obscure. When Hippocratic texts contradicted each other and Galen, which authority could tell the physician how to select the site for venesection, how much blood to take, how rapidly bleeding should proceed, and how often to repeat the procedure? Struggling with these questions, Vesalius began to ask whether facts established by anatomical investigation could be used to test the validity of hypotheses. Unable to ignore the implications of his anatomical studies and clinical experience, Vesalius became increasingly critical of the medical humanists. He could not tolerate the way they ignored the true workings of the human body while they debated "horse-feathers" and trifles.

The Fabric of the Human Body was a revolutionary attempt to describe the human body as it really is without deferring to Galen when the truth could be learned through dissection. Vesalius also demonstrated how well the truth could be conveyed in words and illustrations. About 250 blocks were painstakingly prepared for incorporation into the text. Vesalius sent detailed notes to his publisher with instruction on how the illustrations were to be placed so that they would complement and clarify matters described in the text. Ironically, critics of Vesalian anatomy attacked the *Fabrica* on the grounds that the illustrations were false and misleading and would seduce students and anatomists away from dissection and direct observation. Actually, the importance of dissection is emphasized throughout the text and careful instructions were given on the preparation of bodies for dissection and the instruments needed for precise work on specific anatomical materials. The *Fabrica* was intended for serious anatomists, but Vesalius simultaneously brought out a short text, known as the *Epitome*, so that students too could appreciate the "harmony of the human body." The *Epitome* contained 11 plates showing the bones, muscles, external parts, nerves, veins, and arteries, and pictures of organs that were meant to be cut out and assembled by the reader. The texts and illustrations were widely plagiarized and disseminated, often in the form of inferior translations and abstracts that failed to credit the source of the text and illustrations.

In response to his critics, Vesalius denounced the "self-styled Prometheans" who claimed that Galen was always right and argued that the alleged errors in his texts were proof that the human body had degenerated since the classical era. Galenists, Vesalius declared, could not distinguish between the fourth carpal bone and a chickpea, but they wanted to destroy his work just as their predecessors had destroyed the works of Herophilus and Erasistratus. Recalling how he had once been under Galen's influence, Vesalius admitted that he used to keep the head of an ox handy to demonstrate the *rete mirabile*, a network of blood vessels which Galen placed at the base of the human brain. Unable to find the *rete mirabile* in human cadavers,

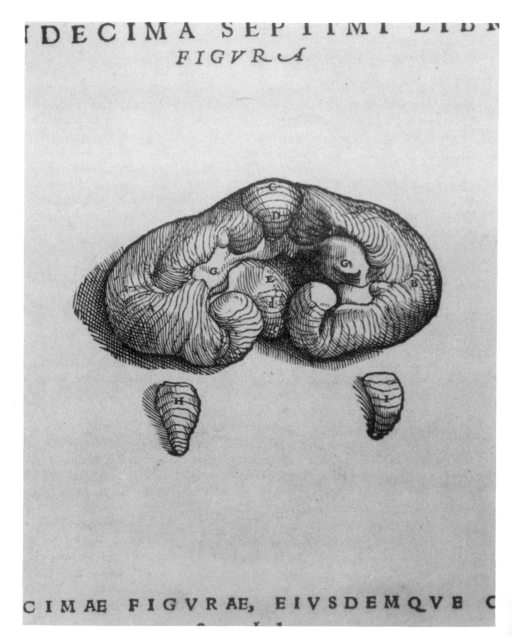

Inferior view of the cerebellum as depicted in *De humani corporis fabrica*, 1543

anatomists rationalized this inconsistency by asserting that, in humans, the structure disappeared very soon after death. When Vesalius finally came to terms with Galenic fallibility, he openly declared that such a network was not present in humans. In contrast to his revolutionary treatment of anatomy, Vesalius did not go much further than Galen and Aristotle in physiology and embryology. He gave an exhaustive description of the structure of the heart, arteries, and veins, and was skeptical of the Galenic claim that the blood moved from right heart to left heart through pores in the septum, but the motion of the blood remained obscure. Thus, while Galen was challenged on anatomical details, his overall teleological system remained intact. For example, having ruled out the presence of the *rete mirabile* in humans, Vesalius had to find an alternative site for the generation of the animal spirits. Since Galen seemed to say that only part of the process that generated the animal spirits occurred in the *rete mirabile* and suggested that the final modifications involved the brain and its ventricles, Vesalius could ascribe the function of the lost network to the cerebral arteries. To complete his anatomical triumph, while preserving Galenic physiology, Vesalius could say that God had demonstrated more ingenuity than Galen could have imagined when he created the human apparatus as opposed to that of the ox used by Galen.

Since the sixteenth century, anatomical research has been the cornerstone of Western medicine. However, we need not suffer through a catalogue of the parts of the body and the post-Vesalian anatomists who discovered them. Instead, let us take a slight digression and consider some general problems of anatomy and medical education: the need for cadavers and the persistent prejudice against human dissection.

Until recent times, anatomists were often forced into dangerous and illegal methods of obtaining human bodies. As a medical student in Paris, Vesalius fought off savage dogs while collecting human bones from the Cemetery of the Innocents. In Louvain he stole the remains of a robber chained to the gallows and brought the bones back into the city hidden under his coat. Grave-robbing incidents were reported wherever Vesalius conducted his famous lecture-demonstrations. One ingenious group of medical students obtained a corpse, dressed it, and "walked" their prize into the dissecting room as if it were just another drunken student being dragged into class. Anatomists too timid to obtain cadavers themselves turned to entrepreneurs known as "Resurrectionists" or "Sack-Em-Up Men," who obtained bodies by grave-robbing, extortion, and murder. In England, under the Murder Act of George II the bodies of criminals considered vile enough to be worthy of death and dissection were awarded to the Royal College of Surgeons as "a peculiar mark of Infamy added to the Punishment." The association between anatomists, hangmen and graverobbers was humiliating and dangerous to anatomists. Long after most European nations had made legal provisions for anatomical studies, body-snatching provided the bulk of the teaching material for gross anatomy in Great Britain, Canada, and the United States. Advocates of improved medical and surgical training were obliged to remind legislators and laymen that if doctors did not practice on cadavers they would learn the art at the expense of their patients.

MEDICINE AND SURGERY

In at least one important area Galen and Vesalius were in full agreement. Both argued that medicine and anatomy had degenerated because physicians had given up the practice of surgery and dissection. During the Middle Ages, the distinction between theoretical and practical medicine had been exaggerated by learned physicians, and power plays within university faculties exacerbated this tension. To enhance the dignity of the medical faculty, theoretical, logical, and universal ideas concerning the nature of human beings were emphasized at the expense of empirical and mechanical aspects of the healing art.

Although surgery and medicine could not be totally disentangled, traditions and laws delineated the territorial rights of practitioners. As a general rule, surgeons were expected to deal with the *exterior* and physicians with the *interior* of the body. Surgeons dealt with wounds, fractures, dislocations, bladder stones and other disorders of the urinary tract, amputations, skin diseases, and syphilis. Surgeons performed bleedings under the direction of physicians, but were expected to defer to physicians in the prescription of postoperative care. Surgical practice was itself divided into separate areas of status, competence, and privilege among surgeons, barber-surgeons, and barbers. Of course, the education, training, status, and legal standing of surgeons and physicians varied considerably throughout Europe. But almost everywhere, warfare provided golden opportunities for enterprising surgeons; the battlefield has always been the ultimate medical school. In such an environment, it was possible for Ambroise Paré, an "unlettered" barber-surgeon, to think his own thoughts, learn by experience, and demonstrate the value and dignity of the art of surgery.

AMBROISE PARÉ

To Ambroise Paré (1510–1590) surgery was a divine calling, despite the lowly status of its practitioners. Described by his contemporaries as independent, original, kind, gentle, impetuous, and ambitious, Paré was honest enough to admit that his major contributions to surgery were simple and not necessarily original. Nevertheless, his willingness to break with tradition and courageously follow methods suggested by his own observations pointed the way towards a general renaissance in surgery. Unlike previous generations of innovative craftsmen, Paré and other sixteenth-century guildsmen could emerge from obscurity because the printing press allowed them to publish popular texts in the vernacular. Paré's writings were collected and reprinted many times during his lifetime and translated into Latin, German, English, Dutch, and Japanese. Always willing to learn from ancient authorities, contemporary physicians, and surgeons, or even quacks with a promising remedy, Paré was a deeply religious man, who acknowledged only one final authority.

Little is known about Paré's background and early life. Even the date of his birth and his religion are unknown. Paré rarely discussed his training and apprenticeship, other than the fact that he had lived in Paris for 3 years during the 9 or 10 years he had studied surgery. Although apprenticeship was ostensibly a time for learning, pupils were all too often exploited by cruel masters who neglected their obligation to teach. To obtain more practical experience, Paré worked at the Hôtel Dieu, a hospital that provided examples of a great variety of disorders, as well as opportunities to participate in autopsies and anatomical demonstrations. Conditions at the hospital were so miserable that during one winter four patients had the tips of their noses frozen and Paré had to amputate them.

Paré's surgical texts provide vivid and moving accounts of the horrors of warfare, as well as the kinds of wounds caused by various weapons. After a battle, the stench of rotting corpses seemed to poison the air, wounds became putrid, corrupt, and full of worms. Often injured soldiers died from lack of food and attention, or from the economy measures used to treat them. For example, surgeons believed that mild contusions were best treated with bed rest, bleeding, wet cupping, and sweat-inducing drugs. Such gentle and time-consuming treatments were fine for officers and nobels, but a common soldier was more likely to be wrapped in a cloth, covered with a little hay, and buried in manure up to his neck to encourage sweating.

Gunpowder weapons were, as Francis Bacon noted, among the world-shaking inventions unknown to Hippocrates and Galen. Although gunpowder was referred to in Europe as early as the thirteenth century, it was not until the fourteenth century that pictures of primitive cannons appeared. Thus, to rationalize the treatment of gunpowder wounds, physicians had to argue from analogies. John of Vigo (1460–1525), one of the first to write specifically on the surgical problems of the new warfare, argued that wounds made by firearms were poisoned. Traditionally, poisoned wounds, such as snake bites, were neutralized by cauterization. Therefore, to reach and thoroughly cauterize deep, penetrating gunpowder wounds Vigo recommended boiling oil. When Paré began his career in military surgery, he followed Vigo's methods until his supply of oil was exhausted and he was forced to treat the rest of his patients with a wound dressing made of eggs, oil of roses, and turpentine. In comparing the courses of recovery, he found that the patients who had received the mild dressing were healing better than those treated with boiling oil. Based on these observations, he promised himself that he would never again rely on books when he could learn from experience; in his writings he urged other surgeons to follow his example. When cauterization was necessary, Paré preferred the "actual cautery" (red hot irons) to the "potential cautery" (strong acids or bases, boiling oil, etc.). To aid the healing of burned flesh, Paré recommended a dressing of raw onions and salt, or his famous "puppy oil balm," a secret recipe he had procured at great trouble and expense and then openly published for the benefit of all surgeons and patients. To prepare puppy oil dressing, the surgeon began by cooking two newly born puppies in oil of lilies until the bones dissolved. The oil was mixed with turpentine, a pound of earthworms, and then cooked over a slow fire. Paré was convinced that puppy oil soothed pain and promoted healing.

When the Faculty of Physicians challenged Paré to explain why many men died of rather minor gunpowder wounds, Paré examined the components of gunpowder to see whether the ingredients contained a special venom or fire. He concluded that there was neither fire nor venom in gunpowder. Indeed, soldiers, blessedly ignorant of medical theory, drank gunpowder in wine to stimulate healing, or applied gunpowder to wounds as a drying agent. Quoting Hippocrates' *On Airs, Places, and Waters*, Paré argued that the noxious air of the battlefield corrupted the blood and humors so that after a battle even small wounds became putrid and the patient died. Finally, Paré suggested that many of these deaths were due to the will of God. If it seems unfair for Paré to blame wound infection on God, it should be remembered that when a patient recovered, Paré invariably said that he dressed the wound, but God healed the patient.

Battlefield surgery often included the amputation of arms or legs, an operation that could lead to death from hemorrhage. Many patients died after amputations because cauterization destroyed the flaps of skin needed to cover the amputation site and increased the danger of infection. The use of the ligature for the repair of torn blood vessels was an old but neglected technique when Paré brought it to the attention of his contemporaries and demonstrated its value in amputations. If the surgeon had performed his task with skill, wealthy patients could be fitted with ingenious and beautifully ornamented devices that allowed for various degrees of movement. Paré also devised wooden legs suitable for the poor.

When Paré suffered a compound fracture of the leg he was fortunate to avoid the usual treatment, which was amputation. (In a simple fracture there is no external wound. Compound fractures involve a break in the skin; the existence of this external wound often leads to complications.) In 1561, Paré was kicked by his horse; two bones of his left leg were broken. Afraid of being kicked again, he stepped back and fell to the ground, causing the fractured bones to break through flesh, hose, and boot. The only medicaments that could be found in the village—egg whites, wheat flour, oven soot, and melted butter—did nothing to assuage the excruciating pain which Paré suffered with quiet dignity. Knowing the usual course of such injuries, Paré feared that he must lose his leg to save his life, but the fracture was reduced, the wound bandaged, the leg splinted, and rose ointment was applied until the abscess drained.

Despite Paré's reputation for kindness, he had a consuming curiosity that made him willing to use human subjects in scientific tests. For example, when Charles IX praised the virtues of a bezoar stone (stone or hairball found in the intestinal tract of animals) he had received as a gift, Paré argued that such stones were not really effective antidotes to poisons. To settle the argument, one of the King's cooks, who was about to be hanged for stealing two silver plates, was allowed to participate in Paré's experiment. The condemned man was given the bezoar stone and a poison provided by the court apothecary. Unfortunately for the cook, Paré was correct. Paré contended that many other widely prescribed and fearfully expensive "remedies"—such as unicorn horn and mummy powder—were as useless as bezoars. Noblemen drank from vessels made of unicorn horn and carried unicorn horn with them when traveling in order to ward off illness, much as modern tourists rely on quinine, Dramamine, and Kaopectate. True unicorn horn was very expensive because the bashful creature could only be captured by a beautiful virgin, but the major source of "unicorn horn" was the rhinoceros or narwhale.

Expressing skepticism about the existence of the unicorn, Paré conducted a series of experiments on alleged unicorn horns, such as examining the effect of unicorn horn on the behavior and survival of venomous spiders, toads, scorpions, and poisoned pigeons. In no case did unicorn horn have any medicinal virtues. Despite Paré's work and the questions raised by other skeptics, apothecaries vigorously defended the virtues of "true" (high quality, high price) unicorn horn. On aesthetic and medical grounds, Paré rejected the use of mummy powder; he said it was shameful for Christians to consume remedies allegedly derived from the bodies of dead pagans.

Opposing the use of orthodox remedies required courage and independence. When Paré published his studies of poisons and antidotes, he was attacked by physicians and apothecaries for trespassing on their territory. One critic claimed that we must believe in the medical virtues of unicorn horn because all the authorities had proclaimed its efficacy. Paré replied that he would rather be right even if that required standing all alone rather than join with others in their errors. Ideas that had been accepted for long periods of time were not necessarily true, for they were often founded upon opionions rather than facts.

THE OCCULT SCIENCES: ASTROLOGY AND ALCHEMY

Historians generally emphasize the artistic and scientific triumphs of the Renaissance, but it was also an age in which superstition and the occult sciences flourished. Medicine, along with the other arts and sciences, remained entangled with astrology, alchemy, and other varieties of mysticism. Out of this mixture of art, science, and magic arose new challenges to medical theory, philosophy, and practice. Astrological medicine was based on the assumption that human affairs and health were influenced by the motions of the heavenly bodies. In practice, astrological medicine required knowing the exact time at which the patient became ill; with this information and a study of the heavens, the physician could prognosticate the course of illness with mathematical precision and avoid dangerous tendencies. In therapeutics, astrological considerations influenced the nature and timing of treatments, the selection of drugs, and the use of charms. For example, the sun ruled the chronic diseases, Saturn was blamed for melancholy, and the moon, which governed the tides and the flow of blood in the veins, influenced the outcome of surgery, bleeding, purging, and acute illness. However, the presumed relationships between the heavenly bodies and the human body were so complex, numerous, and contradictory that in practice it was impossible to carry out any operation without breaking some rule. While medical astrology occupies a prominent place in the Renaissance, it can be seen as a continuity of popular medieval doctrines which were not necessarily linked to high medical culture. Physicians continued to study medical astrology in Renaissance universities, but many Renaissance medical treatises ignore or even explicitly condemn medical astrology. Even in the twentieth century, astrology remains orders of magnitude more popular than astronomy. Chemists, secure in their knowledge that alchemy has few devotees today, have long been amused at the continuous battle against superstition waged by astronomers. Alchemists, however, occupy an ambiguous position in the history of science, alternatively praised as pioneers of modern chemistry and damned as charlatans.

It is generally assumed that the primary goal of alchemy was to transform base metals into gold, but alchemy is a term that encompasses a broad range of doctrines and practices. As we have seen in our discussion of Chinese medicine, the art also included the search for the elixirs of health, longevity, and immortality. In Western history, the idea that the task of alchemy was not to make gold or silver, but to prepare medicines, is most closely associated with Philippus Aureolus Theophrastus Bombastus von Hohenheim, alchemist, physician, and pharmacologist. Fortunately, he is generally referred to as Paracelsus (higher than Celsus), the term adopted by the Paracelsians of the seventeenth century who believed that therapeutics could be revolutionized by the development of chemical or "spagyric" drugs. (Spagyric comes from the Greek words meaning "to separate" and "to assemble.") Paracelsus rejected anatomical research as irrelevant to understanding the most profound questions of life and disease and attempted to substitute the idea that the vital fuctions of the body depended on a mysterious force called the *archaeus*, a sort of internal alchemist.

After a brief period as a student at the University of Basel, Paracelsus turned to the study of alchemy as an apprentice in the mines of the Tyrol. In search of further enlightenment, he wandered through Germany, Spain, France, and perhaps beyond. Explaining his wanderlust, he called Nature a book which the seeker of knowledge must tread with his feet, learning the secrets of alchemists, astrologers, gypsies, magicians, and peasants. Paracelsus bestowed upon himself the title "double doctor," presumably for honors conferred on him by God and Nature, but there is no evidence that he was in the formal sense even a "single doctor." In 1526, Paracelsus returned to Switzerland and secured an appointment as Professor of Medicine and city physician of Basel, where he revealed a genius for staging media events. To show his contempt for ancient dogma, he burned the works of Avicenna and Galen while denouncing orthodox pharmacists and physicians as a "misbegotten

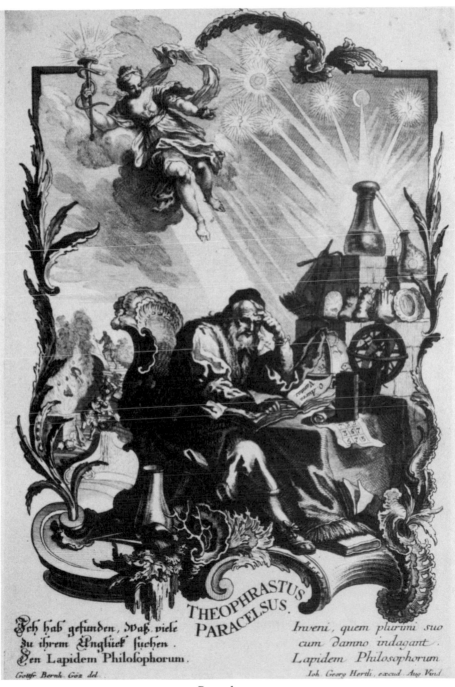

Paracelsus

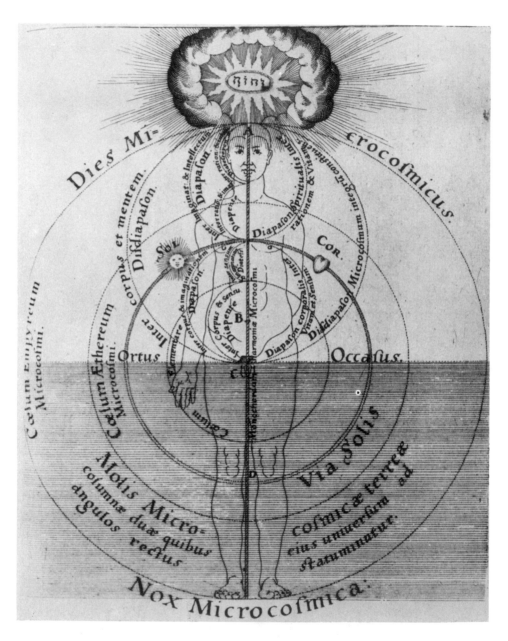

The microcosm (a seventeenth century alchemical chart showing the human body as world soul)

crew of approved asses.'' Wearing the alchemist's leather apron rather than academic robes, he lectured in the vernacular instead of Latin. Although these public displays enraged his learned colleagues, it was a dispute over a fee for medical services that forced him to flee from Basel. His enemies happily noted that he died in a mysterious, but certainly unnatural fashion when only 48, while Hippocrates and Galen, founders of the medical system he despised, had lived long, productive lives.

In opposition to the concept of humoral pathology, especially the doctrines presented by Galen and Avicenna, Paracelsus attempted to substitute the doctrine that the body was essentially a chemical laboratory. Disease was, therefore, the result of derangements in the chemical functions of the body rather than a humoral disequilibrium. Because life and disease were chemical phenomena, specific chemical substances must serve as remedies. The specific healing virtue of a remedy would depend on its chemical properties, not on the qualities of moistness, dryness, and so forth, associated with humoral theory. The challenge of finding a specific remedy for each disease seemed overwhelming, not because of a scarcity of medicines, but because nature was one great apothecary shop. In a burst of optimism, Paracelsus declared that all diseases could be cured when, through alchemy, we came to understand the essence of life and death. Confronting Nature's embarrassment of riches, the alchemist could be guided by the method of separation, the Doctrine of Signatures, and the astrological correspondences among the seven planets, seven metals, and the parts of the body.

Rejecting the Galenic principle that contraries cure, Paracelsus favored the concept that like cures like. However, the true virtues of a crude or complex remedy could only be revealed by alchemically separating the pure from the impure, the useful from the useless. Within the vast *materia medica* poisons had always been of particular interest; Paracelsus argued that alchemy made it possible to separate out the curative virtues hidden within these powerful substance. But determining the therapeutic virtues of new chemical remedies could be very dangerous. Fortunately, many toxic materials cause such rapid purgation that not enough was absorbed to kill the patient. In some cases the purification procedure actually removed everything but the solvent. In place of complex herbal preparations, Paracelsus and his followers favored the use of purified drugs, especially minerals such as mercury, antimony, iron, arsenic, lead, copper, and their salts, and sulfur. Not all the Paracelsian drugs were derivatives of toxic metals; his ''laudanum,'' a preparation used to induce restful sleep and ease pain, contained opium and wine.

Although Paracelsus ridiculed traditional uroscopy, he accepted the underlying idea that since urine contains wastes collected from the whole body it must harbor valuable diagnostic clues. Instead of uroscopy by ocular inspection, he proposed diagnosis by chemical analysis, distillation, and coagulation tests. However, given the state of qualitative and quantitative analysis, his chemical dissection of urine was likely to be about as informative as ocular inspection. In urine analysis, as in studies of potential remedies, many Paracelsians ignored the important residues and concentrated all their attention on the distillate.

To replace humoral categories of disease, Paracelsus attempted to develop a system based on analogies to chemical processes. While generally obscure and inconsistent, his chemical concepts were, however, peculiarly appropriate to metabolic diseases, dietary disorders, and certain occupational diseases. For example, in classifying gout as a ''tartaric disease,'' he had indeed provided an example of a metabolic disease in which body chemistry has gone wrong. That is, in gouty individuals a metabolic product forms local deposits, primarily in the joints, in a manner very roughly analogous to the way in which tartar sediments out of fermenting wine. He also pointed to a relationship between cretinism and goiter, which is due to the lack of iodine in the diet. According to Paracelsus, miners, smelter workers, and metallurgists exhibited a variety of symptoms because their lungs and skin absorbed dangerous combinations of unwholesome airs and clouds of poisonous dust. This noxious chemical melange generated internal coagulations, precipitations, and sediments. Such examples can create the impression that Paracelsus had valid reasons for his attack on Galenism and actually held the keys to a new system of therapeutics, but it is easy to read too much into the Paracelsian literature and confuse obscurity with profundity. Nevertheless, in the hands of his followers Paracelsian medicine served as a useful stimulus to pharmacology and physiology, diagnostics and therapeutics.

SYPHILIS, THE SCOURGE OF THE RENAISSANCE

The changing pattern of epidemic disease or diagnostic categories is a remarkable phenomenon. Although leprosy did not entirely disappear, and waves of plague continued to break over Renaissance Europe, diseases previously rare, absent, or unrecognized—such as syphilis, typhus, smallpox, and influenza—became major public health threats. Many diseases are worthy of a full biography, but none raises more intriguing questions than syphilis, the ''Scourge of the Renaissance.'' Because syphilis is a sexually transmitted disease, it is a particularly sensitive tracer of the obscure pathways of human contacts throughout the world, as well as the intimate links between social and medical concepts.

In mocking tribute to Venus, the goddess of love, the term *venereal* has long served as a euphemism in matters pertaining to sex. But in an era that prides itself on having won the sexual revolution, the more explicit term *sexually transmitted disease* (STD) has been substituted for *venereal disease* (VD). Any disease that can be transmitted by sexual contact may be considered a venereal disease; a more restricted definition includes only those diseases that are never, or almost never, transmitted by any mechanism other than sexual contact. Syphilis and gonorrhea are the major venereal diseases in the wealthy, industrialized nations, but the so-called minor venereal diseases, chancroid, lymphogranuloma venereum, and granuloma inguinale, also

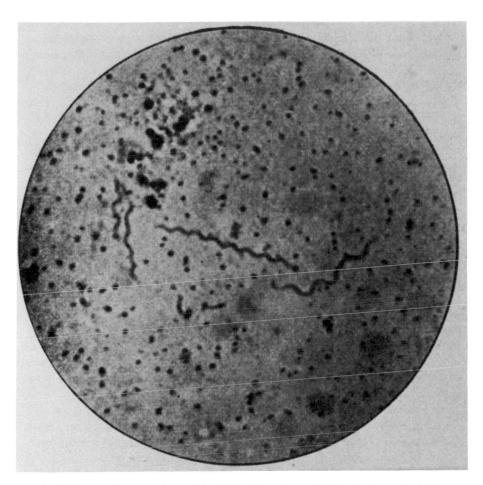

Syphilis spirochaetae as depicted by F. R. Schaudinn and P. E. Hoffmann in 1905

cause serious complications. Scabies and crab lice gain membership in the club if a less rigorous definition of STD is accepted. Additional modern members of the STD club are genital herpes, trichomoniasis, nongonococcal urethritis, and AIDS. Genital herpes was winning the battle to become the most feared venereal disease in the United States until the 1980s when AIDS emerged as the great modern plague.

Despite the antiquity of references to venereal diseases, many Renaissance physicians were convinced that syphilis was unknown in Europe until the end of the fifteenth century; others argued that there was one venereal scourge as old as civilization which appeared in many guises, including gonorrhea and syphilis. The confusion is not surprising, as a brief overview of the natural history of the major venereal diseases will indicate. Diagnosis of syphilis and gonorrhea cannot be based on symptoms alone. In the modern laboratory, a tentative diagnosis of syphilis can be confirmed by the Wassermann blood test, but for gonorrhea confirmation requires identification of *Neisseria gonorrhoeae*, the bacillus discovered by Albert Neisser (1855–1916) in 1879.

Symptoms of gonorrhea usually appear about 3 days after infection, but the incubation period may be as long as 10 days. Pain and the discharge of pus from the urethra is usually the first symptom noticed in males. Eventually, inflammation may obstruct the flow of urine and lead to a life-threatening stricture of the urethra. Surgeons attacked the problem with sounds (curved metal rods) to stretch the narrowed channel and catheters to provide relief from retention of urine. Avicenna introduced medicines into the bladder with a silver syringe, and for good measure inserted a louse in the urethra. (If a louse was not available, a flea or bug might do equally well.) Many patients treated for arthritis and gout were probably suffering from gonococcal infections. In women gonorrhea is often a silent infection that insideously attacks the internal organs, leading to peritonitis, endocarditis, arthritis, spontaneous abortion and stillbirths, or sterility. Infants can acquire gonorrheal infection of the eyes during birth; the instillation of silver nitrate or penicillin into the eyes immediately after delivery can prevent this form of blindness. Public health authorities once thought that penicillin would eradicate gonorrhea, but in the late twentieth century gonorrhea was still the most common venereal disease and the most prevalent bacterial disease on earth. Trends in the development of antibiotic-resistant strains of the gonococcus provide no grounds for optimism; new "superstrains" of antibiotic-resistant gonococci have appeared throughout the world.

In contrast to gonorrhea, untreated syphilis progresses through three stages of increasing severity. A small lesion known as a chancre is the first sign. The chancre may become ulcerated or disappear altogether. The second stage may include fever, headache, sore throat, a localized rash, gumma, skin lesions, patchy bald spots, swollen and tender lymph nodes, sore mouth, and inflamed eyes. Symptoms may appear within weeks or months after infection and subside without treatment. During the third stage, chronic obstruction of small blood vessels, abscesses, and inflammation result in permanent damage to the cardiovascular system and other major organs. Neurosyphilis causes impaired vision, loss of muscular coordination, paralysis, and insanity. A syphilitic woman may experience miscarriages, stillbirths, or bear a child with impaired vision, deafness, mental deficiency, and cardiovascular disease. Syphilis has been called the "great mimic" because in the course of its development it simulates many other diseases. Syphilitic lesions can be confused with those of leprosy, tuberculosis, scabies, fungal infections, and various skin cancers. Before the introduction of specific bacteriological and immunological tests, the great imitator was such a diagnostic challenge that it was said that whoever knows all of syphilis knows all of medicine.

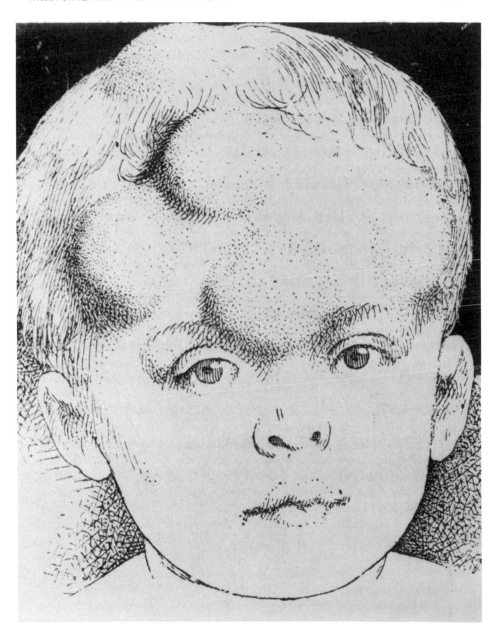

Congenital syphilis (young child with cranial gummata, 1886)

If diseases were catalogued in terms of etiological agents instead of means of transmission, the venereal scourge would be described as a member of the treponematosis family. The treponematoses are diseases caused by members of the *Treponema* group of spirochetes (corkscrew-shaped bacteria). Although these microbes grow slowly, once established in a suitable host they multiply with inexorable patience and persistence. Syphilis is one of four *clinically* distinct human treponematoses; the others are known as pinta, yaws, and bejel. In terms of microbiological and immunological tests, the causative organisms are virtually identical; distinct differences are readily revealed in naturally occurring infections. Some bacteriologists believe that the causative agents of pinta, yaws, bejel, and syphilis are variants of an ancestral spirochete which adapted to different patterns of climate and human behavior. According to what is generally known as the *unitary theory*, the nonvenereal treponematoses are ancient diseases generally transmitted between children. As people migrated to temperate areas and covered themselves with clothing, nonvenereal transmission was inhibited. Under these conditions, many people reached adulthood without acquiring the immunity common in more primitive times. Pinta, a disease endemic in Mexico and Central America, is characterized by skin eruptions of varying color and severity. Until *Treponema carateum* was discovered, pinta was classified among the fungal skin diseases. Yaws, a disease caused by *Treponema pertenue*, flourishes in hot, moist climates. Like syphilis, yaws leads to destruction of tissue, joints and bone. Bejel, or nonvenereal endemic syphilis, is generally acquired in childhood, among rural populations living in warm, arid regions. Like syphilis, bejel has a latent phase, and afflicted individuals may be infectious for many years.

Despite advances in understanding the treponematoses, medical historians are no closer to a definitive account of the origin of syphilis than medical authorities are to eradicating STDs. Reliable accounts of syphilis first appeared in the sixteenth century when the plague that marked its victims with loathsome skin eruptions was known by many names. The French called it the "Neapolitan disease," the Italians called it the "French disease," the Portuguese called it the "Castillian disease"; in India and Japan it was called the "Portuguese disease," and the names "Canton disease, "Great Pox," and "*lues venereum*" were also used. The name used today was invented by Girolamo Fracastoro (Latinized as Fracastorius; 1478–1553), an Italian physician, scientist, mathematician, astronomer, geologist, and poet. In his treatise on *Syphilis, or the French Disease* (1530), Fracastoro created the story of Syphilis the shepherd, who brought about the first outbreak of the scourge by cursing the sun. To punish human beings for this blasphemy, the sun shot deadly rays of disease at the earth. Syphilis was the first victim of the new pestilence, but the affliction soon spread to every village and city, even to the king himself.

Examining the historical evidence concerning the origin of the "venereal scourge" is like entering a labyrinth. If we include the speculations of Fracastoro, his contemporaries, and subsequent medical writers, we come up with many theories but no definitive answer to the question raised in the sixteenth century: What causes presided at the origin of syphilis? Perhaps a better question might be: What factors account for the persistent, perhaps obsessive, fascination with the origin of syphilis? In a story reminiscent of astrological accounts of the origins of the Black Death, sixteenth-century medical astrologers traced the origins of this vile disease to a malign conjunction of Jupiter, Saturn, and Mars in 1485 that produced a subtle poison which spread throughout the universe, unleashing a terrible plague upon Europe. Followers of astrology even today might argue that this theory has never been disproved, but more scientifically plausible theories are still hotly debated.

The so-called Columbus Theory of the origin of syphilis is based on the idea that the New World was the source of new diseases as well as new plants and animals. Many Renaissance physicians assumed that the "great pox" was one of the gifts imported from the New World to the Old World by Columbus and his crew. The fifteenth century was a time of great voyages, commercial expansion, and warfare, during which previously isolated peoples were suddenly immersed in a globalized germ pool. Many epidemic diseases flourished under these conditions, but it was syphilis that has become known as the "calling card of civilized man." Much circumstantial evidence supports the Columbus Theory: the timing of the voyages, the dispersal of the crew, their transformation from sailors to soldiers, their presence in areas where the disease was first reported, the testimony of physicians, the subsequent spread of syphilis, and its changing clinical pattern. While evidence for the Columbus Theory can be assembled in a fairly convincing package, it is important to remember that *coincidence* must not be confounded with *cause*. Moreover, the diagnostic value of documents designed to link "evil pocks" to immorality, human afflictions, and messages from God is somewhat suspect.

Rodrigo Ruiz Diaz de Isla (1462–1542), a Spanish physician, was probably the first to assert that syphilis had been imported to Europe from the West Indies by members of the crew of Columbus. In a book not published until 1539, de Isla claimed to have treated several sailors who returned to Barcelona in 1493 with a strange disease characterized by loathsome skin eruptions. Additional support for the Columbus Theory is found in reports written in 1525 by Gonzalo Hernandez de Oviedo y Valdez, Governor of the West Indies. According to Oviedo, sailors infected in the New World had joined the army of Charles VII at the siege of Naples (1494). When the French army was driven out of Italy in 1495, infected troops and camp followers sparked epidemics throughout Europe.

The Columbus Theory requires, at the very least, conclusive proof of the existence of syphilis in the New World *before* 1492. Unequivocal evidence of syphilis in Europe before the voyages of Columbus would disprove this theory. However, given the difficulties inherent in paleopathology, the diagnostic evidence for syphilis in pre-Columbian America and Europe remains problematic and the debate among historians continues. The problem is compounded by a recent tendency to blur distinctions between syphilis and nonvenereal treponemal infections.

The so-called Leprosy Theory is based on the possibility that syphilis might have hidden itself among the legions of medieval lepers. References to "venereal leprosy" and "congenital leprosy" in Europe before 1492 are compatible with this theory, but all medieval allusions to a connection between leprosy and sex must be examined cautiously. To determine whether some lepers were actually syphilitics, scientists have looked for syphilitic lesions in bones found in leper cemeteries; at present, the evidence remains ambiguous. Another dubious sixteenth-century tradition suggested that the new venereal scourge was a hybrid produced by sexual intercourse between a leper and a prostitute with gonorrhea.

Another hypothesis known as the African or Yaws Theory essentially reverses the Columbus Theory: according to this theory, syphilis was one of the many disasters Europeans brought to the New World by merging the germ pools of Africa and Europe in the Americas. With native Americans perhaps brought to the verge of extinction by smallpox and other foreign diseases, Europeans were importing African slaves into the New World within 20 years of the first contacts. If Africans taken to Europe and the New World were infected with yaws, changes in climate and clothing would have inhibited nonvenereal transmission of the spirochete. Under these condition, yaws could only survive by becoming a venereal disease. If true, the African Theory would explain the apparent relationship between the appearance of syphilis and the adventures of Columbus and his crew. It would also provide a form of intercontinental microbiological retribution with a fitting lesson about the evils of slavery. However, this theory is based on rather weak circumstantial evidence. Given the antiquity of interchanges between Europe and Africa, yaws could have been introduced into Egypt, Arabia, Greece, and Rome from Africa centuries before the voyages of Columbus. Therefore, some other spark must have been needed to trigger the sixteenth-century conflagration. Partisans of various theories present many ingenious arguments, but the evidence for any one theory does not yet seem to be totally convincing.

Whatever the source of syphilis, Fracastoro believed that in its early stage the disease could be cured by a carefully controlled regimen, including exercises that provoked prodigious sweats. Once the disease had taken root in the viscera, a cure required remedies almost as vile as the disease. In another flight of fancy, Fracastoro told the story of a peaceful gardener named Ilceus who was stricken with a terrible disease as punishment for killing a deer sacred to Apollo and his sister Diana. The gods had sworn that no remedy would be found within their empire, so Ilceus journeyed to a cavern deep within the bowels of the earth. Here he was cured when the resident nymphs plunged him into a river of pure quicksilver (mercury). Unlike the nymphs, doctors liked to combine mercury with other agents, such as lard, turpentine, incense, lead, and sulfur. Perhaps the most bizarre prescription was that of Giovanni de Vigo who added live frogs to his quicksilver ointment. Fracastoro preferred a remedy rich in mercury, black hellebore, and sulfur. Covered with this mixture, the patient was wrapped in wool and kept in bed until the disease was washed out of the body in a flood of sweat and saliva. An alternative method of cure by emaciation included starvation diets, purges, sudorifics, and salivation induced by mercury. If this 30-day regimen did not cure syphilis, it would certainly do wonders for obesity.

Mercury became so intimately linked to the venereal scourge that quacksalvers used mercury as an operational definition for syphilis; if mercury provided a cure, the patient was syphilitic. The link between syphilis and mercury probably resulted from the belief that mercury cured diseases of the skin. Reasoning by analogy from the effectiveness of mercurial ointments for scabies and other skin disorders, doctors assumed that mercury would also triumph over syphilitic ulcers. In any case, syphilis made it possible for quacksalvers to achieve the dream of the alchemists, the transmutation of mercury into gold. Patients undergoing mercury inunction sat in a tub in a hot, closed room where they could be rubbed with mercury ointments several times a day. Those who would rather read Shakespeare than ancient medical texts will find many references to the torments of syphilis and the "tub of infamy." Other references to "rubbing and tubbing" indicate that this form of treatment was very well known. If the association between syphilis and mercury inunction had not been so completely forgotten by the 1980s, the Moral Majority would certainly demand censorship of the Mother Goose rhyme: "Rub-a-dub-dub, three men in a tub . . ."

Unequivocal proof of mercury toxicity is rather recent, but suspicions about the dangers of quicksilver were not uncommon among Renaissance practitioners. Bernardino Ramazzini (1633–1714) devoted a chapter of his great treatise *On the Diseases of Workers* to "Diseases of those who give mercurial inunction." As Ramazzini so aptly put it, mercury inunction was performed by the lowest class of surgeons because the better class of doctors would not practice "a service so disagreeable and a task so full of danger and hazard." Realizing that no fee could compensate for loss of their own health, some surgeons made their patients rub each other with mercurial ointments. By the early nineteenth century, some critics of mercurial remedies realized that excessive salivation and ulcers in the mouth were signs of "morbid mercurial irritation" rather than part of the cure.

Even physicians who regarded mercury as a marvelous remedy were not about to let patients escape from their full therapeutic arsenal. Syphilitics were dosed with brisk purgatives, clysters, sudorifics, and tonics, and subjected to bizarre dietary restrictions. Many therapeutic regimens, including that of Fracastoro, emphasized heat, exercise, and sweating. Indeed, therapeutic hyperthermia (fever therapy) was used for both syphilis and gonorrhea well into the twentieth century; experiments on therapeutic hyperthermia utilized tuberculin, bacterial vaccines, malaria, and fever cabinets. Theories of fever have undergone many changes since antiquity, but the significance of fever in disease is still an enigma. However, the rationale for fever therapy is that high body temperature is a defense mechanism which might destroy or inhibit the activities of pathogenic parasites. Elevation of body temperature is not without risk. Not surprisingly, after undergoing therapeutic hyperthermia for the treatment of venereal disease, many patients suffered disorientation and various unpleasant side effects.

During the first phase of the syphilis epidemic, the only serious challenge to mercury was a remedy known as guaiac, or "Holy Wood." Guaiac was obtained from evergreen trees indigenous to South America and the West Indies. According to the Doctrine of Signatures, if syphilis originated in the New World, the remedy should be found in the same region. Imported Holy Wood became the remedy of physicians and their wealthy clients, while mercury remained the remedy of the poor. Paracelsus complained that his work on the therapeutic virtues of mercury had been suppressed by wealthy merchants and physicians who were deluding the sick by promoting expensive and useless guaiac treatments. One of the most influential and enthusiastic of the early anti-mercurialists, Ulrich Ritter von Hutten (1488–1523) was a victim of both the venereal disease and the noxious cures prescribed by his physicians. In 1519 von Hutten published a very personal account of guaiac and syphilis. Having suffered through 11 cures by mercury in 9 years, von Hutten claimed that guaiac had granted him a complete and painless cure. He enthusiastically urged all victims of the venereal scourge to follow his example. However, he died only a few years after his cure, perhaps from the complications of tertiary syphilis. Fracastoro, who had recommended vigorous exercise, sweating, and mercury, also provided an appropriate myth about a group of Spanish mariners who observed a ceremony performed by the natives of the New World in which syphilis was cured with Holy Wood.

Of course there were many minor challenges to mercury and Holy Wood, including preparations based on gold, silver, arsenic, lead, and dozens of botanicals. Holy Wood retained its popularity for little more than a century, but mercury was still regarded as an anti-syphilitic in the 1940s. As humoral pathology gradually gave way to a pathology of solids based on anatomical investigations, copious salivation was no longer interpreted as a sign of efficacy, and milder mercurial treatments gained new respect. Because of the unpredictable course of the disease, case histories could be found to prove the efficacy of every purported remedy.

Perhaps the medical use of mercury proves nothing but the strong bond between therapeutic illusions and the almost irresistible compulsion to do something. Four hundred years of mercury therapy for syphilis have been summed up as probably the most colossal hoax in the history of medicine. With the medical community and the public convinced that mercury cured syphilis, it was almost impossible to conduct clinical trials in which patients were deprived of this remedy. However, William Fergusson, Inspector General of Hospitals of the Portuguese Army, noticed an interesting unplanned "clinical test" during British military operations in Portugal in 1812. Portuguese soldiers with syphilis generally received no treatment at all, while British soldiers were given vigorous mercury therapy. Fergusson thought that the Portuguese soldiers recovered more rapidly and completely than the British. About 100 years later Norwegian investigators provided further support for therapeutic restraint in a study of almost 2000 untreated syphilitics. In 1929, follow-up studies of subjects in the 1891–1910 Oslo Study indicated that at least 60% of the untreated syphilitics had experienced fewer long-term problems than patients subjected to heroic mercury treatments.

Evaluating remedies for venereal disease was complicated by the confusion between gonorrhea and syphilis. In the eighteenth century, John Hunter (1728–1793) attempted to untangle the problem by injecting himself (or, according to a less heroic version of the story, his nephew) with pus taken from a patient. Unfortunately, Hunter's results increased the confusion, because he concluded that gonorrhea was a symptom of syphilis. His results are best explained by assuming that his patient had both syphilis and gonorrhea. Philippe Ricord (1800–1889) is generally regarded as the first to separate syphilis and gonorrhea. His work brought the term syphilis into greater use as a replacement for the nonspecific *lues venerea*. All lingering doubts as to the distinction between syphilis and other venereal diseases were settled at the beginning of the twentieth century with the discovery of the "germ of syphilis" and the establishment of the Wassermann reaction as a diagnostic test.

In 1905 Fritz Richard Schaudinn (1871–1906) and Paul Erich Hoffmann (1868–1959) identified the causal agent of syphilis, *Spirochaeta pallida*, later renamed *Treponema pallidum*. The discovery was soon confirmed by Hideyo Noguchi (1876–1928). Diagnostic screening was made possible in 1906 when August von Wassermann (1866–1925) discovered a specific blood test for syphilis. The Wassermann reaction redefined the natural history of syphilis, especially secondary and tertiary stages, latent and congenital syphilis. Wassermann and his co-workers, who embarked on their research with assumptions that later proved to be quite incorrect, have been compared to Columbus, because in a search for "their own 'India,' they unexpectedly discovered a new 'America'." When Noguchi demonstrated *Treponema pallidum* in the brains of paretics (patients suffering from paralytic dementia), the natural history of syphilis was complete, from initial chancre to paralytic insanity and death.

Shortly after identification of the microbial agent and the discovery of a sensitive diagnostic test, new drugs allowed public health officials to launch a campaign to eradicate the venereal diseases. Prevention through chastity had, of course, always been a theoretical possibility, but in practice, this approach has never prevailed over the venereal diseases. Condoms had been promoted as implements of safety since the seventeenth century, but these devices were said to be "gossamer against disease" and "leaden against love." In 1910 when Paul Ehrlich (1854–1915) introduced the arsenical drug Salvarsan, a remedy that seemed to be more safe and effective than any previous form of treatment for syphilis, it became easier to see the disease as a microbial threat to the public health, rather than divine retribution for illicit sex. With Salvarsan restoring syphilitics to good health, the righteous worried that God would have to find some other punishment for immorality. According to those who persist in seeing disease as punishment for individual and collective sin, genital herpes and AIDS, viral diseases beyond the reach of antibiotics, were sent to serve this purpose.

The trade name Salvarsan reflected the high hopes the pharmaceutical industry and the medical community had for the new remedy. Moralists, quacks, and those who made fortunes by defrauding victims of venereal diseases denounced Ehrlich's "modified poison." The majority of physicians, however, welcomed Salvarsan along with mercury as "destroyers of spirochetes." Though some physicians optimistically predicted that Salvarsan would eradicate the disease, more cautious or prescient observers warned that syphilis was likely to thwart such therapeutic illusions.

After a significant decline in the incidence of syphilis during the 1950s, rates of syphilitic infection began to climb again in the 1960s. While AIDS hysteria eclipsed other public health problems in the 1980s, the Centers for Disease Control continued to report an increase in primary and secondary syphilis. Certainly, the persistence of gonorrhea and syphilis—despite Salvarsan, penicillin, comprehensive wartime venereal disease programs, repression of prostitution, case-finding and tracing of sexual contacts, premarital testing, endless moralizing and preaching, and educational campaigns—does not promote optimism about the possibility for control of AIDS, the new "venereal scourge." Both AIDS and syphilis present fascinating biological puzzles that require an understanding of social and environmental forces, as well as microbiology and immunology. Indeed, it is almost impossible to resist drawing parallels between syphilis, with its 500-year history, and AIDS, which has been known as a diagnostic entity only since the 1980s. Fear, prejudice, lack of effective or enlightened medical and public responses typify the reaction to both diseases. In particular, the history of the infamous Tuskegee Study is indicative of the way in which deep social and cultural pathologies are revealed through the stigmata of specific diseases.

In 1932, the United States Public Health Service initiated a study of the natural history of untreated syphilis very loosely modeled on the Oslo Study. Conducted in Macon County, Alabama, with the assistance of personnel at the Tuskegee Institute, the Veterans' Administration Hospital in Tuskegee, the Macon County Health Department, and others, the experiment is known as the Tuskegee Study, although in the 1970s the Tuskegee Institute claimed to have had little or no contact with the experiment after the 1930s. Six hundred impoverished black men were recruited for the study with promises of free medical care and money for burial (after autopsy): 400 were diagnosed as syphilitic at the beginning of the study and 200 were selected to serve as uninfected controls. Published reports of the study appeared with some regularity from 1936 into the 1960s. Throughout the course of the experiment, the physicians conducting the study deliberately withheld available therapy and deceived the participants by assuring them that they were receiving appropriate medical care for "bad blood." In 1970 an official of the Public Health Service declared that the Tuskegee Study was incompatible with the goal of controlling venereal disease because nothing that had been learned in the course of this poorly planned and badly executed experiment would ever "prevent, find or cure" a single case of syphilis. But it was not until 1972, when investigative reporters brought the experiment to public attention, that the study was terminated. The Tuskegee Study revealed nothing of value about the natural history of the syphilis, but told a disturbing story of racism, poverty, and ignorance. Official investigations have generally focused on the question of why the study was allowed to continue after the 1940s when penicillin became the drug of choice in treating the disease. The assumption was often made that withholding treatment during the 1930s was justifiable on the grounds that the treatments available at the time were both worse than the disease and ineffective. During the 1930s, physicians were no longer praising Salvarsan as a miracle cure for syphilis, but they were subjecting patients to long, expensive, painful treatment programs involving numerous intramuscular injections of Salvarsan in combination with applications of mercury or bismuth ointments. Perhaps ethical questions about the treatment of the well-to-do, as well as the withholding of treatment from the poor are applicable to the time period preceding the introduction of penicillin.

In the sixteenth century therapeutics lagged further and further behind other aspects of medical theory and practice. As teachers and writers, learned physicians of the sixteenth century believed that they were making a break with the medieval and Arabic past, primarily by recapturing and assimilating pristine Greek knowledge. Many scholars were convinced that, despite evidence of intellectual continuity, medicine was undergoing rapid and significant changes. Physicians were acquiring the anatomical and pharmacological knowledge and ideas that promoted increasingly novel and sophisticated debates about the nature and cause of disease; this did not automatically change the nature or efficacy of their prescriptions, but it made the search for further knowledge possible and highly desirable.

SUGGESTED READING

Baker, Brenda J., and Armelagos, George J. (1988). The Origin and Antiquity of Syphilis: Paleopathological Diagnosis and Interpretation. *Current Anthropology* 29: 703-737.

Barzun, Jacques, ed. (1974). *Burke and Hare: The Resurrection Men*. Metuchen, NJ: The Scarecrow Press.

Belt, Elmer (1955). *Leonardo the Anatomist*. Lawrence, KS: University of Kansas Press.

Brandt, Allan M. (1978). Racism and Research: The Case of the Tuskegee Syphilis Study. *Hastings Center Report* 8(#6): 21-29.

Brandt, Allan M. (1987). *No Magic Bullet: A Social History of Venereal Disease in the United States Since 1880. With a New Chapter on AIDS*. New York: Oxford University Press.

Braudel, Fernand (1976). *Capitalism and Material Life 1400-1800*. Trans. Miriam Kochan. London: Weidenfeld and Nicolson.

Bynum, W. F., and Nutton, Vivian, eds. (1981). *Theories of Fever from Antiquity to the Enlightenment*. London: Wellcome Institute for the History of Medicine.

Caius, John (1912). *The Works of John Caius, M.D.*. Ed. E. S. Roberts. Cambridge, England: Cambridge University Press.

Capp, Bernard (1979). *English Almanacs, 1500-1800: Astrology and the Popular Press.* Ithaca, NY: Cornell University Press.

Carmichael, Ann G. (1986). *Plague and the Poor in Renaissance Florence.* New York: Cambridge University Press.

Choulant, Johann Ludwig (1962). *History and Bibliography of Anatomical Illustration.* Trans. and annotated by Mortimer Frank, repr. with additional essays. New York: Hafner.

Cipolla, Carlo M. (1969). *Literacy and Development in the West.* Baltimore, MD: Penguin Books.

Cipolla, Carlo M. (1976). *Public Health and the Medical Profession in Renaissance Italy.* New York: Cambridge University Press.

Crosby, Alfred W. (1986). *Ecological Imperialism: The Biological Expansion of Europe, 900-1900.* New York: Cambridge University Press.

Culliton, Barbara J. (1976). News and Comment: Penicillin-Resistant Gonorrhea: New Strain Spreading Worldwide. *Science* 194: 1395–1397.

Cushing, Harvey (1962). *A Bio-Bibliography of Andreas Vesalius.* New York: Schuman.

Debus, Allen G. (1978). *Man and Nature in the Renaissance.* New York: Cambridge University Press.

Debus, Allen G. (1986). *Chemistry, Alchemy, and the New Philosophy, 1500-1700.* London: Variorum.

Debus, Allen G., ed. (1972). *Science, Medicine and Society in the Renaissance.* New York: Neale Watson Academic Publications. 2 volumes.

Doe, Janet (1937). *A Bibliography of the Works of Ambroise Paré.* Chicago: University of Chicago Press.

Eisenstein, Elizabeth (1983). *The Printing Revolution in Early Modern Europe.* Abridged. ed. New York: Cambridge University Press.

Elliott, David C., Baehr, George, Schaffer, Loren W., Usher, Glenn S., Lough, S. Allan (1941). An Evaluation of the Massive Dose Therapy of Early Syphilis. *JAMA* 117: 1160-1166.

Ewalt, J. R. and Ebaugh, F. G. (1941). Treatment of Dementia Paralytica: A Five-Year Comparative Study of Artificial Fever and Therapeutic Malaria in 232 Cases. *JAMA* 111: 2474-2477.

Fee, Elizabeth, and Fox, Daniel, eds. (1988). *AIDS. The Burdens of History.* Berkeley: University of California Press.

Fico, Marsilio (1989). *Three Books on Life.* A Critical Edition and Translation with Introduction and Notes by Carol V. Kaske and John R. Clark. Medieval & Renaissance Texts & Studies. Binghamton, NY: The Renaissance Society of America.

Fierz, Marcus (1983). *Girolamo Cardano (1501-1576): Physician, Natural Philosopher, Mathematician, Astrologer, Interpreter of Dreams.* Boston, MA: Berkhauser.

Fleck, Ludwik (1979). *Genesis and Development of a Scientific Fact.* Ed. by T. J. Trenn and R. K. Merton; trans. by F. Bradley and T. J. Trenn; Foreword by T. S. Kuhn. Chicago: University of Chicago Press.

Forty Years of Federal Experiments on Victims of Syphilis. Senate Hearings, July 26, 1972. *Congressional Record:* pp. S11854-11855.

Fracastoro, Girolamo (1984). *Fracastoro's "Syphilis".* Trans, intro. Geoffrey Eatough. Liverpool, England: Francis Cairns.

Goldwater, L. J. (1972). *Mercury, a History of Quicksilver.* Baltimore, MD: Fork.

Grendler, Paul F. (1989). *Schooling in Renaissance Italy. Literacy and Learning, 1300-1600.* Baltimore, MD: Johns Hopkins Press.

Grmek, Mirko (1990). *History of AIDS.* Princeton, NJ: Princeton University Press.

Hamby, W.B. (1960). *The Case Reports and Autopsy Records of Ambroise Paré.* Springfield, IL: Charles C. Thomas.

Hartmann, Franz (1973). *The Prophecies of Paracelsus.* New York: Rudolf Steiner Publications.

Hudson, Ellis Herndon (1965). Treponematosis in perspective. *Bulletin of the World Health Organization* 32: 735-748.

Imhof, Arthur E. (1985). From the Old Mortality Pattern to the New: Implications of a Radical Change from the Sixteenth to the Twentieth Century. *Bulletin of the History of Medicine* 59: 1-19.

Jones, James H. (1981). *Bad Blood: The Tuskegee Syphilis Experiment.* New York: The Free Press.

Keele, Kenneth D. (1983) *Leonardo da Vinci's Elements of the Science of Man.* New York: Academic Press.

Kerrigan, William, and Braden, Gordon (1989). *The Idea of the Renaissance.* Baltimore, MD: Johns Hopkins University Press.

Kluger, Matthew J., Ringler, Daniel H., and Anver, Miriam R. (1975). Fever and Survival. *Science* 188: 166-168.

Leifer, William, Chargin, Louis, and Hyman, Harold Thomas (1941). Massive Dose Arsenotherapy of Early Syphilis by Intravenous Drip Method. Recapitulation of the Data (1933-1941). *JAMA* 117: 1154-1160.

Lind, L. R. (1974). *Studies in Pre-Vesalian Anatomy: Biography, Translations, Documents.* Philadelphia, PA: American Philosophical Society.

Lind, L. R. and Asling, C. W., trans. (1969). *The Epitome of Andreas Vesalius.* Translated from the Latin, with introduction and anatomical notes. Cambridge, MA: MIT Press.

Lindeboom, G. A. (1975). *Andreas Vesalius and His Opus Magnum: A Biographical Sketch and an Introduction to the Fabrica.* Netherlands, Nieuwendijk: de Forel.

MacCurdy, Edward (1956). *The Notebooks of Leonardo da Vinci.* London: Jonathan Cape.

Maclean, Ian (1983). *The Renaissance Notion of Woman. A Study in the Fortunes of Scholasticism and Medical Science in European Intellectual Life.* New York: Cambridge University Press.

Malgaigne, J. F. (1965). *Surgery and Ambroise Paré.* Trans. W.B. Hamby. Norman, OK: University of Oklahoma Press.

Mathias, Andrew (1811). *The Mercurial Disease. An Inquiry into the History and Nature of the Disease Produced in the Human Constitution by the Use of Mercury: With Observations on Its Connexion with the Lues Venerea.* Philadelphia: Edward Parker.

McAuliffe, C. A., ed. (1977). *The Chemistry of Mercury.* Toronto: Macmillan.

McKeown, Thomas (1979). *The Role of Medicine. Dream, Mirage, or Nemesis?* Princeton, NJ: Princeton University Press.

McKnight, Stephen A. (1989). *Sacralizing the Secular: The Renaissance Origins of Modernity.* Baton Rouge, LA: Louisiana State University Press.

McVaugh, Michael, and Siraisi, Nancy G., eds. (1990). *Renaissance Medical Learning. Evolution of a Tradition. Osiris,* 2nd series, volume 6.

O'Malley, C. D. (1964). *Andreas Vesalius of Brussels, 1514-1564.* Berkeley: University of California Press.

O'Malley, C. D. (1965). *English Medical Humanists: Thomas Linacre and John Caius.* Lawrence, KS: University Kansas Press.

O'Malley, C. D. and Saunders, J. B. de C. M., eds. (1952). *Leonardo da Vinci on the Human Body.* New York: Schuman.

Pagel, Walter (1958). *Paracelsus: An Introduction to Philosophical Medicine in the Era of the Renaissance.* Basel: S. Karger.

Pagel, Walter (1984). *The Smiting Spleen. Paracelsianism in Storm and Stress.* Basel: Karger.

Paracelsus (1941). *Four Treatises of Theophrastus von Hohenheim Called Paracelsus.* Baltimore, MD: Johns Hopkins Press.

Paracelsus (1951). *Paracelsus: Selected Writings.* Intro. by J. Jacobi; Trans. by N. Guterman. New York: Pantheon Books.

Parascandola, John (1981). The Theoretical Basis of Paul Ehrlich's Chemotherapy. *JHMAS* 36: 19–43.

Paré, Ambroise (1969). *Ten Books of Surgery.* Trans. by R. W. Linker and N. Womack. Athens, GA: University of Georgia Press.

Paré, Ambroise (1982). *Ambroise Paré on Monsters and Marvels.* Trans., Intro., and Notes by Janis L. Pallister. Chicago: University of Chicago Press.

Park, Katherine (1985). *Doctors and Medicine in Early Renaissance Florence.* Princeton, NJ: Princeton University Press.

Plesset, Isabel (1980). *Noguchi and His Patrons.* Rutherford, NJ: Fairleigh Dickinson University Press.

Quétel, Claude (1990). *The History of Syphilis.* Trans. J. Braddock and Brian Pike. Baltimore, MD: Johns Hopkins University Press.

Ramazzini, Bernardini (1940). *De morbis artificum diatriba. Diseases of Workers.* The Latin Text of 1713. Trans. and notes by Wilmer Cave Wright. Chicago: University of Chicago Press.

Richardson, Ruth (1987). *Death, Dissection and the Destitute.* London, England: Routledge and Kegan Paul.

Rosebury, T. (1973). *Microbes and Morals: The Strange Story of Venereal Disease.* New York: Ballantine Books.

Saunders, J. B. de C. M., and O'Malley, Charles D. (1947) *Andreas Vesalius Bruxellensis: The Bloodletting Letter of 1539.* New York: Henry Schuman.

Shumaker, Wayne (1972). *The Occult Sciences in the Renaissance.* Berkeley, CA: University of California Press.

Siraisi, Nancy G. (1987). *Avicenna in Renaissance Italy. The Canon and Medical Teaching in Italian Universities.* Princeton, NJ: Princeton University Press.

Temkin, Owsei (1977). Therapeutic Trends and the Treatment of Syphilis Before 1900. In *The Double Face of Janus.* Baltimore, MD: Johns Hopkins University Press.

Vesalius, Andreas (1949). *The Epitome of Andreas Vesalius.* Translated from the Latin, with introduction and anatomical notes by L. R. Lind and C. W. Asling. Cambridge, MA: MIT Press.

Vickers, Brian, ed. (1984). *Occult and Scientific Mentalities in the Renaissance.* Cambridge, England: Cambridge University Press.

Wear, Andrew, French, Roger, K., and Lonie, I., eds. (1985). *The Medical Renaissance of the Sixteenth Century*. New York: Cambridge University Press.

Webster, Charles (1975). *The Great Instauration: Science, Medicine and Reform, 1626-1660.* New York: Holmes & Meier.

Webster, Charles, ed. (1979). *Health, Medicine, and Mortality in the Sixteenth Century*. New York: Cambridge University Press.

Willcox, R. R., and Guthe, T. (1966). *Treponema Pallidum: A Bibliographical Review of the Morphology, Culture, and Survival of T. Pallidum and Associated Organisms*. Geneva: World Health Organization.

Wrigley, E. A. and Schofield, R. S. (1981). *The Population History of England 1541-1871*. Cambridge, MA: Harvard University Press.

8

THE SCIENTIFIC REVOLUTION AND THE CIRCULATION OF THE BLOOD

The Scientific Revolution is generally thought of as the great transformation of the physical sciences that occurred during the sixteenth and seventeenth centuries, and is primarily associated with Nicolaus Copernicus (1473-1543), Galileo Galilei (1564-1642), and Isaac Newton (1642-1727). We can, however, by shifting the focus of concern from physics and astronomy to medicine and physiology, search for new ways of understanding and integrating science and medicine into the context of political, religious, and social change. In the sixteenth century, as we have seen, Vesalius and Paracelsus challenged ancient ideas about the nature of the microcosm, the little world of the human body. In the seventeenth century, William Harvey's discovery of the circulation of the blood transformed ways of thinking about the meaning of the heartbeat, pulse, and movement of the blood. Revolutionary insights into the microcosm reinforced the shock waves created when the earth was removed from its place at the center of the universe by Copernicus, Kepler, and Galileo. While Harvey's work can be seen as part of the scientific revolution, that is, primarily medical research as *science*, it also reflects continuing and consuming problems of medical practice and medical philosophy, such as the uses of venesection, the distribution and nature of the spirits, and the relationship between the soul and the body.

BLOOD IN MYTH AND MEDICINE

Blood has always conjured up mysterious associations far removed from the physiological role of this liquid tissue. Blood has been used in religious rituals, fertility rites, charms, and medicines, and no horror film would be complete without buckets of blood. Strength, courage, and youthful vigor were thought to reside in the blood. Even Renaissance physicians and theologians believed in the medicinal power of youthful blood. The physicians of Pope Innocent VIII are said to have prescribed human blood as a means of reviving the dying Pope. How the blood was to be administered is unclear, but the results were predictable. The three young donors died, the Pope died, and the physicians vanished.

With philosophers, physicians, and ordinary people sharing a belief in the power of blood, the nearly universal enthusiasm for therapeutic bloodletting seems paradoxical to the twentieth-century mind. For hundreds of years, Galenic theory and medical practice demanded and rationalized therapeutic and prophylactic bloodletting as a means of removing corrupt humors from the body. According to the Roman encyclopedist Pliny the Elder (23-79), even wild animals practiced bloodletting. Phlebotomists attacked the sick with arrows, knives, lancets, cupping vessels, and leeches. Indeed, until rather recent times, the surgeon was more commonly employed in spilling blood with leech and lancet than staunching its flow.

DISCOVERY OF THE MINOR OR PULMONARY CIRCULATION

Although Renaissance anatomists rejected many Galenic fallacies concerning the *structure* of the human body, their concepts of *function* had undergone little change. Ancient dogmas served as a defensive perimeter for physicians confronting professional, political, intellectual, and theological minefields. Even Vesalius avoided a direct attack on Galenic physiology and was rather vague about the whole

Discovery of the minor and major circulation

question of the distribution of the blood and spirits. When scientific inquiry led to the brink of heresy, Vesalius found it expedient to cite the ancients and marvel at the ingenuity of the Creator. Nevertheless, despite the delicate issue of the relationship between the movement of the blood and the distribution of the spirits, other sixteenth century scientists were able to challenge the Galenic shortcut between the right side and the left side of the heart.

Michael Servetus (1511–1553), the first European to describe the pulmonary circulation, was a man who spent his whole life struggling against the dogmatism and intolerance that permeated the Renaissance world. If any man died twice for his beliefs it was Servetus. His attacks on orthodoxy were so broad and blatant that he was burned in effigy by the Catholics and in the flesh by the Protestants. While challenging religious dogma, Servetus proved that contemporary anatomical information was sufficient to allow a heretic to elucidate the pathway taken by the blood in the minor, or pulmonary circulation.

Servetus left his native Spain to study law, but like Paracelsus he soon joined the ranks of the wandering geniuses and mavericks destined to spend their lives disturbing the universe. After his first major treatise, *On the Errors of the Trinity* (1531), was published, both Catholic and Protestant theologians agreed that the author was a heretic of the worst sort. Finding it necessary to go underground, Servetus established a new identity as "Michael Villanovanus." Under this name, he attended the University of Paris before moving to Lyons where he published a new edition of the *Geographia* of the second century astronomer and geographer Ptolemy of Alexandria. Even when editing a classic of such antiquity Servetus could not resist the opportunity to express dangerous opinions. While describing France, Servetus referred to the ceremony of the Royal Touch in which the king miraculously cured victims of scrofula. "I myself have seen the king touch many attacked by this ailment," Servetus wrote, "but I have never seen any cured."

Returning to the University of Paris to study medicine, Servetus supported himself by lecturing on mathematics, geography, and astronomy. When he stepped over the line that Christian doctrine had drawn between acceptable areas of astrology and the forbidden zone of judicial astrology (essentially fortune-telling), he was threatened with excommunication. Attacks on judicial astrology can be traced back to the time of St. Augustine (354–430), but the theological opposition and philosophical skepticism seem to have intensified by the end of the fifteenth century. Although his first impulse was to defend his actions, his case was hopeless and Servetus returned to his underground life. The separation between medicine and astrology among learned circles in France has been attributed the the attack of the medical faculty of Paris on an astrologer named Villanovanus in 1537.

As if looking for more trouble, Servetus entered into a correspondence with John Calvin (1509–1564), the French Protestant reformer who founded a relgious system based on the doctrines of predestination and salvation solely by God's grace. In addition to criticizing Calvin's *Institutiones*, Servetus sent him an advance copy of

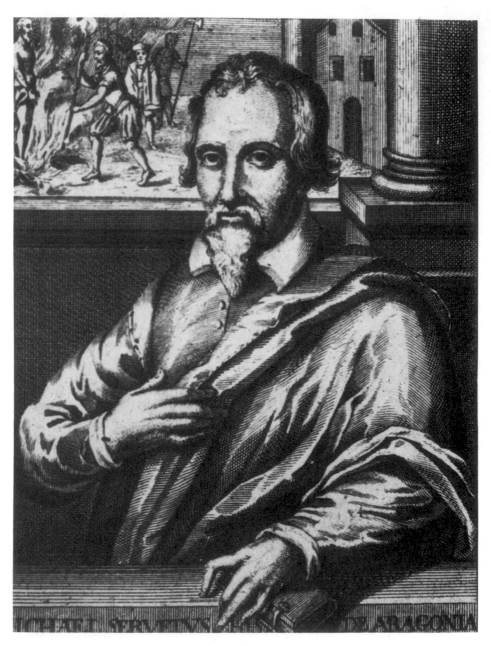

Michael Servetus

his radical treatise, *On the Restitution of Christianity* (1553). Calvin responded by sending pages torn from the *Restitution* to the Catholic Inquisition with the information that Servetus had printed a book full of scandalous blasphemies. Servetus was arrested and imprisoned, but managed to escape before he was tried, convicted, and burned in effigy. Four months later, Servetus surfaced in Calvin's Geneva, where he was arrested and condemned to burn "without mercy." Attempts to mitigate the sentence to burning "with mercy" (strangulation before immolation) were unsuccessful. Almost all the newly printed copies of The *Restitution* were added to the fire. In 1903 the Calvinist congregation of Geneva expressed regrets and erected a monument to the martyred heretic. Moreover, a review of his case revealed that the death sentence had been illegal, because the proper penalty should have been banishment.

Given the fact that Servetus' account of the pulmonary circulation is buried within the 700-page *Restitution*, it is clear that his inspiration and motives were primarily religious, not medical or scientific. According to Servetus, to understand the relationship between God and humanity, and to know the Holy Spirit, one must understand the spirit within human beings through knowledge of the human body, especially the blood, for as stated in Leviticus "the life of the flesh is in the blood." Prevailing knowledge of what we might call the plumbing arrangements of the cardiovascular system could be traced to Galen, but Servetus argued that the fact that more blood was sent to the lungs than was necessary for their own nourishment indicated that passage of blood through pores in the septum was not the major path by which blood entered the left side of the heart. Servetus contended that the change in the color of the blood indicated that aeration took place in the lungs rather than in the left ventricle. Then, charged with the vital spirit formed by the mixing of air and blood in the lungs, bright red blood was sent to the left ventricle. Servetus did not go on to consider the possibility of a systemic blood circulation; he was satisfied that he had reconciled physiology with his theological convictions concerning the unity of the spirit.

What effect did Servetus have on sixteenth-century science? In retrospect, Servetus seems a heroic figure, but if his contemporaries knew of his work they were unlikely to admit to being in sympathy with the ill-fated heretic. Moreover, only three copies of the *The Restitution* are known to have survived the flames. It is unlikely that Servetus influenced anatomists any more than Ibn an-Nafis, who had described the pulmonary transit in the thirteenth century. However, there is always uncertainty about the actual diffusion of ideas and information—especially that which might be considered heretical, dangerous, and subversive—as opposed to the survival of documentary evidence. Whatever influence Servetus did or did not have on progress in physiology, his career remains a fascinating revelation of the dark underside of the Renaissance and religious intolerance. His *Restitution* proves that in the sixteenth century a man with rather limited training in medicine and anatomy could understand the pulmonary circulation.

While in no way as colorful a figure as Servetus, Realdo Colombo (Realdus Columbus; ca. 1510–1559) was a more influential scientist and teacher. Colombo, the son of an apothecary, served as apprentice to Giovanni Antonio Lonigo, an eminent Venetian surgeon, for 7 years before he began his studies of medicine, surgery, and anatomy at the University of Padua. In 1538, Colombo was noted in the records of the University as an outstanding student of surgery. When Vesalius, who had served as professor of anatomy and surgery since 1537, left the University in 1542 to supervise the publication of the *Fabrica*, Colombo was appointed as his replacement. Although Colombo had attended Vesalius' course of dissections, he always referred to Lonigo as his most important mentor. Colombo was appointed to the professorship on a permanent basis in 1544 after the resignation of Vesalius. Displaying little reverence for his predecessor, Colombo became one of the most vociferous critics of the *Fabrica* and the former colleagues became bitter enemies. From the time of his public demonstrations of 1543 to his death, Colombo drew attention to errors in the work of Vesalius and boasted of his own skills in surgery, autopsy, dissection, and vivisection. However, Colombo's plans to create an illustrated anatomical treatise that would supercede the *Fabrica* were thwarted when it became clear that Michelangelo, with whom Colombo expected to collaborate, would be unable to work on the project because of advancing age and infirmity. In 1545, Colombo left Padua to take a professorship at Pisa. Three years later, he settled permanently in Rome. Vesalius described Colombo as a scoundrel and an ignoramus. Later, the anatomist Gabriele Fallopio accused Colombo of plagiarizing discoveries made by himself and other anatomist.

Colombo may have been demonstrating the pulmonary circulation as early as 1545, but his anatomical treatise, *De re anatomica*, was not published until 1559. Calling upon the reader to confirm his observations by dissection and vivisection, Colombo boasted that he alone had discovered the way in which the lungs serve in the preparation and generation of the vital spirits. Air was received by the lungs where it mixed with blood brought in by the pulmonary artery from the right ventricle of the heart. Blood and air were taken up by the branches of the pulmonary vein and carried to the left ventricle of the heart to be distributed to all parts of the body. Although Ibn an-Nafis and Michael Servetus had also described the pulmonary circulation, Colombo apparently had no knowledge of their work and made the discovery through his own dissections and vivisection experiments. Moreover, because Colombo's formal training and scholarship was inferior to that of Vesalius he apparently was less familiar with certain aspects of Galen's writings on the lungs, heart, and blood. Despite his professions of originality and daring, Colombo was rather conservative in his discussion of the functions of the heart, blood, and respiration. In any case, Galenic dogma was still too firmly entrenched for relatively modest inconsistencies and corrections to cause a significant breach in its defenses.

The difficulty of establishing the relationship between a scientific discovery, or a specific observation, and the conversion of physicians and scientists to a new theory is very well illustrated in the case of Andrea Cesalpino (1519–1603; Andreas Cesalpinus). Celebrated as the discoverer of both the minor and major circulation by certain admirers, Cesalpino, Professor of Medicine and Botany at the University of Pisa, was a learned man who combined a great reverence for Aristotle with an appreciation of Renaissance innovations. His medical views were based on the Aristotelian philosophical framework established in his *Quaestionum peripateticarum* (1571). While he also wrote several books on practical medicine, his major work was in botany.

Certainly, Cesalpino had a gift for choosing words like *circulation* and *capillary vessels* that ring with remarkable prescience in the ears of posterity, at least in translation. His descriptions of the valves of the heart, the blood vessels that link the heart and the lungs, and the pulmonary circulation were admirable. However, Cesalpino also spoke of the heart as the fountain from which four great veins irrigated the body "like the four rivers that flow out from Paradise." While his contemporaries generally ignored Cesalpino's ideas about the heart, modern champions of Cesalpino have devoted much effort to finding his references to the circulation and arranging these gems into patterns that escaped the notice of less devoted readers. Like Servetus, Cesalpino is worth studying as a reflection of the range of ideas available to anatomists in the sixteenth century. Cesalpino was preoccupied with Aristotelian ideas about the primacy of the heart and the movement of innate heat. As Aristotle's champion, Cesalpino attacked Galenic concepts with philosophic arguments and anatomical evidence. For this work, Cesalpino deserves a place in the history of physiology, but not the place properly occupied by William Harvey.

GIROLAMO FABRICI AND THE VENOUS VALVES

Because William Harvey suggested that the demonstration of the venous valves by Girolamo Fabrici (Hieronymus Fabricius; ca. 1533–1619), his teacher at the University of Padua, had been a major factor in making him think the blood might travel in a circle, the discovery of these structures occupies an important place in the story of the circulation. Many other anatomists described the venous valves at about the same time, but we shall examine only the work of the man who directly inspired Harvey.

After earning his doctorate at the University of Padua, Fabrici established a lucrative private practice and gave lessons in anatomy. Eventually he replaced Gabriele Fallopio (1523–1562) as professor of surgery and anatomy. Teaching anatomy was a difficult and unpleasant proposition and Fabrici, like Fallopio, seems to have evaded this responsibility whenever possible. Sometimes he disappeared before completing the course, angering students who had come to Padua to learn from the great anatomist. Fabrici saw teaching as drudgery which conflicted with his research and private practice. Students complained that he was obviously bored and indifferent when teaching. Presumably, they thought it more natural for the teacher to be enthusiastic and the students to be bored and indifferent.

On the Valves of the Veins was not published until 1603, but Fabrici noted that he had been studying the structure, distribution, and function of the venous valves since 1574. Fabrici assumed that nature had formed the valves to retard the flow of blood from the heart to the periphery so that all parts of the body could obtain their fair share of nutrients. Arteries did not need valves because the continuous pulsations of their thick walls prevented distention, swelling, and pooling. If a ligature is tied around the arm of a living person with moderate tightness as in bleeding, little knots are seen along the course of the veins. These swellings correspond to the location of the valves as revealed by dissection. Intrigued by Fabrici's demonstrations of the venous valves, Harvey repeated these experiments and again observed that when the ligature was in place it was not possible to push blood past the valves. Fabrici believed that the little structures in the veins acted like the floodgates of a millpond which regulate volume, rather than valves which regulated direction. Unlike Fabrici, Harvey realized that the venous blood was directed towards the heart, not to the periphery.

WILLIAM HARVEY

William Harvey (1578–1657) was the eldest of seven sons born to Thomas Harvey, and the only member of this family of merchants and landowners to become a physician. After receiving the Bachelor of Arts from Caius College, Cambridge, in 1597, Harvey followed the footsteps of the great English humanist-scholars to Padua. In 1602, Harvey returned to England and established a successful medical practice. His marriage to Elizabeth Browne, the daughter of Lancelot Browne, physician to Queen Elizabeth I and James I, gave him access to the highest court and professional circles. In rapid succession, Harvey was elected Fellow of the College of Physicians (1607), appointed Physician to St. Bartholomew's Hospital (1609), Lumleian Lecturer for the College of Physicians (1615–1656), and physician extraordinary to James I (1618). Harvey retained the latter position when Charles I became king in 1625 and was promoted to physician in ordinary in 1631 and senior physician in ordinary in 1639. (As strange as it may seem, *ordinary* in the court medical hierarchy was more prestigious than *extraordinary*.) As one of the king's physicians, Harvey was charged with some peculiar assignments, such as the diagnosis of witchcraft, an area of considerable interest to James I. Harvey's duties also entailed extensive travels with King Charles and service during the Civil War. It was at the request of the King that Harvey performed one of his most unusual autopsies, the post-mortem on Thomas Parr who had claimed to be the oldest man in England. Brought to London in 1635, Old Parr was presented to Charles I, and exhibited at the Queen's Head Tavern. Life in London undermined Parr's good health and he soon died, supposedly 152 years old. From the autopsy results, Harvey concluded that pleuropneumonia was the cause of death, but others thought it might have been old age.

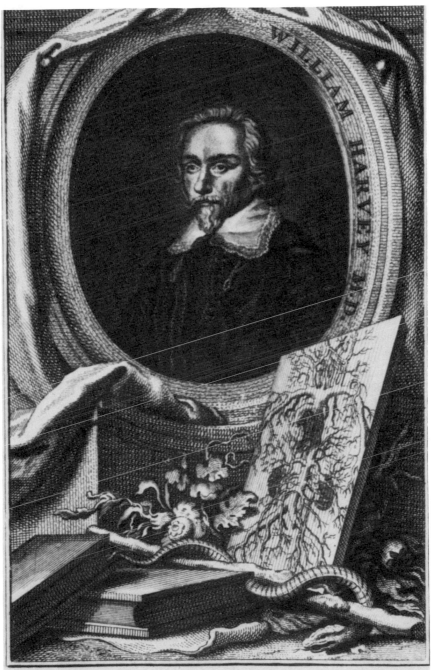

For J. Hinton at the King's Arms in Newgate Street

William Harvey

Harvey may have inspired a revolutionary approach to experimental biology and human physiology, but professionally and socially he was a man of a rather conservative disposition. Throughout the battles between the followers of King Charles I and the Parliamentary forces under Oliver Cromwell (1599–1658), Harvey remained loyal to his king. After the Royalists were defeated and King Charles was publicly beheaded in 1649, Harvey retired to live with his brothers in the countryside near London. Tormented by gout and deteriorating health, he apparently became addicted to opium and may have attempted suicide more than once.

Harvey seems to have arrived at an understanding of the motion of the heart and blood before he had assembled all his final proofs and well before 1628 when *An Anatomical Treatise on the Motion of the Heart and Blood in Animals* (usually referred to as *De motu cordis*) was published. Perhaps Harvey delayed publication because, as he confessed in his book, his views on the motions of the blood were so novel and unprecedented that he was afraid of the probable repercussions and expected that he might "have mankind at large for my enemies."

Considering that Harvey, like all medical students for hundreds of years, had been force-fed a steady diet of Galenism, and that conformity was generally the ticket to success and advancement within an extremely conservative profession, how was it possible for Harvey to free himself from the past? Rather than finding it remarkable that generations of physicians had meekly accepted Galenism, we should be moved to wonder how Harvey was able to realize that the grand and elegant doctrines he had been taught about the motion and function of the heart and blood were wrong. When reading *De motu cordis*, one is struck most by the thought that *in principle*, Harvey's experiments and observations could have been performed hundreds of years before. During the seventeenth century new instruments, such as the telescope and microscope, literally opened up new worlds to science and imagination, but Harvey's work was performed without the aid of the microscope.

Like Aristotle, whom he greatly admired, Harvey asked seemingly simple but truly profound questions in the search for final causes. In thinking about the function of the heart and the blood vessels, he moved closer to Aristotle's idea that the heart is the most important organ in the body while he revealed the errors in Galen's scheme. Harvey wanted to know why the two structurally similar ventricles of the right and left heart should have such different functions as the control of the flow of blood and of the vital spirits. Why should the artery-like vein nourish only the lungs, while the vein-like artery had to nourish the whole body? Why should the lungs appear to need so much nourishment for themselves? Why did the right ventricle have to move in addition to the movement of the lungs? If there were two distinct kinds of blood—nutritive blood from the liver distributed by the veins and blood from the heart for the distribution of vital spirits by the arteries—why were the two kinds of blood so similar? Such questions were not unlike those Harvey's contemporaries were prepared to ask and debate.

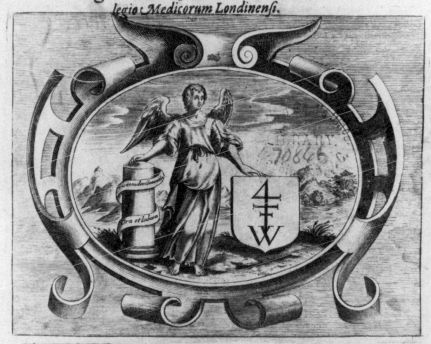

De motu cordis (courtesy of the National Library of Medicine)

Using arguments based on dissection, vivisection, and the works of Aristotle and Galen, Harvey proved that in the adult all the blood must go through the lungs to get from the right side to the left side of the heart. He proved that the heart is muscular and that its important movement is the contraction, rather than the dilation. But his most radical idea was that it was the beat of the heart that produced a continuous circular motion of the blood.

In warm-blooded animals, the systole (contraction) and diastole (expansion) of the heart are so rapid and complex that Harvey at first feared that the motion of the heart could be understood only by God. But he solved this problem by using animals with simpler cardiovascular systems and a slower heartbeat, such as snakes, snails, frogs, and fish. With cold-blooded animals or dogs bled almost to death, Harvey was able to create model systems in a kind of slow motion. When observations and experiments were collated, it was apparent that the motion of the heart was like that of a piece of machinery in which all parts seemed to move simultaneously, until one understood the individual parts.

Harvey also posed a question of child-like simplicity that modern readers find most compelling and that, if overemphasized, tends to take Harvey out of his seventeenth-century context and makes him appear more modern in outlook and approach than

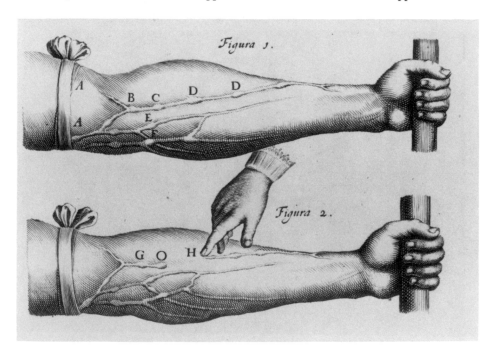

William Harvey's demonstration of the circulation of the blood

is really appropriate. Harvey asked himself: How much blood is sent into the body with each beat of the heart? Even the most cursory calculation proves that the amount of blood pumped out of the heart per hour exceeds the weight of the entire organism. If the heart pumps out 2 ounces of blood with each beat and beats 72 times per minute, 8640 ounces ($2 \times 72 \times 60$), or 540 pounds of blood are expelled per hour. Whether calculated for humans, sheep, dogs, or cattle, the amount of blood pumped out of the heart in an hour always exceeds the quantity of blood in the whole animal, as demonstrated by exsanguination. Indeed, the reader is advised to go to a butcher shop and watch an experienced butcher exsanguinate an ox; by opening an artery in a live animal, the butcher can rapidly remove all the blood.

It is all too easy to assume that these arguments should have provided an immediate death blow to the Galenic system. However, the kind of evidence that appears most compelling and unequivocal today did not necessarily appeal to Harvey's contemporaries. Arguing from experimental and quantitative data in physiology was remarkable in an era when even physicists were more likely to speculate than to weigh and measure. Moreover, opponents of Harvey's work presented what seemed to be quite logical alternatives, at least in light of accepted Galenic theory. For example, some critics argued that the heart attracted only a small amount of blood from the liver where sanguification (the formation of blood) occurred. This blood foamed and expanded to such a great extent under the influence of the heat of the heart that the heart and arteries appeared to be full. Furthermore, multiplying the putative volume of blood discharged by the heart by the number of heartbeats per minute was meaningless, because it was not necessary to assume that blood was driven from the heart with each heartbeat.

Having solved the mechanical problem of the motion of the heart and blood and demonstrated the true function of the venous valves, Harvey generally avoided arguments about the generation and distribution of the various kinds of spirits. Harvey had demonstrated the errors in Galen's system and had discovered essentially all that could be known about the structure and function of the cardiovascular system without the use of the microscope. Thus, one of the major gaps in Harvey's work was his inability to identify the structures joining the arterial and the venous system. He was forced to close this gap with hypothetical "anastomoses" or "pores in the flesh." As scientists like Marcello Malpighi (1628–1694) extended the limits of anatomical study with the microscope, the capillary network completed the cardiovascular system.

Also unfinished at the time of Harvey's death was a book he planned to publish about his ideas on disease. The manuscript for this book may have been among those destroyed during the Civil War. Because of this loss, Harvey's concept of how knowledge of the circulation might solve many questions about disease and medical practice must be constructed by piecing together comments made in his surviving works. *De motu cordis* promised that the new understanding of the circulation would solve many mysteries in medicine, pathology, and therapeutics. In later works Harvey alluded to his "Medical Observations," but no such book was ever published.

Replacing the Galenic system that had so thoroughly, if incorrectly, explained such mysterious vital phenomena as the *purpose* of the heart, lungs, liver, veins, arteries, and spirits was completely beyond Harvey's technical and theoretical methods and goals. For seventeenth century physicians, the new theory of the circulation raised more questions than it answered. If Harvey was correct, how could all the vital phenomena that Galenism had dealt with so long and so well be explained? For example, if the blood was not consumed by the tissues, how did they secure their nourishment? If the blood was not continuously formed from food by the liver, how was it synthesized? If the blood moved in a closed, continuous circle, what was the purpose of the arterial and venous systems and how did the body accomplish the generation and distribution of the vital spirit and the innate heat? If the venous blood did not originate in the liver, which played such a central role in the Galenic system, what was the function of this organ? If vital spirit was not produced by the mixture of air and blood either in the lungs or in the left ventricle of the heart, what was the function of respiration? What was the difference between arterial and venous blood if the whole mass of the blood was constantly recirculated? If Galen was incorrect about the anatomy and physiology of the human body, what principles would guide medical practice?

Like almost all fundamental discoveries, Harvey's work provoked an avalanche of new questions and a storm of controversy. Many critics were unable or unwilling to understand the implications of Harvey's work; others found it impossible to give up the old Galenic system that had provided all encompassing rationalizations for health and disease, diagnosis and therapeutics. How could medicine be saved if Galen was sacrificed for the sake of Harvey's radical theory? The theory of the continuous circulation raised many disturbing questions for which Harvey provided no answers. Such questions stimulated Harvey's admirers to embark on new experimental ventures, while critics denounced his theory as useless, false, impossible, absurd, paradoxical, and harmful. For some scholars, revolutionary ideas about the movement of the blood, the respiration, and the distribution of spirits were so painful that they tried to force the new ideas backwards into ancient Greek works by remarkably convoluted arguments.

Well aware of the revolutionary nature of his work, Harvey predicted that no one under 40 would understand it. His work constituted a revolution in science worthy of comparison to that launched by Sir Isaac Newton. Although illness, age, and loss of precious materials and manuscripts during the Civil War prevented Harvey from accomplishing all his goals, he did live to see his followers establish a new experimental physiology inspired by his ideas and methods. The questions raised by Harvey's work provided the "Oxford physiologists"—men such as Robert Boyle, Robert Hooke, Richard Lower, John Mayow, and Christopher Wren—with a new research program for attaining a better understanding of the workings of the human body.

HARVEY'S PARADOXICAL INFLUENCE: THERAPY BY LEECH AND LANCET

Harvey's work opened up new fields of research and ignited violent controversies, but it certainly did not threaten the livelihood of phlebotomists. While provoking new arguments about the selection of appropriate sites for venesection, the discovery of the circulation seemed to stimulate interest in bloodletting and other forms of depletion therapy. Not even Harvey seemed to worry about the compatibility, or incompatibility, of venesection with the concept of a closed, continuous circulation. Indeed, Harvey defended venesection as a major therapeutic tool for the relief of diseases caused by *plethora*. Long after accepting Harvey's theory, physicians praised the health-promoting virtues of bloodletting with as much (if not more) enthusiasm as Galen.

In addition to prescribing the amount of blood to be taken, the physician had to select the optimum site for bleeding. Long-standing arguments about site selection became ever more creative as knowledge of the circulatory system increased. Many physicians insisted on using distant sites on the side opposite the lesion. Others chose a site close to the source of corruption in order to remove putrid blood and attract good blood for repair of the diseased area. Proper site selection was supposed to determine whether the primary effect of bloodletting would be evacuation (removal of blood), derivation (acceleration of the blood column upstream of the wound), or revulsion (acceleration of the blood column downstream of the wound). Debates about the relative effects of revulsion and derivation are at the heart of François Quesnay's physiocratic system, the first so-called scientific approach to economics. (The term physiocracy refers to the idea that society should allow natural economic laws to prevail.) The debate between Quesnay, Professor of Surgery and physician to Louis XV, and the physician Jean Baptiste Silva began with conflicting ideas about medical issues involved in bloodletting and culminated in rationalizations of social and economic theories.

Bleeding was recommended in the treatment of inflammation, fevers, a multitude of disease states, and hemorrhage. Patients too weak for the lancet were candidates for milder methods, such as cupping and leeching. Well into the nineteenth century, no apothecary shop could be considered complete without a jar of live leeches, ready to do battle with afflictions as varied as epilepsy, hemorrhoids, obesity, tuberculosis, and headaches (for very stubborn headaches leeches were applied inside the nostrils). Enthusiasm for leeching reached its peak during the first half of the nineteenth century. By this time, leeches had to be imported because the medicinal leech, *Hirudo medicinalis*, had been hunted almost to extinction by about 1800 throughout Western

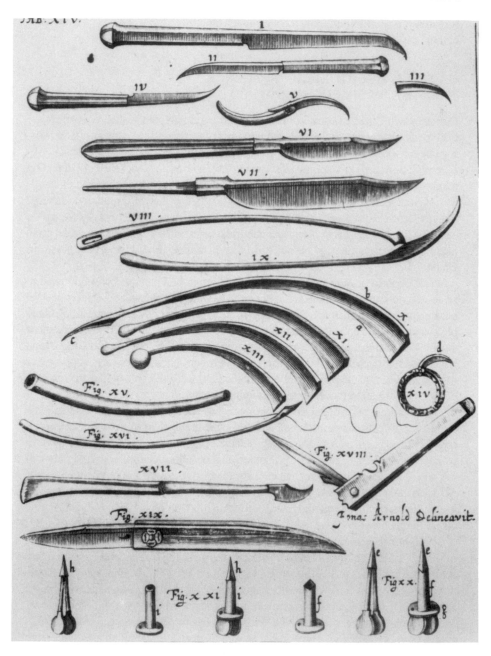

Bloodletting instruments as depicted in a 1666 text by Johann Schultes (1595–1645)

Europe. François Joseph Victor Broussais (1772–1838), an influential French physician, was the undisputed champion of medicinal leeching. Broussais believed that almost all diseases were caused by an inflammation of the digestive tract which could be relieved by leeching. Perhaps the most bizarre use of leeches was the case of a young woman who attempted to commit suicide with the aid of 50 leeches.

Leeches make their living by sucking blood and will generally attach themselves to almost any available animal, be it fish, frog, or human. On the positive side, leeches are excellent fish bait and they probably control the snail population in lakes and ponds. Moreover, unlike snails (the vector of schistosomiasis, or snail fever), leeches do not play a significant role as intermediate hosts of human parasites. The leech has become a favorite experimental animal among neurobiologists, who consider its ganglion a thing of beauty. In comparison to many other medical procedures, leeching was at least essentially painless. The amount of blood taken was controlled by prescribing the appropriate number of leeches. It should be noted that plastic and reconstructive surgeons in the 1980s rediscovered the usefulness of leeching; the anticoagulant action of leech saliva improves local blood flow and thus aids healing. Indeed, the success of leech therapy created a new era of leechmania as scientists in 1990 gathered together to present papers on the Biomedical Horizons of the Leech. Researchers reported that leeches produce a remarkable array of enzymes, anticoagulants, antibiotics, and anesthetics. Moreover, patients, especially children, become fascinated by these living medical instruments. In the not too distant future, the best of the leech proteins will probably appear as pure and very expensive drugs, synthesized by the powerful new techniques of molecular biology and patented by innovative pharmaceutical companies.

For hundreds of years after the death of Galen, physicians warned their patients about the dangers posed by a plethora of blood. If a plethora of blood caused disease, venesection was the obvious remedy; thus, spontaneous hemorrhages and venesection were as natural and helpful to the maintenance of life as the menstrual purgation was in healthy women. Bleeding was a perfectly rational means of treatment within this theoretical framework. To explain the persistence of bloodletting, physicians have tried to find modern explanations for the success stories of their predecessors. For example, in patients with congestive heart failure, bleeding might provide some relief because *hypervolemia* (an excess quantity of blood) is a component of this condition. But well into the nineteenth century many physicians believed that a ''useless abundance of blood'' was a principal cause of all disease.

Vigorous therapeutics, including copious bleeding and massive doses of drugs, formed the basis of the ''heroic'' school of American medicine, best exemplified by the death of George Washington in 1799. Under the supervision of three eminent physicians, Washington was bled, purged, and blistered until he died, about 48 hours after complaining of a sore throat. Across the Atlantic, the eminent Edinburgh surgeon John Brown (1810–1882) treated his own sore throat by applying six leeches and a mustard plaster to his neck, and 12 leeches behind the ear and, for good measure, removing 16 ounces of blood by venesection.

Questioning the validity of bloodletting required a large dose of skepticism and courage. Jan Baptista van Helmont (1579–1644), physician and chemical philosopher, was one of the rare individuals who dared to protest against the "bloody Moloch" presiding over medicine. van Helmont's assault on bloodletting as a dangerous waste of the patient's vital strength was one of the most controversial ideas to confront seventeenth-century doctors. Not only did van Helmont reject bloodletting as a medical treatment, he denied the doctrine that plethora was the cause of disease. In answer to attacks on his position launched by orthodox physicians, van Helmont proposed putting the question to a clinical test. This suggestion for a clinical trial involving large numbers of matched, but randomly selected patients may be the real measure of his originality. To demonstrate that bloodletting was *not* beneficial, van Helmont suggested taking 200 to 500 poor people and dividing them into two groups by casting lots. He would cure his allotment of patients without phlebotomy, while his critics treated the other half with as much bloodletting as they thought appropriate. The number of funerals in each group would be the measure of success or failure.

Unfortunately, this kind of test of phlebotomy was not carried out until the nineteenth century when the French physician Pierre Charles Alexandre Louis (1787–1872) used his numerical system—the collection of facts from studies of large numbers of hospitalized patients—to evaluate therapeutic methods. Even Louis's statistical studies of the efficacy of venesection failed to cause the typical physician to change his methods. This was especially true of the American students who admired Louis's research, but not his therapeutics. Critics of the numerical system charged Louis's followers with excessive zeal in the art of diagnosis, and negligence in healing the sick. Many doctors believed that Louis's attempt to evaluate the efficacy of bloodletting was a rash, reckless rejection of the wisdom of the ages. Even admirers of the numerical system were reluctant to modify their therapeutic habits and were skeptical of applying facts obtained in Parisian hospitals to other environments. Louis's studies indicated that bloodletting did not affect the course of pneumonia, a condition in which venesection was thought to be particularly beneficial. Some physicians argued that Louis's data actually proved that venesection was ineffective when performed too conservatively; this inspired tests of multiple bleedings in rapid succession in the treatment of endocarditis, polyarthritis, pneumonia, typhoid fever, and other diseases. Anecdotal evidence of patient survival, not statistical data, was taken as proof of efficacy.

Unconvinced by skeptics or statistics, most physicians continued to believe that bleeding was one of the most powerful therapeutic methods in their time-honored system. Only a learned physician could judge whether to bleed from veins or arteries, by leech, lancet, or cupping. Advocates of bloodletting argued that more patients were lost through timidity than through the loss of blood. Two hundred years after Harvey discovered the circulation of the blood, medical authorities were still instructing their students to treat hemorrhage by bleeding to syncope (fainting, or collapse), because venesection encouraged coagulation of the blood and arrested hemorrhage.

It is generally assumed that the practice of therapeutic bloodletting had become extinct by the end of the nineteenth century, and that physicians had put away the magic wand of the "dark ages of medicine" forever, but according to the 1923 edition of Sir William Osler's *Principles and Practice of Medicine*, the "Bible" of medicine for generations of American doctors, after a period of relative neglect, bleeding was returning to favor in the treatment of cardiac insufficiency and pneumonia. Indeed, a renaissance of bloodletting had begun about 1900, particularly for pneumonia, rheumatic fever, cerebral hemorrhages, arterial aneurysms, and epileptic seizures that were thought to be correlated with menstruation. Bloodletting was said to be effective in relieving pain, difficulty in breathing, and lowering temperature. From a practical point of view, bleeding convinced doctor, patient, and family that something important, something supported by hundreds of years of learned medical theory, was being done. Those who have observed the quiet prevailing among blood donors might also consider the fact that a quiet patient, especially one brought to a state of fainting, will get more rest and be less of a nuisance to caretakers than a restless, delirious, and demanding one.

BLOOD TRANSFUSION

As a scientist, Harvey demonstrated admirable skepticism towards dogma and superstition, but he was not especially innovative as a practitioner and he does not seem to have considered the possibility of therapeutic blood transfusions. However, Harvey's disciples were soon busily injecting drugs, poisons, nutrients, pigments, and blood itself into animal and human veins. The transfusion and infusion of medicinal substances into the bloodstream did not become part of the standard therapeutic arsenal for many years, but seventeenth century experimentalists did raise many intriguing possibilities. Interest in transfusion was high from 1660 until about 1680, when various countries began to outlaw this dangerous, experimental practice. Unfortunately, many of the early therapeutic experiments based on the theory of the circulation appear as paradoxical as the continued enthusiasm for bloodletting.

Although the first transfusion experiments generated great expectations, blood transfusion did not begin to satisfy the four cardinal virtues of a successful medical technique—simplicity, certainty, safety, and efficacy—until after World War I. The immunological mechanisms that guard the body against foreign invaders and distinguish between self and nonself provided the major obstacles to successful blood transfusion. Unlike twentieth-century transplant surgeons, seventeenth-century physicians had no theoretical framework concerning immunological barriers between different individuals and species. Why should they expect differences of blood type when four elements and four humors were sufficient to explain macrocosm and microcosm?

The avalanche of experiments on blood transfusion that followed acceptance of Harvey's theory led to competing claims for priority. However, the first significant studies of blood transfusion were performed by Christopher Wren, Richard Lower, and Robert Boyle in England, and by Jean Denis in Paris. According to Thomas Sprat's *History of the Royal Society* (1667), Christopher Wren was the first to carry out experiments on the injection of various materials into the veins of animals. During experiments exhibited at meetings of the Royal Society, experimental animals were purged, vomited, intoxicated, killed, or revived by the intravenous injection of various fluids and drugs. Dogs, birds, and other animals were bled almost to death and sometimes revived by the injection of blood from another animal. Reasoning that the nature of blood must change after it has been removed from the living body, Richard Lower decided to transfer blood between living animals by connecting the artery of the donor to the vein of the recipient. During a demonstration performed at Oxford in February 1666, Lower removed blood from a medium-sized dog until it was close to death. Blood taken via the cervical artery of a larger dog revived the experimental animal. Using additional donors, Lower was able to repeat this procedure several times. When the recipient's jugular vein was sewn up, it ran to its master, apparently none the worse for its bizarre experience. These remarkable experiments led observers to speculate that someday blood transfusions could cure the sick by improving their bad blood with blood from a more robust donor and that it might even be used to improve temperament, perhaps by injecting the blood of a Quaker into an Archbishop.

At about the same time that Lower was engaged in blood transfusion experiments in animals, Jean Baptiste Denis (or Denys, ca. 1625–1704), Professor of Philosophy and Mathematics at Montpellier and physician to Louis XIV, was already crossing the species barrier in preparation for therapeutic experiments on humans. In March 1667, after 19 successful transfusions from dog to dog, Denis transfused blood from a calf into a dog. Observing no immediate adverse effect, Denis concluded that animal blood could be used to treat human diseases. Denis suggested that animal blood might be a better remedy than human blood, because animal blood would not be corrupted by passion, vice, and other immoral human traits. Humans were well nourished by the flesh of animals; thus, it was reasonable to assume that animal blood could also be well assimilated by human beings. As a practical matter, animal blood could be transfused directly from an artery. With the help of Paul Emmerez, a surgeon and teacher of anatomy, Denis tested his methods on a 15-year-old boy who had suffered from a stubborn fever. To reduce excessive heat, his doctors had performed 20 therapeutic bleedings in 2 months. Dull, drowsy, and lethargic from the combined effects of illness and medical attention, the patient had been pronounced incredibly stupid and unfit for anything. On June 15, 1667, Emmerez drew off about 3 ounces of blood from a vein in the boy's arm and Denis injected about 10 ounces of arterial blood from a lamb. The operation caused a marvelous transformation: the boy regained his former wit, cheerfulness, and appetite. The only adverse effect was a sensation of great heat in his arm.

After this happy outcome, Denis injected about 20 ounces of lamb's blood into a healthy 45-year-old paid volunteer. Again, except for a sensation of warmth in the arm, no ill effects were reported. In another experiment, a patient suffering from a frenzy was given a large transfusion of calf's blood. Though cured of his frenzy, the patient experienced pains in the arm and back, rapid and irregular pulse, sweating, vomiting, diarrhea, and bloody urine. Given the poor man's state of health and previous treatments, Denis saw no compelling reason to blame the patient's physical problems on the transfusion. However, a fatality in another patient effectively ended the first phase of experimental blood transfusions. A 34-year-old man who had been suffering attacks of insanity for about 8 years improved after two transfusions of calf's blood. When the madness reappeared, treatment was resumed, and the patient died. Certainly the death of a patient following the ministrations of a flock of physicians was not without precedent, but this case precipitated a violent controversy and an avalanche of pamphlets. At first, Denis blamed the patient's death on overindulgence in wine, women, and tobacco, but he later suggested that the widow had deliberately poisoned his patient. Although the courts did not convict Denis of malpractice, to all intents and purposes, blood transfusion was found guilty. Denis and Emmerez abandoned experimental medicine and returned to conventional careers.

English scientists were quite critical of the experiments performed by Denis, but they too were experiencing mixed success in blood transfusions. About 6 months after Denis' first human transfusion, Richard Lower and his associates hired Arthur Coga, a man described as debauched, frantic, and somewhat cracked in the head, as a test subject. Some of Lower's colleagues were skeptical, but others believed that transfusion might cool Mr. Coga's blood and rid him of his frenzy. Apparently there was no debate as to whether the experiment might be dangerous; the only issue of interest was whether it would be effective. After the injection of about 12 ounces of sheep's blood, Mr. Coga reported feeling much improved. Unfortunately, after a second transfusion Coga's condition deteriorated. Rumors circulated that his bad behavior had been deliberately engineered by parties trying to discredit the Royal Society and make the experiment look ridiculous. The learned Fellows of the Royal Society were justified in their fear of ridicule. Their reports provided satirists like Jonathan Swift (1667–1745) and Thomas Shadwell (1641–1692) with ample raw material. In Shadwell's comic play *The Virtuoso,* amateur scientist Sir Nicholas Gimrack transfuses 64 ounces of sheep's blood into a maniac. After the operation, the patient became so wholly sheepish that he bleated perpetually, chewed his cud, and sprouted a magnificent coat of wool while a sheep's tail emerged from his "human fundament." Sir Nicholas planned to transfuse many more lunatics so that he could harvest the wool.

Safe blood transfusions were made possible when the immunologist Karl Landsteiner (1868–1943) demonstrated the existence of distinct blood group types.

In 1930, Landsteiner was awarded the Nobel Prize for his studies of blood group factors. Landsteiner found that all human beings belong to one of four different blood groups, designated O, A, B, and AB. Blood group typing also provides information useful in criminal cases, paternity suits, genetics, and anthropology. Indeed, so much information can be gleaned from the blood that patients hospitalized for several weeks might begin to think phlebotomy is once again an integral part of medical care.

Despite the fact that blood transfusion has become a routine procedure, myths and superstitions continue to flourish in one form or another, making many people reluctant to donate or accept blood. Of course, not all fears about the safety of blood transfusion are unjustified. Unless blood is properly tested, recipients of blood and blood products are at risk for diseases like syphilis, malaria, hepatitis, and AIDS. Inevitably, the need to detect and exclude unhealthy donors creates conflicts between public health concerns and individual liberty. Denying a person the right to donate blood may not seem a great infringement of personal liberty, but being labeled as a carrier of the hepatitis virus or HIV (the AIDS virus) may have very serious consequences.

NEW HEARTS FOR OLD

The emergence of cardiovascular disease as the major cause of death in the industrialized nations is a recent phenomenon, but deaths due to heart attack and stroke have long been of interest to physicians and scientists. Unfortunately, the approaches to the treatment of heart disease that have seized the most media attention—heart transplant surgery and the artificial heart—are methods that are unlikely to have commensurate effects on morbidity and mortality. The first human heart transplant operation was performed by South African surgeon Christiaan Barnard in December 1967. In the wake of Barnard's emergence as a world-class celebrity, other daring heart surgeons were soon performing equally dramatic operations. Some of most daring and unsuccessful operations in the 1960s and 1970s involved the transplantation of the hearts of chimpanzees, baboons, and sheep and artificial hearts into moribund patients. Ten years after Christiaan Barnard triggered an era of boundless excitement and fierce competition among surgical centers, the heart transplant industry experienced a wave of disappointment and disillusionment.

In retrospect, it is clear that the great expectations generated by heart transplants were based solely on the boldness of the surgical feat, rather than any rational hopes of long-term success. The same problem that defeated Denis three centuries before—the body's rejection of foreign materials—insured the failure of heart transplantation. However, unlike Denis, doctors in the 1960s were well aware of the body's immunological barriers. Even with drugs that suppressed the patient's immune system and attempts to provide some degree of tissue matching, the risk of tissue rejection and infection were virtually insurmountable obstacles. Optimistic surgeons pointed out that blood transfusion had once faced seemingly impossible obstacles and predicted that organ transplants would one day be as commonplace as blood transfusions. Advocates of organ transplants even managed to ignore the obvious objection that while blood is a renewable resource, hearts are not. If the interval between the first heart transplant and the new transplant era occurs in one-tenth the time it took to make blood transfusion routine, much of the credit will belong to a remarkable drug called cyclosporin, which suppresses the immune response. As surgeons proclaimed a new era in which organ transplants would be routine rather than experimental, health-care prophets warned that in the not too distant future the supply of money rather than hearts might become the rate-limiting factor. Given the tremendous toll taken by cardiovascular diseases, some researchers argue that prevention rather than treatment is our most pressing need. High risk, high cost therapy is likened to fighting poliomyelitis by developing more sophisticated artificial lung machines instead of preventive vaccines. Unfortunately, prevention lacks the glamour and excitement of surgical intervention.

SANTORIO SANTORIO AND THE QUANTITATIVE METHOD

All too often Harvey's success is simplistically attributed to his ingenious use of the quantitative method. But as the career of Santorio Santorio (Sanctorius, 1561–1636) indicates, painstaking experimentation and precise measurements are not enough to answer fundamental questions belonging to quite a different sphere. Many seventeenth-century scientists welcomed the idea of extending medical knowledge through the quantitative method, but no one transformed this goal into a way of life with the dedication of Santorio, physician and philosopher. In Italy he is honored as the founder of quantitative experimental physiology. Santorio established a successful private practice after graduating from the University of Padua in 1582. In 1611, he was appointed to the Chair of Theoretical Medicine at the University of Padua, but by 1624 his students were charging him with negligence on the grounds that his private practice often took precedence over his teaching duties. Although he was found innocent, Santorio resigned from the University in 1629 in order to return to Venice.

In addition to medical practice, Santorio became intimately involved in research concerning "insensible perspiration." According to classical theory, a kind of respiration taking place through the skin produced imperceptible exhalations known as *insensible perspiration*. Santorio believed that he could reduce the problem of insensible perspiration to purely mechanical processes which could be studied by exact measurements. In order to do so he invented a special balance, a chair suspended from a steelyard, in which he measured his body weight after eating, drinking, sleeping, resting, and exercising, in health and disease for more than 30 years. Santorio published his results as a series of aphorisms in a small book entitled *Ars de statica medicina* (*Medical Statics*, 1614). The book went through at least 30 editions and was translated into several languages; the first English translation appeared in 1676. Santorio was rather vague about his experimental methods, but

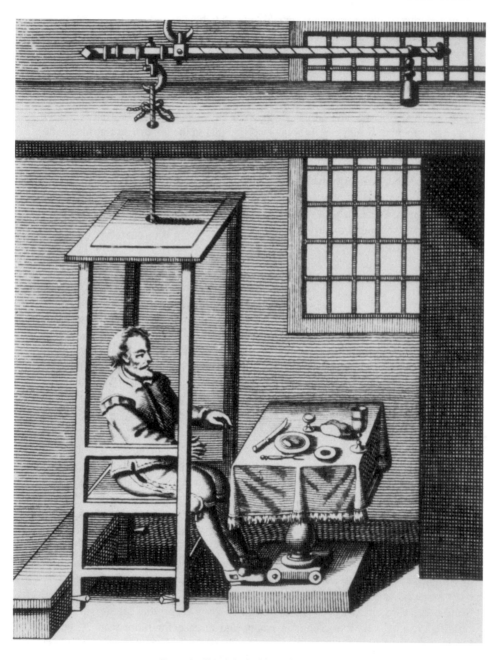

Santorio Santorio in his weighing chair

each aphorism was presented as a deduction from measurements. Nevertheless, he boasted that he had accomplished something new and unprecedented in medicine, that is, the exact measurement of insensible perspiration by means of reasoning and experimentation. Santorio suggested that readers might like to emulate the quantitative lifestyle by taking meals sitting on a balance which would provide a warning when the proper amount of food had been consumed.

Taking the position that measuring insensible perspiration was essential to medical progress, Santorio argued that physicians who did not understand quantitative aspects of insensible perspiration could not cure their patients. In answer to Santorio's claim that he could measure the amount of insensible perspiration, critics charged that even if the quantity of vapors could be measured it was their quality, not their quantity, that was significant in pathological phenomena.

Medical Statics was only one of several books written by Santorio. The others reveal that despite his obvious innovations he was still working and thinking in terms of seventeenth-century medicine's Galenic heritage. As a whole, his life and work were devoted to reason, experience, and the study of Hippocrates, Galen, and Avicenna. While accepting the fact that Renaissance anatomists had contradicted Galen on particular points, Santorio did not regard this as a major problem for the theory and practice of medicine. Quantitative studies of metabolism, not unlike those of Santorio, were still being carried out in the nineteenth century when the great French physiologist, Claude Bernard (1813–1878), denounced such experiments as attempts to understand what occurred in a house by measuring who went in the door and what came out the chimney. On the other hand, Santorio was successful in inventing or improving several instruments capable of making measurements useful in medical practice and scientific investigation, including a clinical thermometer, hygrometer, pulsimeter, a water bed, specialized tables, beds, baths, chairs, enemas, and various surgical tools. Moreover, Santorio was a champion of scientific medicine and an opponent of the superstitious, mystical, and astrological influences so common in his era. The spirit of invention and experiment was marvelously developed in this physician, even if his results were not commensurate with the painstaking nature of his investigations. Santorio did not reject the legacy of Hippocrates and Galen. He did not expect his measuring instruments and quantitative experiments to create a break with the past, but rather to provide more certain means of supporting the practice of Galenic medicine. After all, Galen himself had set an example of life-long dedication to experiment and observation.

SUGGESTED READINGS

Adelmann, H. B. (1942). *The Embryological Treatises of Hieronymus Fabricius of Aquapendente*. Ithaca, NY: Cornell University Press.

Arcieri, G. P. (1945). *The Circulation of the Blood and Andreas Cesalpino of Arezzo*. New York: S. F. Vanni, Publishers.

Arcieri, G. P. (1947). Passages where Andrea Cesalpino of Arezzo (Cesalpinus) describes and demonstrates the blood circulation. *ALCMAEON* Vol. IX, No. 3.

Bainton, Roland H. (1960). *Hunted Heretic: The Life and Death of Michael Servetus, 1511–1553*. Boston: Beacon Press.

Boas, M. (1962). *The Scientific Renaissance, 1450–1630*. New York: Harper & Row.

Bonelli, M. L. R., and Shea, W. R. (1975). *Reason, Experiment, and Mysticism in the Scientific Revolution*. New York: Science History.

Brown, Theodore M. (1977). Physiology and the Mechanical Philosophy in Mid-Seventeenth Century England. *Bulletin of the History of Medicine* 51: 25–54.

Bylebyl, Jerome J., ed. (1978). *William Harvey and His Age. The Professional and Social Context of the Discovery of the Circulation*. Baltimore, MD: Johns Hopkins Press.

Castiglioni, Arturo (1931). The Life and Work of Santorio Santorio (1561–1636). Trans. by Emilie Recht. *Medical Life* n. s. 38 (12): 729–785.

Comrie, Julius H. (1983). *Exploring the Heart: Discoveries in Heart Disease and High Blood Pressure*. New York: Norton.

Davis, Audrey B. (1973). *Circulation Physiology and Medical Chemistry in England 1650–80*. Lawrence, KS: Coronado Press.

Dickinson, C. J., and Marks, J., eds. (1978). *Developments in Cardiovascular Medicine*. Lancaster, England: MTP Press.

Fabrizzi, Girolamo (1933). *De Venarum Ostiolis. By Fabricius ab Aquapendente*. Facsimile, with English trans., ed. by K. J. Franklin. Springfield, IL: Charles C. Thomas.

Farr, A. D. (1980). The first human blood transfusion. *Med. Hist.* 24: 143–162.

Fishman, A. P., and Dickinson, Woodruff Richards, eds. (1964). *Circulation of the Blood. Men and Ideas*. New York: Oxford University Press.

Foster, M. (1901). *Lectures on the History of Physiology during the Sixteenth, Seventeenth and Eighteenth Centuries*. Cambridge, England: Cambridge University Press. (New York: Dover, 1970.)

Fox, Renee C., and Swazey, Judith P. (1978). *The Courage to Fail: A Social View of Organ Transplants and Dialysis*. 2nd ed. Chicago: University of Chicago Press.

Frank, Robert G., Jr. (1980). *Harvey and the Oxford Physiologists. Scientific Ideas and Social Interactions*. Berkeley, CA: Univeristy of California Press.

French, Roger, and Wear, Andrew, eds. (1989). *The Medical Revolution of the Seventeenth Century*. New York: Cambridge University Press.

Fulton, John F. (1953). *Michael Servetus, Humanist and Martyr*. New York: Reicher.

Hackett, Earle (1973). *Blood, The Paramount Humor*. London: Jonathan Cape, Ltd.

Harris, Charles R. S. (1973). *The Heart and the Vascular System in Ancient Greek Medicine from Alcmaeon to Galen*. Oxford, England: Clarendon Press.

Harvey, William (1976). *An Anatomical Disputation Concerning the Movement of the Heart and Blood in Living Creatures*. Trans. G. Whitteridge. Oxford, England: Blackwell Scientific.

Harvey, William (1961). *Lectures on the Whole of Anatomy*. Annotated trans. by C. D. O'Malley, F. N. L. Poynter, and K. F. Russel. Berkeley: University of California Press.

Hoff, Hebbel, and Guillemin, Roger (1963). The First Experiments on Transfusion in France. *JHMAS* 18: 103–124.

Hunter, Michael (1981). *Science and Society in Restoration England*. New York: Cambridge University Press.

Jarcho, Saul (1980). *The Concept of Heart Failure from Avicenna to Albertini.* Trans., commentaries, and essay by Saul Jarcho. Cambridge, MA: Harvard University Press.

Keele, Kenneth David (1965). *William Harvey: The Man, the Physician, and the Scientist.* London: Nelson.

Keynes, G. L., ed. (1949). *Blood Transfusion.* Bristol, England: John Wright and Sons, Ltd.

Keynes, G. L. (1966). *The Life of William Harvey.* Oxford, England: Clarendon.

Landsteiner, Karl (1962). *The Specificity of Serological Reactions.* Rev. ed. New York: Dover.

Louis, P. C. A. (1836). *Researches on the Effects of Bloodletting in Some Inflammatory Diseases, and on the Influence of Tartarised Antimony and Vesication in Pneumonias.* Trans. C. G. Putnam. Preface and Appendix by James Jackson. Boston: Hilliard, Gray & Co.

Niebyl, Peter H. (1977). The English Bloodletting Revolution, or Modern Medicine before 1850. *Bulletin of the History of Medicine* 51: 46–83.

O'Malley, C. D. (1953). *Michael Servetus. A Translation of His Geographical, Medical and Astrological Writings with Introductions and Notes.* Philadelphia, PA: American Philosophical Society.

Osler, William, and McCrae, Thomas (1923). *The Principles and Practice of Medicine.* New York: Appleton.

Pagel, Walter (1982). *Jan Baptista Van Helmont: Reformer of Science and Medicine.* Cambridge, England: Cambridge University Press.

Pagel, Walter (1976). *New Light on William Harvey.* Basel: S. Karger.

Payton, Brian (1981). History of Medicinal Leeching and Early Medical References. In K. J. Muller et al. *Neurobiology of the Leech.* Cold Spring Harbor, New York: Cold Spring Harbor Laboratory.

Rapaport, Felix T., and Dausset, Jean, eds. (1968). *Human Transplantation.* New York: Grune & Stratton.

Reece, R. (1966). George Washington: His Death and His Doctors. *Minnesota Medicine* 49: 1185–1190.

Risse, Gunter B. (198). The Renaissance of Bloodletting: A Chapter in Modern Therapeutics. *JHMAS* 34: 3–22.

Sanctorius (1720). *Medicina statica*: Being the Aphorisms of Sanctorius, Trans. into English with large Explanations. 2nd ed. To which is added Dr. Keil's *Medica statica Britannica . . .* by John Quincy, MD. London: Printed for W. & J. Newton in Little-Britain.

Saunders, J. B. (1978). The history of the venous valves. In C. J. Dickinson and J. Marks, eds. *Developments in Cardiovascular Medicine.* Lancaster, England: MTP Press, pp. 335–351.

Sigerist, H. E. (1933). *The Great Doctors: A Biographical History of Medicine.* Trans. E. and C. Paul, 1958. Garden City, NY: Doubleday.

Singer, C. (1957). *A Short History of Anatomy and Physiology from the Greeks to Harvey.* New York: Dover.

Wangensteen, Owen Harding, and Wangensteen, Sarah D. (1978). *The Rise of Surgery from Empiric Craft to Scientific Discipline.* Minneapolis, MN: University of Minnesota Press.

Wardrup, James (1837). *On the Curative Effects of the Abstraction of Blood: With Rules for Employing Both Local and General Blood-Letting In the Treatment of Diseases.* Philadelphia: A Waldie.

Warner, John Harley (1985). The Selective Transport of Medical Knowledge: Antebellum American Physicians and Parisian Medical Therapeutics. *BHM* 59: 213–231.

Wear, Andrew, French, Roger, and Lonie, I. M., eds. (1985). *The Medical Renaissance of the Sixteenth Century*. New York: Cambridge University Press.

Webster, Charles (1976). *The Great Instauration: Science, Medicine and Reform, 1626–1660*. New York: Holmes and Meier.

Whitteridge, G. (1971). *William Harvey and the Circulation of the Blood*. New York: American Elsevier.

Willus, F. A., and Keys, T. E., eds. (1961). *Classics of Cardiology*. 2 vols. New York: Dover.

Wintrobe, Maxwell M. (1985). *Hematology, The Blossoming of a Science: A Story of Inspiration and Effort*. Philadelphia, PA: Lea & Febiger.

SELECTED ASPECTS OF CLINICAL AND PREVENTIVE MEDICINE: FROM SYDENHAM TO SMALLPOX

T he sixteenth century was a time of almost universal expansion throughout Europe, but it was followed by an era of political, social, and spiritual unrest. The seventeenth century was a time of bitter controversies in medicine and science, religion, and politics; it was a time of warfare and revolution, Reformation and Counter-Reformation. An increasingly literate public was becoming skeptical of ancient medical dogma; chemical remedies were challenging traditional Galenicals, and instruments like the telescope, microscope, barometer, thermometer, and pulse clock were providing new means of investigating the natural world.

England's own philosopher of science and Lord High Chancellor, Francis Bacon (1561–1626), called for a more pragmatic approach to medicine and nature. Bacon urged physicians to collect data empirically, without regard to ancient theory, in order to form new theories, make new discoveries, prolong life, and understand the workings of the body in health and disease. Bacon's vision of the "Grand Instauration" that would reorder the sciences and improve the human condition helped inspire the establishment of new scientific societies and novel medical philosophies.

Changes in medical philosophy and practice probably affected few patients directly. Learned physicians served only the rich; the bulk of the population lived and died without the assistance of physicians or surgeons. Seeking medical attention was impossible for impoverished peasants and workers, who could afford neither the physician's fees nor the elaborate remedies he prescribed. It was not the physician who dealt with the afflictions of the common people, but the great army of "irregular practitioners''—barber-surgeons, apothecaries, herbalists, midwives, empirics, and peripatetic quacks.

Pretentious physicians, more interested in their purses than their patients, provided a favorite target for satirists. The physician with his fancy wig, ornate velvet coat, buckled shoes, and gold-handled cane made a pretty picture. At least the hollow handle of the cane had a practical purpose; stuffed with smelling salts and perfume, it provided an antidote to the aroma of the sickroom. The average physician resembled Molière's caricature of the pompous snob whose prescription for any illness was always "clyster, bleed, purge," or "purge, bleed, clyster." (*Clyster* is an old word for enema.) In Molière's play *Love's the Best Doctor*, we learn that "we should never say, such a one is dead of a fever," because, to tell the truth, the patient died of "four doctors and two apothecaries." However, physicians were mastering the art of using new drugs, such as quinine, ipecac, and valerian, while the introduction of New World foods, especially potatoes and corn, had a remarkable effect on health and population growth. The potato became the staple food of the poor in northern Europe, the British Isles, and Ireland. A one-acre plot of potatoes could feed a family of six all year. Maize, or "Turkish wheat" (corn), provided plenty of calories, but also made pellagra an endemic disease in many areas. Some New World plants, such as tobacco, were simultaneously credited with medicinal virtues and condemned as poisons.

Although mortality rates for this period are generally crude estimates, interest in the accurate measurement of births and deaths was growing. John Graunt (1620–1674), author of *Observations upon the Bills of Mortality* (1662), the first book on vital statistics, attempted to derive general trends from the "Bills of Mortality" (weekly lists of burials) and the records of marriages and baptisms kept by parish clerks. He noted that the urban death rate was greater than that of rural areas. Infant mortality, a good index of general health and sanitation, was very high: probably 40% of all infants died before reaching their second birthday. Renowned astronomer Edmond Halley (1656–1742), who was also interested in the theory of annuities and mortality rates, noted that those who reached maturity should not complain about the shortness of their lives, because half of all those born seemed to die within 17 years. Nevertheless, science had been revolutionized, and it seemed reasonable to expect a similar revolution in medicine. To this end, physicians devoted to scientific research developed elaborate theories which had little to do with the practical details of patient care. Thomas Sydenham, who has been honored as the English champion of clinical, or bedside medicine, provides an instructive example of a physician who recognized the growing tension between medicine as science and medicine as care of the sick.

THOMAS SYDENHAM

Thomas Sydenham (1624–1689) epitomized the reaction of the clinician to abstract and speculative medicine and to the pretensions of physicians who behaved as if their scientific research was more significant than medicine practiced at the bedside of the

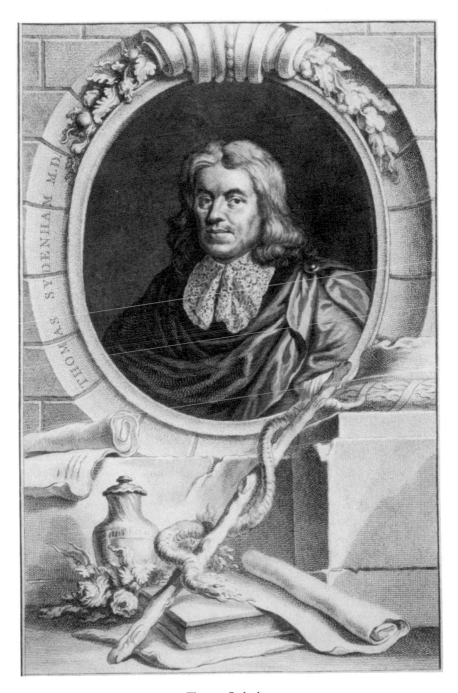

Thomas Sydenham

patient. When scientific medicine was generally practiced in the autopsy room, the physician whose major interest was his research might well be frustrated by patients with long, lingering illnesses. Like Hippocrates, Sydenham believed that it was the task of the physician to assist the body's natural healing processes while searching for the causes of disease. Since clinical medicine was an art which demanded acute observation, experience, and balanced judgment, the true physician should dedicate himself to useful techniques, common sense, and the principles of Hippocrates. Revered as the "English Hippocrates," Sydenham was eulogized as "the great representative of the practical medicine of practical England" and the man who recognized "the priority of direct observation, and its paramount supremacy to everything else."

Politically, as well as professionally, Sydenham was William Harvey's opposite. Indeed, Sydenham's goals and achievements have been ascribed to the events that made him a highly politicized person; his attempts to reform medicine were apparently inseparable from his political stance. Thomas and his brothers fought as soldiers in the Parliamentary Army; their mother was killed in a Royalist raid. Several close encounters with death during the war convinced Sydenham that a special providence had spared his life. After the Royalists were defeated, Sydenham resumed his studies at Oxford and was granted a bachelor of medicine in less than 2 years. When hostilities began again, Sydenham rejoined the army. In 1655, Sydenham resigned his Oxford fellowship and established a private practice in an aristocratic London neighborhood close to the malarial marshes that generated a steady supply of fever patients. He also attended the sick poor at various London hospitals. While Sydenham became a Licentiate of the Royal College of Physicians in 1663, he was never granted the honor of becoming a Fellow of that prestigious association. In an age where personal abuse was a common form of professional discourse, Sydenham was always ready to return real or imagined insults. Defensive about the deficiencies in his formal education, Sydenham boasted of his ability to "think where others read." His enemies tried to rescind his license and banish him from the College of Physicians for medical heresy and irregular practice.

Puritan principles, especially the idea that increasing useful knowledge was a paramount religious duty, guided Sydenham's approach to medicine. Studying cadavers was useless, because death was an admission of defeat, or proof of inadequate care. Sydenham argued that medical education could take place only at the bedside of the sick, not in the classroom, library, or anatomy theater. Despite his admiration for Hippocrates, he insisted that experience had been his only teacher. Many of the anecdotes treasured by Sydenham's followers reflect this attitude. For example, when Richard Blackmore asked Sydenham to recommend the best books for learning medicine, he replied: "Read 'Don Quixote'; it is a very good book; I read it myself still." Perhaps this retort reflected his opinion of both young doctor Blackmore and the medical literature of his time, along with microscopy and pathological anatomy.

Although Sydenham ridiculed attempts to study the ravages of disease through post-mortems, he considered close study of the natural history of disease among hospital patients valuable training. According to Dr. Robert Pitt, by carefully studying the course of disease in a hospital for the "meaner class" of patients, Sydenham was able to determine whether a fever could be cured by "Natural Power" or whether "it required Bleeding, Vomiting, Purgatives . . . before risking the lives of people of quality." When accused of diminishing the dignity of the healing art by recommending plain and simple medicines, Sydenham countered that wise men understood that "whatever is useful is good." Not only were simple remedies useful, they were safer than the fashionable "superfluous and over-learned medicines" which were likely to aggravate the disease until the tormented patient "dies of his doctor." Recommending moderation in all things, Sydenham prescribed appropriate diets, drugs, exercise, and opium, the drug God had created for the relief of pain. However, Sydenham noted that a rag dipped in rosewater, applied to the forehead, often did more good than any narcotic.

In 1665, the year of the Great Plague and Fire, Sydenham and his family fled from London. In the countryside, he found the time to complete his *Medical Observations Concerning the History and Cure of Acute Diseases*. As an admirer of the rapidly developing science of taxonomy, Sydenham prescribed analogous methods for the study of the natural history of disease. Combining direct observations and Robert Boyle's chemical theories, Sydenham suggested that subterranean effluvia generated disease-causing miasmata when they came in contact with "corpuscles" in the air. As the atmosphere became "stuffed full of particles which are hostile to the economy of the human body," each breath drew into the body "noxious and unnatural miasmata" which mixed with the blood and engendered acute epidemic diseases.

In his attempt to extend scientific taxonomy to medicine, Sydenham envisioned disease as an entity existing independently of the person who might become its victim, a concept generally referred to as the ontogenic concept of disease. Acute diseases caused by changes in the atmosphere which affected great numbers of people were called epidemics; other acute diseases attacked only a few people at a time and could be called intercurrent or sporadic. Physicians had long been content with vague designations of diseases in terms of major symptoms, but Sydenham believed that the physician must learn to distinguish between different diseases with similar symptoms. For example, the fevers were vaguely classified as continued, intermittent, and eruptive. Typhus was the most common of the continued fevers, malaria was the prime example of an intermittent fever, and smallpox was the most dreaded eruptive fever. Smallpox, which Sydenham carefully distinguished from scarlet fever and measles, was so common in the seventeenth century that, like Rhazes, Sydenham regarded it as essentially part of the normal maturation process. Physicians generally kept smallpox patients confined to bed under a great weight of blankets and prescribed heating cordials to drive out diseased matter. Sydenham contended that the orthodox "heating regimen" caused excessive ebullition of the blood, which led to improper fermentation, confluent pustules, brain fever, and death. To assist nature, Sydenham prescribed a simple and moderate "cooling regimen" featuring light covers, moderate bleeding, and a liberal allowance of fluids.

Sydenham's short treatise on mental illness has been called the most important seventeenth-century work on psychological disorders and their treatment. According to Sydenham, psychological disorders were as common as physical complaints. Moreover, hysteria, a disorder the ancients attributed to the wanderings of the uterus, seemed to be the most common of all chronic diseases. Perhaps it was no surprise that hardly any women were wholly free of this disorder, but it was certainly remarkable to learn that men were also subject to hysterical complaints. Faced with the challenge of determining a new etiology, Sydenham ascribed hysteria to disordered animal spirits. Time, the prince of physicians, healed many of these patients, but "steel syrup" (iron filings steeped in wine) and horseback riding were also therapeutic. For both mental and physical complaints, Sydenham was as enthusiastic about horseback riding as modern health gurus are about jogging. Some patients had to be tricked into health-restoring exercise. For example, in dealing with a patient who stubbornly refused to get well, Sydenham suggested a consultation with the wonder-working Dr. Robinson at Inverness. The patient made the long trip on horseback only to find that there was no such doctor, but, as Sydenham expected, anticipation, exercise, and anger effected a cure.

Some of Sydenham's most vivid writings are those describing the onset, pain, and progress of gout. Sydenham confessed that he had endured the agonies of gout for 34 years without discovering anything useful about its nature or treatment. For gout, stone, and chronic hematuria (which he bluntly referred to as "a great pissing of blood"), his only antidote was opium and more opium. Little could be added to Hippocrates' observation that gout generally attacked young adult males, while sparing women and eunuchs. Victims of the disease were thought to be men who had indulged in heavy wines, rich foods, premature venery, and those with an "unhappy hereditary tendency." Today, primary gout is described as an inherited disorder of purine metabolism which results in the accumulation of uric acid; secondary gout is a condition apparently caused by lead or various drugs. Gout attacks are not fatal, but they are so painful that some victims have been driven to suicide. An attack usually begins with exquisite pain in the great toe, chills, shivers, restlessness, and fever. Eventually, gout cripples the major joints and results in the chronic torment of kidney stones. Sometimes the stones killed the patient "without waiting for the gout." Living with fear, anxiety, and pain, the victim's mind "suffers with the body; and which suffers most" Sydenham could not say. The only comfort Sydenham had to offer was the thought that gout "kills more rich men than poor, more wise men than simple." Nature, Sydenham said, balanced her accounts by giving those she had favored an affliction to produce an appropriate mixture of good and evil; gout was the disease of kings, emperors, admirals, and philosophers. Despite Sydenham's belief that gout reflected divine justice, the relationship between gout and genius is simply an artifact of our interest in the medical problems of the rich and famous and indifference to the innumerable impoverished victims of disease who suffered the torments of gout without benefit of medical or biographical attention.

Physicians traditionally attacked gout with bleeding, sweating, purges, cathartics, emetics, diuretics, blisters, massage, and cauterization. From his own experience, Sydenham could testify that none of these methods worked any better than ancient Roman charms and incantations. Abstinence in diet and drink was advisable, but in Sydenham's experience: "If you drink wine you get gout—if you do not, gout gets you!" Unfortunately, Sydenham failed to appreciate the value of colchicum, the one remedy that could have mitigated his sufferings. Colchicum, a crude extract of the autumn crocus, was used in many purges. The Doctrine of Signatures provided a tenuous link between colchicum and gouty arthritis by associating the shape of the flower with that of the crippled hand. Although the drug was reputed to have aphrodisiac properties, it also caused unpleasant side effects, including stomach irritation, nausea, and death. Nevertheless, colchicum generally produces dramatic relief from the pain of gout, as the success of the secret remedies of various quacks and empirics demonstrated. By the eighteenth century, physicians had joined the quacks in recommending colchicum for the relief of gout, but the mechanism by which colchicine, the active ingredient in colchicum, relieves gout attacks is still obscure. Colchicine was first isolated in 1820 by Pierre Joseph Pelletier (1788–1842) and Joseph Bienaimé Caventou (1795–1877), the founders of alkaloid chemistry. In addition to its therapeutic virtues, colchicine is invaluable to cell biologists and horticulturists, because it arrests mitosis at metaphase. This causes polyploidy (an increase in chromosome number) in plants and can create new varieties.

QUININE AND MALARIA

As wrong as Sydenham was in his assessment of colchicine for gout, he was right in his masterful studies of quinine for malaria, the debilitating fever still worthy of the title "million-murdering Death" in the twentieth century. If we consider the impact of diseases on populations over time as measured by the greatest harm to the greatest number, malaria has been the most devastating disease in history. Malaria seems to have achieved its widest distribution in Europe during the seventeenth century, but it was not uncommon even in the nineteenth century.

One of the great accomplishments of seventeenth-century medical science was the discovery that quinine could be used as a specific remedy for malaria. Quinine is the active ingredient in cinchona (also known as Peruvian bark, Jesuits' bark, or Devil's bark), a traditional Peruvian remedy for fevers supposedly named after the Countess of Chinchon, wife of the Governor of Peru. The story of the feverish Countess appears to be pure fiction, but, with or without her blessings, the New World remedy spread quickly throughout Europe. As demand for the wonder-working bark drove its price higher and higher, charlatans amassed great fortunes selling secret remedies containing Peruvian bark and imitations which mimicked quinine's bitter taste, but had no anti-malarial properties. By the end of the 1660s, confidence in Peruvian bark had dropped precipitously because many physicians claimed that the drug was responsible for dangerous relapses and sudden deaths. Careful study convinced Sydenham that the bark was safe and effective; adverse reactions were due to improper use rather than to any evil in the drug itself.

Peruvian bark was important not only as a remedy for malaria, but also for its symbolic value in challenging the ancient foundations of pharmacology. Medical dogma called for remedies that were complex and purgative, but Peruvian bark cured malaria without purgation. Orthodox medical theory condemned the new remedy as "irrational" because it was theoretically impossible for healing to occur without the expulsion of morbid matter. Therefore, while the bark seemed to interrupt cycles of intermittent fevers, it must be acting by trapping dangerous materials within the body. Sydenham argued that experience was more compelling than theory; the drug was safe and effective if dosage, timing, and duration of treatment were carefully regulated. In terms of medical practice and theory, quinine was as revolutionary as gunpowder had been to the art of warfare.

Despite Sydenham's conviction that the bark was harmless, quinine actually causes some very unpleasant side effects, such as vomiting, headache, rashes, and deafness. Indeed, some physicians used complaints about ringing in the ears to determine optimum dosage. Because few practitioners, or patients, could accept the concept of specificity in diseases and remedies, Peruvian bark was freely prescribed for fevers, colds, flu, seasickness, headache, and hangover. But quinine is a specific remedy for the intermittent fever we call malaria; its use as a general febrifuge and tonic exposed many people to risks without benefits. Peruvian bark prepared Europe for a new relationship with malaria. For hundreds of years, malaria and other murderous diseases kept Europeans from penetrating the vast African continent. Thus, quinine was to become one of the tools that made European exploitation of Africa, and much of Asia, possible. In areas where malaria is endemic, slight genetic variations may provide a powerful evolutionary advantage. The prevalence of genes for disorders known as sickle cell anemia and thalassemia suggests such an evolutionary pattern. Biologists as well as anthropologists are fascinated by the relationships between the genes for abnormal hemoglobins and resistance to malaria. Quinine was isolated in 1820. Within 10 years the purified drug was being produced in large quantities. Until the 1850s, the forests of Peru, Bolivia, and Colombia were the only sources of the bark, but the Dutch and British established cinchona plantations in Indonesia and India. Intensive experimentation led to significant increases in the yield of alkaloids. By the turn of the century, the Dutch had captured more than 90% of the world market. The Dutch monopoly on this vital drug was not broken until the 1940s with the Japanese conquest of Indonesia and the European development of synthetic antimalarial drugs.

Malaria is caused by a minute protozoan with a complex life cycle which includes phases in the human blood stream and in the female Anopheles mosquito. The mosquito transmits the parasite to new victims. Because anopheline mosquitoes prefer to lay their eggs in stagnant waters, malaria becomes endemic in marshy areas. As we have seen, the ancients noted the connection between malaria and marshes, but the basis of this relationship was not discovered until the end of the nineteenth century. During the first half of the twentieth century, the conquest of malaria seemed to be a real possibility, but the optimism raised by the anti-malaria campaigns of the 1950s and 1960s ended in the 1970s as the resurgence of malaria became obvious. Resistance of the mosquito vectors to pesticides was only part of the problem; socioeconomic and geopolitical issues were more significant. Malaria flourished because global recessions, political upheavals, and large-scale population migrations militated against the high levels of financial and administrative support, sophisticated organizational infrastructure, and international cooperation needed to sustain anti-malarial campaigns.

In the 1980s, the hope that malaria could be eradicated by pesticides and drugs had been abandoned; malaria was still causing 2–4 million deaths a year, afflicting about 300 million people, and putting 2 billion people at risk. To reverse this trend, the World Health Organization established special programs to support research on malaria, schistosomiasis, trypanosomiasis, leishmaniasis, filariasis, and leprosy in areas where the diseases are endemic. Because of recent advances in molecular biology, parasitology—once known as tropical medicine—has become an attractive and challenging area of biomedical research. Since the 1970s basic research on the biology and immunology of malaria has raised hopes for the development of anti-malaria vaccines. Certainly Sydenham would pronounce such research both good and useful.

While scientific assaults on the malaria plasmodium were becoming increasingly sophisticated, scientists learned that their naiveté about economic factors and geopolitics might destroy efforts to launch a malaria vaccine. Disputes between the World Health Organization and the biotechnology companies that have the technical competence to manufacture novel vaccines were the 1980's version of the central problem in tropical medicine, the tension between the underdeveloped nations, which need the remedies, but lack the resources to develop them, and the developed nations, which could develop the remedies, but do not need them. Given the role malaria has played in history, it would be ironic indeed if the question of whether or not it is possible to develop a malaria vaccine is subverted by the problem of whether it is politically or economically expedient to do so.

THE EIGHTEENTH-CENTURY FOUNDATIONS OF MODERN MEDICINE

The eighteenth century has been called the adolescence of modern medicine, the era in which the foundations of scientific medicine were first established. During this period the ideas of the great philosophical movement known as the Enlightenment inspired the search for rational systems of medicine, practical means of preventing disease, improving the human condition, and disseminating the new learning to the greatest number of people possible. This era boasts a prodigious who's who of physicians and scientists, easy to list, but impossible to discuss in the detail they deserve. A few of the leading lights of clinical medicine will have to serve as exemplars of their age.

Just as Thomas Sydenham is honored for following Hippocrates in his emphasis on patient care and epidemiological observations, Hermann Boerhaave (1668–1738) is remembered for his role in revitalizing clinical medicine. Teacher, writer, and chemist, Boerhaave was probably the most influential physician of the eighteenth century; his contemporaries thought of him as the "Newton of Medicine." Boerhaave drew his inspiration from the work of Hippocrates, Bacon, and Sydenham; indeed, in deference to the "English Hippocrates," he doffed his hat every time Sydenham's name was mentioned. Like Sydenham, he suffered the torments of gout. As a student, Boerhaave immersed himself in chemistry, medicine, botany, philosophy, and languages. Certainly he commanded boundless energies as well as erudition to hold, simultaneously, Professorships of Botany, Chemistry, Clinical Medicine, and Medicine at Leiden.

By establishing a hospital especially for teaching purposes, Boerhaave was able to combine theoretical and practical instruction at the patient's bedside. "Bedside instruction," the reform of one of the greatest deficiencies of academic medicine, made Leiden a major center of medical education—at least until Boerhaave's disciples succeeded in bringing clinical instruction to other schools. *Bedside medicine* prepared the way for the *hospital medicine* which developed during the last years of the eighteenth century and flourished in the first half of the nineteenth century. No major discovery can be attributed to Boerhaave, but medical students were taught to think of his system as "perfect, complete and sufficient" and powerful enough to fill the void created by abandoning Galen. Those who dared to differ from the great Boerhaave were denounced as medical heretics. Through lectures faithfully recorded by his disciples, Boerhaave became teacher to the world. The books that expressed Boerhaave's ideas, *Institutiones medicae* (1708), *Book of Aphorisms* (1709), *Index plantarum* (1710), and *Elementia chemiae* (1732), remained in use for almost 100 years. Unfortunately, like Galenism, Boerhaave's beautifully crafted system so thoroughly satisfied his contemporaries that it tended to stifle curiosity and imagination. Nevertheless, Boerhaave impressed upon medical philosophers and scientists the necessity to ground all inquiries and explanations of human health and disease on anatomy and physiology, chemistry and physics.

The great virtue, and fault, of Boerhaave's system was the way he integrated classification and natural science with considerations of the nature, causes, and treatment of disease. For example, eighteenth-century physiologists regarded the study of the chemistry of digestion as part of a deep philosophical argument about life; if one could understand how the dead matter of plant and animal foods could nourish living tissue one would discover the secret of life. According to Boerhaave, if the digestive processes were inadequate, various foods gave rise to acids. Since acids were supposedly foreign to bodily humors, "acid acrimony" produced disorders of the intestinal tract which affected the blood, milk, skin, and brain. Obviously, such disorders should be treated with "anti-acids" such as meat, fish, leafy vegetables, and alkaline powders. The chemistry of Boerhaave's medical system is intriguing, but often confusing, because terms that seem familiar to modern chemists had quite a different meaning. For example, "earth" signified an inert material that could not be liquefied by fire or dissolved in water. A "salt" was a substance that dissolved in water and was liquefied by fire. "Sulfur" and "oil" were substances that melted and burned, but could not mix with water. Eventually the deficiencies and failures of eighteenth-century medical philosophical systems became all too apparent. New discoveries and unlovely facts would force nineteenth-century physicians to confine themselves to formulating more modest and limited explanatory frameworks.

MORBID ANATOMY AND LOCALISM

The eighteenth century is also notable for the work of Giovanni Battista Morgagni (1682–1771), author of the masterpiece of pathological anatomy, *On the Seats and Causes of Disease* (1761). After studying medicine in Bologna, Morgagni became Professor of Theoretical Medicine and Anatomy at the University of Padua. The work he carried out for the next half century was to bring the University almost as much glory as his predecessor Andreas Vesalius. Morgagni's attempt to find correlations between clinical symptoms and post-mortem findings was based on over 600 dissections. Careful observation of the appearance and course of various diseases was essential to Morgagni's research program, as were dissections and experiments on various animals as a means of understanding clinical patterns of disease in humans. Convinced that normal human anatomy had been well established, Morgagni focused his considerable energies on exploring the origin and seat of diseases that caused pathological changes observable in the cadaver. The longest section in Morgagni's treatise deals with disorders of the belly. After carefully describing each case history, Morgagni attempted to correlate observations of the course of illness with his findings at autopsy. Autopsies sometimes revealed errors in diagnosis and treatment which led to the death of the patient. In one case, the attending physician had diagnosed a stomach complaint, but the post-mortem revealed that the patient had a normal stomach and diseased kidneys.

Autopsies sometimes revealed sad and bizarre behaviors. For example, in discussing findings related to the suppression of urine, Morgagni noted several cases where girls had damaged the bladder by introducing needles or pins into the urethra. Some girls claimed to have swallowed these items, but others tried to conceal their injuries, even if it meant death. He also reported strange cases of males who died with needles in their urinary organs. Morgagni boasted that he had dissected more male urethras than any other anatomist, but he complained that he had not found as many cases of damage to the urethra due to gonorrhea as he had expected. He was unsuccessful in discovering the seat of gonorrhea in males and females, but dissections did prove that over the course of many years the disease insidiously made its way throughout the body. In compiling case studies, the morbid anatomist needed a healthy dose of skepticism. Colleagues offered him reports of bizarre hungers brought on by lice growing in the stomach and worms in the appendix. Morgagni was quite suspicious of the first, but thought that the second seemed plausible. In discussing various kinds of fluxes (diarrheas), he urged his readers to view with skepticism all accounts of the ingestion or excretion of frogs, toads, lizards, etc. The anatomist must examine the physical evidence and determine what kind of bodily parts were actually involved.

Morgagni is regarded as a pioneer of morbid anatomy and a guide to a new epoch in medical science. Even though Morgagni remained essentially a humoralist, his work marked a trend away from general humoral pathology towards the study of localized lesions and diseased organs. By encouraging physicians to think of disease in terms of localized pathological changes rather than disorders of the humors, Morgagni's work encouraged a new attitude towards specific diagnostic and surgical interventions. He was the first person to attempt a systematic examination of the connection between the symptoms of disease in the living body and post-mortem results revealed only to the dedicated investigator. Morgagni's work helped to established an anatomical orientation in pathology and the recognition that unseen anatomical changes in the living body were reflected in the clinical picture. Confirmation could be found only in the autopsy room, but recognition of the relationship encouraged interest in finding ways of anatomizing the living—that is, detecting hidden anatomical lesions in living patients. This goal would be realized in Leopold Auenbrugger's studies of chest percussion, the establishment of "hospital medicine" at the Paris Hospital, René Laënnec's invention of the stethoscope, and the remarkable rise of medical instrumentation that followed.

ENLIGHTENMENT PHILOSOPHY AND MEDICAL REFORM

Although elaborate systems fascinated eighteenth century-physicians, this period also produced pragmatic reformers who realized that one could not heal sailors and soldiers or peasants and workers with learned speculations. Social and medical reformers inspired by the Enlightenment belief that it was possible to improve the human condition through the application of reason to social problems turned their attention to public health and preventive medicine. In the eighteenth century, to an unprecedented extent, the ship, the army barrack, the factory, the prison, the hospital, and the boarding school were closed worlds in which unrelated people were confined, sharing unhygienic conditions, unhealthy diets, and communicable diseases. Reformers and philanthropists argued that scientific investigations of the abominable conditions of cities, navies, armies, prisons, mental asylums, and hospitals could improve the health and prosperity of society as a whole. Sometimes this battle was led by medical men familiar with specific constituencies, such as Sir John Pringle, surgeon general of the British armies, or James Lind, Charles Blane, and Thomas Trotter, pioneers of naval medicine and hygiene. Philanthropists and physicians called for the reform of prisons and mental asylums.

The goals and ideals, as well as the sometimes authoritarian methods embraced by the developing field of public health medicine, are reflected in the work of Johann Peter Frank (1745–1821), a pioneer of what is now called social medicine. His philosophy was encapsulated in his 1790 oration, "The People's Misery—Mother of Diseases," and expounded in great detail in the six volumes of his *System of Complete Medical Police* (1777–1817). This monumental work was a widely known and influential exposition of the social relations between health and disease. Weaving together the noblest ideals of Enlightenment thought, enlightened absolutism, and pragmatic public health goals, Frank devoted his life to teaching Europe's monarchs that the people constitute the state's greatest wealth and that it was in the state's best interest to see that its subjects should be "as numerous, healthy, and productive as possible." Human resources could best be maintained through "rational hygienic measures" by combining the power of the state with the knowledge of the physician. For the welfare of the people, the physician must be responsible for the two branches of "state medicine": forensic medicine and the medical police who enforced the dictates of state medicine.

Even as a student, Frank displayed a profound "inner restlessness." He attended various universities in France and Germany before he obtained his medical degree from Heidelberg in 1766. When Frank became personal physician to the Prince-Bishop of Speyer, he began to test his ideas about a new social medicine by studying the conditions of the serfs and determining how the government could affect the health of its subjects. Among other things, Frank established a school to train midwives, hospitals to serve the poor, and a school of surgery. In 1779, Frank published the first volume of his *Medical Police*. Subjects covered included marriage, fertility, and childbearing. His next two volumes dealt with sexual intercourse, prostitution, venereal diseases, abortion, foundling hospitals, nutrition, clothing, and housing. Although these books made him famous, they did not please the Prince-Bishop. A position in the service of Emperor Joseph II provided better conditions for Frank's studies of medical practitioners and institutions, public health measures, and the condition of working people and peasants.

By the second half of the twentieth century the population explosion was recognized as a major threat to global economic and social welfare, but Frank was most concerned with the opposite problem. *Medical Police* reflects the economic and political concerns of the rulers of Austria, Prussia, France, and Spain, who were convinced that they needed more people for their armies, industries, and farms. The enlightened despot and his enlightened physicians understood that people could only be productive if they were healthy and able-bodied; in other words, the welfare of the people was the welfare of the state. Thus, no detail was too small to escape Frank's attention if it might conceivably affect the future fertility of the state's subjects. Medical police would be authorized to supervise parties, outlaw unhealthy dances like the waltz, enforce periods of rest, and forbid young women to wear corsets and other fashionable articles of clothing that endangered future pregnancies. If Frank's concept of medical police seems harsh, his definition of the qualities of the true physician reflects his belief that the most important qualities of the physician were the love of humanity and the desire to alleviate suffering and provide consolation where there was no cure.

By studying the lives of peasants and workers, Frank hoped to make physicians and philosophers see how diseases were generated by a social system that kept whole classes of people in conditions of permanent misery. Eighteenth-century social classes, as Frank knew them, consisted of the nobility, bourgeoisie, and paupers. The great majority of all people fell into the last class. Frank argued that one of the worst aspects of the impoverishment of the masses was the harshness of the conditions imposed upon peasant women and children. Pregnant women needed care and kindness in order to successfully carry out their duty to the state, that is, producing healthy new workers. Reports of the accidents that maimed and killed children left alone while their mothers worked in the fields prove that the past was not a golden age of prefeminist family life. Babies cried themselves almost to death with fear, hunger, thirst, and filth; sometimes pigs or dogs got into the house and attacked them; sometimes infants wandered out and died by falling into wells, dung pits, or puddles of liquid manure.

Other aspects of medicine and its place in eighteenth-century society are reflected in the changing pattern of medical professionalization in France. France entered the eighteenth century with a medical system steeped in traditional Hippocratic doctrines, which obscured a remarkably broad range of highly individualistic approaches to therapeutics. Dominated by learned physicians who endlessly debated abstract medical philosophies, medicine had changed very little since the Middle Ages. By the end of the century, French medicine had been transformed by two very powerful catalysts: revolution and war. Ignorant of medical philosophy, military men were known to say that many lives could be saved by hanging the first doctor found bleeding the wounded with his right hand and purging them with the left. Promoting the ideology of equality, revolutionary leaders denounced the old medicine as the embodiment of all the worst aspects of the Old Regime from favoritism and monopoly to neglect and ignorance. Ironically, the revolutionary movement that intended to eradicate doctors, hospitals, medical organizations, and institutions generated a new public health policy, better trained doctors, new medical schools, and hospitals which offered unprecedented opportunities for clinical experimentation, autopsies, and statistical studies. Hospital reform was especially difficult, costly, and painful, but the revolutionary era established the hospital as the primary locus of medical treatment, teaching, and research.

NUTRITION, MALNUTRITION, HEALTH, AND DISEASE

Although nutrition is generally regarded as a twentieth-century science, the belief that health and long life depend on the regulation of food and drink is one of the most ancient and universal principles of medical theory. Foods were generally classified in terms of opposing qualities such as hot or cold, moist or dry, which determined whether particular foods would be strengthening, weakening, purgative, or constipating. These concepts were not seriously challenged until well into the eighteenth century when the new chemistry sparked an interest in the *acidity* or *alkalinity* of foods, as we have seen in the work of Boerhaave. By the end of the nineteenth century these chemical distinctions were giving way to a new physiological concept of the role of food components in the animal economy. Since that time, nutrition scientists have lamented that the development of their field has been hampered, not by neglect, but by enormous amounts of misinformation, generated, at least in part, by its uniquely popular appeal.

The modern science of nutrition grew out of efforts to understand and isolate the dietary factors promoting health and preventing disease. Finding the causes of vitamin deficiency diseases was no simpler than unraveling the etiology of infectious diseases; indeed, both kinds of disorders often appeared in the form of devastating plagues and pestilences. Despite the accumulation of empirical evidence that specific foods could cure and prevent specific diseases, scientists could not unequivocally establish the existence of putative micronutrients without substantial progress in chemistry. Nevertheless, James Lind and other pioneers of nutritional science proved it was possible to prevent diseases by specific changes in diet. Although there are many vitamin deficiency diseases, scurvy is of special interest because the experimental foundations of our understanding of the disease are part of the abiding legacy of the eighteenth century. Scurvy may be among the most ancient and ubiquitous pestilences, tormenting its victims with rotting of the gums and teeth, deep aches and pains, blackening of the skin, and an overwhelming lassitude. Seeing whole monasteries, families, or armies afflicted with scurvy, ancient writers variously concluded that the disease was contagious, congenital, inherited, transmitted by scorbutic nurses, or generated by malign combinations of diet and atmosphere. Hermann Boerhaave considered scurvy a very infectious poison.

Scurvy was once known primarily as the devastating army sickness, but as sailing ships replaced oared galleys and long ocean voyages became possible, the old army sickness became the sailors' disease. Nostalgic visions of graceful "tall ships" notwithstanding, these vessels were more accurately called floating hells. The common sailor could expect accommodations that were dirty, damp, vermin-infested, and a moldy, monotonous diet of salt pork, indigestible oatmeal, and ship's biscuits.

Lord George Anson, to whom James Lind dedicated his *Treatise on Scurvy*, lost more than four-fifths of his men to scurvy during his voyage of circumnavigation in 1741. Deaths of mariners were so common that they were hardly worth noting; as long as one in five ships returned to Europe with a cargo of spices, the sponsors of an expedition could make a good profit. Between 1500 and 1800, scurvy killed more sailors than all other diseases and disasters combined; thus, it is not surprising that naval surgeons were among the first to provide good clinical descriptions of the disease and remedies to prevent and cure it.

Before obtaining his M.D. at the University of Edinburgh in 1748, James Lind (1716–1794) served as ship's surgeon on voyages to the West Indies, Guinea, and the Mediterranean. In 1758 Lind was appointed Senior Physician to Haslar Hospital, where he often saw more than 300 scorbutic patients a day. His lesser-known contributions to medicine include observations on tropical medicine, a distillation apparatus for making safe drinking water, and a remedy composed of quinine, spirits, and citrus peel which sounds like the essential summer restorative, the gin and tonic. A practical man, proud of his experience, but well read and reflective, Lind was ready to take exception to the most learned physicians of his day. While his contemporaries deferred to scholars like Hermann Boerhaave, Lind was not equally impressed. After reviewing scholarly writings on scurvy, Lind insisted that theories must stand or fall according to the test of experience. Clearly, Lind saw himself as more original and less gullible than Boerhaave and his disciples, who were censured for recommending a book on scurvy by a writer who claimed the disease was caused by sin and the devil. Scholars who attributed scurvy to a "very infectious poison" could not explain why no officers contracted the disease when it raged with remarkable virulence among common soldiers. Learned men who wrote about scurvy felt obliged to ground their ideas in theoretical rationalizations derived from classical authors. For the scholar, remedies were only of interest if theory explained their action. Similarly, if an idea was theoretically sound, no empirical tests were necessary. For example, according to Boerhaave, the blood serum of patients with scurvy was too thin and acrid, while the material that made up the clot was too thick and viscid. Therefore, it was the physician's delicate task to thicken and neutralize the acridity of the serum while simultaneously thinning the clot-forming portion of the blood.

Although scurvy took many forms, its characteristic signs were putrid, bleeding gums and blue-black spots on the body. Generally, the first signs of the disease were pale and bloated complexion, listlessness, and fatigue. Eventually, internal hemorrhages caused weakness, lethargy, stiffness and feebleness of the knees, swelling of the ankles and legs, chronic sores, putrid ulcers, and breathlessness following any exertion. Advanced cases were marked by coughing and pains in the bones, joints, and chest. Profuse hemorrhages and violent dysenteries reduced the patients to extreme weakness. During the last stage of the disease, Lind noted various anomalous and extraordinary symptoms, such as the breakdown of previously healed ulcers, chest pains, difficult respiration, and sudden death.

During two cruises of 10 and 11 weeks in 1746 and 1747, scurvy attacked the British frigate *Salisbury* with great virulence after only 4 weeks at sea. Although the captain generously provided the sick with fresh provisions, including mutton broth and meat from his own table, 80 of the 350 crewmen suffered from scurvy. Generally, the sailor's diet consisted of putrid beef, rancid pork, moldy biscuits, and bad water. Probably only a liberal allowance of beer, brandy, and rum could make such food palatable. While greens, fresh vegetables, and ripe fruits were regarded as preservatives against scurvy, Lind could not tell whether these foods were needed to counteract the bad effects of the moist sea air, or to correct the quality of hard, dry ship's rations. One hundred years previously, John Woodall (1570–1643), author of *The Surgeon's Mate, or Military and Domestic Medicine* (1636), called attention to the antiscorbutic virtues of lemon juice. Woodall's observations were interesting, but only anecdotal. It was Lind's special genius to test possible antiscorbutics with a controlled dietary experiment. A group of scorbutic sailors were put on a diet of gruel, mutton broth, puddings, boiled biscuits, barley, raisins, rice, currants, and wine. Two of the men were given a quart of cider a day; two were given *elixir vitriol* (sulfuric acid diluted with water and alcohol); two received rations of vinegar; two of the worst patients were given sea water; two received a combination of garlic, mustard seed, balsam of Peru, gum myrrh, and barley water well acidulated with tamarinds and cream of tartar; two others were given two oranges and one lemon per day. Within 6 days one of the sailors who had received oranges and lemons was fit for duty and the other was well enough to serve as a nurse. Lind's experiment not only demonstrated that oranges and lemons cured scurvy, it also showed that it was possible to test alleged remedies.

Proving that lemons and oranges cured scurvy was easier than convincing the authorities to utilize the information. There was no scientific obstacle to the eradication of sea scurvy, but it was essentially impossible for a naval surgeon to force his superiors to abandon the old prejudices and entrenched opinions which had been sanctioned by "time, custom and great authorities." The British Admiralty did not adopt Lind's remedy until 1795 when it proposed that lemon juice should be provided after 6 weeks on standard rations. The British Board of Trade did not require rations of lime juice in the merchant marine until 1865. Lemons did not become part of standard rations in the American Navy until 1812. Even without official blessings, some ship's surgeons included a kind of lemonade in their medical kit, but supplies of antiscorbutics were generally inadequate and unreliable. Army doctors ignored or rejected Lind's work and argued that a great many factors, especially a history of "evil habits," along with fatigue, depression, and bad food, could cause scurvy.

Apathy and ignorance only partially explain the failure of the medical community to call for the universal adoption of Lind's remedy. Although ship's doctors and sailors were well acquainted with the natural history of scurvy, confusion about the nature of the disease persisted into the twentieth century. Moreover, experience seemed to prove that scurvy had no single cause or cure. One argument against the dietary deprivation theory of scurvy was the observation that ship's cooks were often the first to die of scurvy. A certain degree of skepticism is certainly valid in the face of any claim for a cure too wonderful to be true. Indeed, marvelous health-giving fruits seemed more at home in a utopian fantasy such as Francis Bacon's (1561–1626) *New Atlantis* than in a medical treatise. In Bacon's allegory, the sickly crew of a lost British ship that landed in the mythical New Atlantis was cured by a fruit that resembled an orange. Physicians had heard of many equally miraculous cures from sailors and explorers, but some folk remedies were probably quite effective. For example, when Jacques Cartier's expedition in search of a northern route through North America was trapped by the ice during the winter in 1536, his crew was attacked by scurvy. Native Americans showed the French how to make a remedy from the bark and leaves of a certain tree. At first, most of the sick refused to try the Indian remedy, but it was soon in great demand. The French had to admit that all the learned doctors of France could not have restored their health and strength as successfully and rapidly as the Indian remedy. Other seamen and doctors ascribed antiscorbutic virtues to high morale, good food served with French sauces, water distilled over powdered scurvy grass, cleanliness, decent food, dry clothing, wholesome exercise, sour oranges and lemons, oil of vitriol, and periodic access to fresh land air. Many sailors believed that being buried in the earth up to the neck would cure scurvy.

One of the most distinguished and influential of all naval physicians, Sir Gilbert Blane (1749–1834), Physician to the Fleet, and personal physician to Lord Rodney, Commander-in-Chief, was able to implement reforms which ship's surgeons had long desired. Sir Gilbert earned the nickname "Chilblain" because his concern for the welfare of the common sailor was so well hidden by the reserved manner he exhibited towards his social inferiors. Throughout history, it had been taken for granted that armies would lose more men by sickness than by the sword, but in the eighteenth century new approaches to vital statistics provided disconcerting evidence of the human and economic toll. As Physician to the Fleet, Blane received a monthly report of the prevalence of diseases, mortality, and other matters related to health from every ship's surgeon. In order to improve the condition of Britain's sailors, Blane used these data to prepare his first treatise on naval hygiene. Later, in his *Observations on the Diseases of Seamen*, Blane advised the authorities that preserving the health of seamen was not only a matter of sympathy and humanity, but a form of enlightened self-interest spurred by economic and political necessity. As warfare and economic ventures required greater numbers of mariners, statistical methods proved that the state could not afford to waste its valuable stock of able-bodied men who were essential to the public defense and constituted the "true sinews of war." As a nation dependent on her navy, Britain had to realize that even if her officials thought of mariners "merely as a commodity," economic and political necessities should convince them that it was less expensive to maintain life and health than to support invalids and replace the dead. In 1795 Blane became Commissioner of the Board of the Sick and Wounded Sailors. As Commissioner, Blane sponsored many much needed reforms. After 1796, the incidence of sea scurvy declined dramatically.

The inexorable logic of numbers demonstrated that in the years before Blane's reforms were instituted, nearly every seventh British sailor had perished, while many others were permanently disabled. At the beginning of the war in America, one in 2.4 men became ill and one in 42 died; at the end of the Napoleonic wars these rates had been reduced to one in 10.7 sick and one in 143 dead. Blane calculated that if the mortality rate that had prevailed in 1779 had not been reduced, Britain's entire stock of seamen would have disappeared before the defeat of Napoleon. By 1815, although fevers, pulmonary inflammation, and dysentery continued to plague British mariners, sea scurvy had been nearly eradicated. Whatever expenses had been incurred in provisioning ships with citrus fruits were clearly offset by lower manpower costs. Dr. Thomas Trotter (1760–1832), another Physician to the Fleet, continued the battle for improving the health of sailors. In addition to dietary reform, Trotter recognized the value of inoculation against smallpox and became an early champion of vaccination. Indifferent to scholarly theories about scurvy, Trotter simply contended that fresh citrus fruits provided "*something* to the body" that fortified it against the disease and warned his readers to resist "imaginary facts and fallacious conclusions."

Despite lime rations, sporadic outbreaks of scurvy continued to occur at sea, while army surgeons fatalistically accepted scurvy as one of the pestilences of war, along with typhus, typhoid, and dysentery. Nevertheless, when a British naval expedition returned from the arctic in 1876 with the news that half the 120 men had suffered from scurvy, and four had died, the House of Commons called for an inquiry. Similar scandals caused doubt and confusion among scientists as to the nature of scurvy and antiscorbutics. In the 1870s physicians were surprised to find scurvy appearing among the children of middle-class families in London's suburbs. Unlike the poor, who relied on potatoes, wealthy people were likely to feed their children bread and butter and canned milk. In this case, we can see how some medical and hygienic advances solve one problem, but create unforeseen difficulties; the reduction in infantile diarrheas due to sterilization of milk allowed infantile scurvy to flourish. As more families switched to tinned milk, infantile scurvy appeared in both rich and poor families. Problems associated with artificial feeding continue to spread throughout the world as the manufacturers of infant formulas promoted the modern way to feed baby. A new class of adult scorbutics was created in the 1960s as Zen macrobiotic diets became more fashionable and more extreme; some followers of such dietary regimens consumed nothing but brown rice sprinkled with sesame seeds.

Many people living in climates more inhospitable than Europe were able to avoid scurvy through the ingenious use of plant and animal resources. For example, American Indians made teas and tonics from the needles, sap, or bark of appropriate trees, and the native people of Australia used a green plum with a high vitamin C content for medicinal purposes. Although cereals, peas, and beans lack antiscorbutic properties in their dry state, during their sprouting stage they are good sources of vitamin C. The value of bean sprouts has long been appreciated in the Orient. Although some groups of Eskimos were able to gather berries and others ate the vegetable material found in the rumen of caribou, for the most part the Eskimo menu was limited to meat and fish. Since vitamin C is present at low levels in animal tissues, it is possible to avoid scurvy by consuming fresh meat and whole fish without the niceties of cleaning and cooking.

Physicians and scientists generally agreed that the prevalence and severity of scurvy was related to dietary factors, but constitution, contagion, or climate were considered equally important factors. For example, Jean Antoine Villemin (1827–1892) attributed scurvy to a contagious miasma, similar to that which caused epidemic typhus. Villemin argued that even if fresh vegetables and lemons had some curative value, that did not mean that a deficiency of such items caused scurvy any more than a deficiency of quinine caused malaria. Russian physicians expressed a similar belief as late as World War I when they suggested that scurvy was an infectious disease spread by lice. A chemical theory reminiscent of Boerhaave's was proposed by Sir Almroth Wright (1861–1947) who argued that scurvy was caused by acid intoxication of the blood. Wright insisted that the direct administration of anti-scorbutic chemicals, such as sodium lactate, would restore the normal alkalinity of the blood more efficiently than lime juice.

As scientists attempted to determine the antiscorbutic value of various foods, they found that animal experiments often added to the confusion because different animal species vary in their vitamin requirements. An animal model for the systematic evaluation of antiscorbutics was discovered by Axel Holst (1860–1931) and Theodor Frölich (1870–1947) in 1907. Holst, Professor of Hygiene and Bacteriology at the University Christiana, Oslo, had studied bacteriology in France and Germany. He had also visited Christiaan Eijkman's (1858–1930) laboratory in the Dutch East Indies to learn about beriberi, a disease caused by the lack of thiamine in the diet. Searching for a mammalian model for beriberi, Holst tested the guinea pig. When he noted signs of scurvy, he enlisted the assistance of Theodor Frölich, a pediatrician concerned with infantile scurvy. Holst and Frölich demonstrated that scurvy in the guinea pig was induced by diet and cured by diet. If Holst had used the rat as his experimental animal, the story would have been quite different. Although some scientists considered the rat the ideal and universal model for deficiency diseases, unlike guinea pigs and primates, rats do not need vitamin C.

Experiments conducted on human guinea pigs in order to deliberately produce scurvy provided further support for Lind's hypothesis. His contemporary William Stark (1740–1770) was probably the first physician to attempt a systematic series of dietary deprivation experiments. Stark served as his own guinea pig. Weakened by a diet of bread and water, to which he had added tiny amounts of various oils, bits of cooked meat, and honey, Stark, with gums swollen and purple, consulted the great Sir John Pringle (1707–1782), founder of modern military medicine. Although Pringle had considerable experience with scurvy, instead of recommending fruits or vegetables, he advised a reduction in salt intake. Less than 9 months after beginning his experiments, Stark was dead. Had his eminent colleagues suggested oranges and lemons instead of venesection, Start might have recovered and provided further proof for Lind's thesis. In 1940, John Crandon, a young American surgeon, served as his own guinea pig in a study of the relationship between vitamin C deficiency and wound healing. Perhaps the most surprising finding in Crandon's experiment was that signs of scurvy did not appear until he had endured about 19 weeks on a restricted diet. In similar experiments conducted in England during World War II, it took 30 weeks to provoke signs of scurvy. Presumably, the nutritional status of twentieth-century volunteers was very different from that of the wretched sailors Lind described.

Although progress in bacteriology and surgery helped reduce the death toll from battlefield injuries during World War I, dysentery and deficiency diseases rendered some military units totally unfit for any kind of action. Using guinea pigs to test antiscorbutic diets, Harriette Chick (1875–1977) and associates at the Lister Institute carefully measured the antiscorbutic quality of various foods. These experiments finally set to rest many myths about scurvy and antiscorbutics. Surprisingly, not all varieties of lemons and limes were effective; moreover, preserved citrus juices were often totally useless as antiscorbutics. Nevertheless, as late as 1928 scientists still considered it possible that certain foods produced scurvy and that others functioned as antidotes.

Laboratory experiments and historical research on the antiscorbutics that had been used by the Navy helped to explain many paradoxical reports. While it may be true that "a rose is a rose is a rose," we cannot assume that "a lime is a lime is a lime." During the first half of the century, British Naval lime juice usually came from Mediterranean sweet limes or Malta lemons. In the 1860s the Navy began using lime juice from the West Indian sour lime; the antiscorbutic power of this lime is negligible. As a result of progress in nutrition, during World War II discussions about provisions for the armed forces focused on how to allow a safety margin against scurvy rather than emergency measures to combat epidemic scurvy.

Many researchers were actively pursuing the antiscorbutic factor, but it was the biochemist Albert Szent-Györgyi (1893–1986), who was not actually looking for vitamins, who discovered it. Although Szent-Györgyi began his career as a doctor, he had no interest in medical practice. The route that led to Szent-Györgyi's discovery of vitamin C was extremely circuitous. It began with studies of Addison's disease (a metabolic disorder caused by malfunctioning of the adrenal glands). One of the symptoms of this disease is darkening of the skin. Szent-Györgyi associated the bronzing of Addison's disease with the browning of fruits like apples and attempted to isolate the mysterious anti-bronzing factor from lemons and oranges. In 1927, Szent-Györgyi isolated a novel substance which he planned to call "ignose," meaning "I do not know," because it could not be chemically identified. When editors refused to publish a paper about "ignose," Szent-Györgyi suggested "godnose," but he finally had to settle for "hexuronic acid." Nutritional experiments conducted in collaboration with the American biochemist Joseph Svirbely in 1931 demonstrated that hexuronic acid was vitamin C. Szent-Györgyi was awarded a Nobel Prize in 1937 for his work on biological oxidation reactions and vitamin C.

Hexuronic acid was renamed "ascorbic acid" because of its role in the prevention of scurvy. Ascorbic acid plays an essential role in the final stages of the synthesis of collagen, a protein which serves as a kind of intercellular cement and plays a major structural role in connective tissue. Although Lind certainly did not know that vitamin C prevents and cures scurvy, he emphasized the fact that exhaustion, hunger, desperation—factors now known as stress—predisposed sailors to scurvy. The role of vitamin C in preventing scurvy is now clearly established, but the range of activities ascribed to this vitamin and the appropriate daily dosage for human beings have become controversial issues.

The mystique of vitamin C has grown exponentially since 1966 when Irwin Stone, an industrial chemist, made the claim that primates suffer from an inborn error of metabolism which could be corrected by consuming large amounts of vitamin C (about 4000 mg per day for an average man). Megavitamin therapy, also known as orthomolecular medicine, acquired some eminent spokesmen, such as Roger J. Williams, the discoverer of pantothenic acid, and the ingenious chemist and two-time Nobel Laureate, Linus Pauling. Vitamin C enthusiasts claim that it has anti-viral and anti-bacterial activity, lowers blood cholesterol, cures the common cold, and increases mental alertness, intelligence, and general well-being. Predictably, as AIDS hysteria mounted, reports appeared in San Francisco newspapers that the disease could be cured with megadoses of vitamin C. As early as 1982, when awareness of the new plague was just beginning, expensive vitamin preparations called "HIM" (Health and Immunity for Men) were being advertised to the "sexually active male" as a means of maximizing the ability of the immune system to fight infections and maintaining "sexual vitality and potency."

With so many "authorities" pushing megadose vitamin products for mental and physical illness, a hearty dose of skepticism and caution is necessary. The idea that if a little bit is good, a lot must be better does not fit the facts about vitamins; some may be toxic or teratogenic (causing deformity of the fetus) in large doses. Whether nutritional guidelines are based on the tradition of clinical observation or modern laboratory research, the history of scurvy indicates that the well-being of populations depends more on the politics of nutrition than the science of nutrition. The economic and political aspects of nutrition are most apparent in the continual rediscovery of the trinity of malnutrition, poverty, and disease. Advances in the science of nutrition proved that certain diseases, notably scurvy and pellagra, were not due to contagion or microbes and were not, therefore, a direct threat to those with adequate diets. During the late nineteenth century, the threat of infectious diseases and the development of germ theory diverted attention from other kinds of diseases. But today, in wealthy, industrialized nations the growing burden of chronic disorders has overshadowed the threat of infectious disease. By the 1970s the United States Congressional Office of Technology Assessment was chastising researchers for neglecting dietary links to cancer, stroke, hypertension, diabetes, and dental disorders. Although there is general agreement about the importance of nutrition for good health, physicians and researchers remain cautious when confronted with claims that the diet-disease connection provides an immediate panacea for the modern epidemic of killer diseases and chronic degenerative disorders attacking the wealthy industrialized nations.

SMALLPOX: INOCULATION, VACCINATION, AND ERADICATION

In the case of vitamin deficiency diseases, preventive measures were available long before effective means of control were adopted. A similar case can be made for the prevention of smallpox. Smallpox was not attacked on a global scale until the costs of safety for the wealthy exceeded the costs of eliminating the disease among the poor. The origin of smallpox is unknown, but it may have evolved from one of the pox viruses of wild or domesticated animals. Presumably, smallpox smoldered in obscurity for centuries among the innumerable local fevers of Africa or Asia until changing patterns of human migration, warfare, and commerce carried the disease to Persia and Europe, Central Asia and China. Smallpox probably made only sporadic incursions into Europe before the Middle Ages, but by the seventeenth century it had become "the most terrible of all the ministers of death." Smallpox probably accounted for about 10% of all deaths in seventeenth century London. James Jurin, secretary of the Royal Society, calculated that smallpox had killed 1/14 of the inhabitants of the London area during the 42-year period before 1723. While mortality rates were usually about 15 to 25%, during some epidemics 40% of those stricken with smallpox died. About 30% of all children in England died of smallpox before reaching their third birthday; smallpox, along with diarrhea, worms, and teething, was one of the inevitable crises of childhood.

Smallpox is usually contracted through the upper respiratory tract, but the virus may also be transmitted by clothing, blankets, or shrouds contaminated with pus or scabs. During an incubation period lasting about 12 days, the virus spreads to the internal organs and multiplies rapidly. After virus particles are released into the bloodstream, the first vague signs of illness appear. At this stage an accurate diagnosis is almost impossible because many illnesses begin with fever, aches, sneezing, nausea, and fatigue. By the time the characteristic rash appears, the victim may have passed the infection on to others. Within a week the patient may become a "dripping unrecognizable mass of pus," suffering from delirium due to high fever and giving off a putrid, stifling odor. Septic poisoning, broncho-pneumonia, ugly scars, blindness, and deafness were not uncommon complications, but the worst form of the disease, known as black or hemorrhagic smallpox, was almost always fatal. No medicine can cure smallpox once the infection is established, but ever since Rhazes separated smallpox and measles from other eruptive fevers, physicians have added to his ingenious prescriptions. Some physicians recommended opening the vesicles with a golden needle, while others prescribed a dressing of horse or sheep dung for smallpox and goat manure for measles. A few skeptics warned that the physician might be more dangerous than the disease.

Unable to afford the services of a physician, peasants in many parts of Europe attempted to protect their children by deliberately exposing them to a person with a mild case in order to "buy the pox" under favorable conditions. (Those antediluvian fossils who grew up before routine immunization against measles, mumps, and rubella may remember similar attempts to get children to catch these childhood diseases at a favorable time.) However, some folk practices involved methods more daring than passive exposure. Ingrafting involved taking fresh material from smallpox pustules and inserting it into a cut or scratch on the skin of a healthy individual. In China, the "flower-blossom disease" was induced by inhaling a powder made from the crusts of smallpox scabs. Experience taught illiterate practitioners in Africa, Asia, India, and Turkey that deliberately exposing their patients to a significant risk at a propitious time provided long-term benefits, but learned physicians tended to dismiss these practices as barbaric superstitions. During the eighteenth century increasing interest in natural curiosities led to closer scrutiny of many ancient folk practices including inoculation, or variolation ("inoculation" from the Latin *inoculare*, to graft; "variolation," from *variola* the scholarly name for smallpox).

Credit for transforming the so-called Turkish method from a curious "heathen custom" into a fashionable practice among the English elite is traditionally ascribed to Lady Mary Wortley Montagu (1689–1762). Lady Mary's husband Edward Wortley Montagu was appointed Ambassador Extraordinary to the Turkish Court at Constantinople in 1718. Among all the curious customs the inquisitive Lady Mary observed in Turkey, the practice of variolation was especially intriguing. In letters to friends in England, Lady Mary described how people wishing to "take the smallpox" arranged to share a house in the cool days of autumn. An inoculator brought a nutshell full of matter from the very best sort of smallpox and inserted it into scratches made at the appropriate sites. About 8 days after the operation, the patients took the fever and stayed in bed for a few days. To demonstrate her faith in the procedure, Lady Mary arranged to have the operation performed on her 6 year old son. Charles Maitland, the ambassador's physician, and Emanuel Timoni, the Embassy surgeon, were present when young Edward was variolated by an old woman with a rather blunt and rusty needle.

During the smallpox epidemic of 1721, Lady Mary was back in London. When she insisted on having her 4-year-old daughter inoculated, Maitland requested that several physicians be present as witnesses. According to Lady Mary, the physicians observing the inoculation were so hostile she was afraid to leave her child alone with them. After the pocks erupted, one of the physicians was so impressed that he had Maitland inoculate his only surviving child (all the others had died of smallpox). An avalanche of pamphlets and sermons was let loose by clergymen and physicians. In a particularly vicious attack on inoculation, the Reverend Edmund Massey denounced this dangerous and sinful practice as a malicious invention of the Devil. According to Reverend Massey, diseases were a form of "happy restraint" God sent into the world to test our faith and punish our sins. God might sometimes give man the power to cure disease, but the power to inflict them was His own. Reverend Massy feared that members of his flock might be less righteous if they were more healthy. In response to attacks on ingrafting, Lady Mary published "A Plain Account of the Inoculating of the Small Pox" so that ordinary people could learn about the methods practiced in Constantinople. Emphasizing the loss of clients that physicians would suffer if smallpox were eliminated, she argued that physicians considered the Turkish method a terrible plot to reduce their income. A funeral monument for Lady Mary in Lichfield Cathedral, erected in 1789, praised her for introducing her country to the beneficial art of smallpox inoculation.

Another advocate of inoculation, the Reverend Cotton Mather (1663–1728), also became interested in inoculation after learning of its use among "primitive, heathen" people. Mather was the author of about 450 pamphlets and books and the victim of a series of personal tragedies, including the deaths of two wives, the insanity of a third wife, and the deaths of 13 of his 15 children. Insatiable curiosity as well as an obsession with "doing good" drove Mather to seek knowledge of medicine and explanations for the "operations of the invisible world" from unorthodox sources, including Africans, Turks, dreams, and apparitions. In *The Angel of Bethesda*, a medical treatise not published until 1972, Mather suggested that the "animated particles" revealed by the microscope might be the cause of the disease. To maintain a sense of balance, we must also recall Mather's ambiguous role in the Salem witchcraft troubles, and his conviction that while sheep "purles" were medicinal, human excrement was an unparalleled remedy.

By the time John Winthrop's fleet of 17 ships set out for New England in 1630, smallpox had already exerted a profound effect on the peoples of the New World. The Spanish conquistadors had found smallpox a more powerful anti-personnel weapon than gunpowder. Colonists in North America discovered that the threat of smallpox to Europeans was modest in comparison to the devastation it caused among native Americans. Seventeenth-century settlers referred to the terrible toll smallpox took among the Indians as another example of the "wonder-working providences" by which the Lord made room for His people in the New World.

Of course even Old World stock was not exempt from the threat of smallpox. When the disease struck Boston, a city of about 12,000 inhabitants, in 1721, prayers, fast days, quarantines, and travel bans failed to halt the epidemic. Almost half the people of Boston contracted smallpox; of those infected about one in seven died. During this epidemic, Mather initiated the test of inoculation he had been planning since he first heard of the practice. Reverend Mather first heard about inoculation from a young African slave given to him by members of his congregation; Mather named the young man Onesimus. When Mather asked Onesimus if he had ever had smallpox, he answered "yes and no." Showing Mather the scar on his arm, Onesimus explained that in Africa people deliberately took a mild smallpox to avoid the more dangerous natural form. When Mather later read Timoni's account of inoculation in the *Philosophical Transactions of the Royal Society* (1714), he accepted it as confirmation of what he had previously learned from Onesimus. Mather was immediately convinced that he could rid the New World settlements of smallpox if he could secure the cooperation of the doctors. When smallpox appeared in 1721, Mather sent out letters to Boston's doctors asking them to hold a consultation concerning inoculation. Imbued with a firm sense of ministerial privilege, duty, and authority, Mather saw no impropriety in offering advice to townspeople and medical men, but his interference was resented by many New Englanders. The most dramatic statement of displeasure consisted of a "granado" thrown through the pastor's window. By the "Providence of God" the device failed to explode, allowing Mather to read the attached note: "COTTON MATHER, You Dog, Dam you, I'll inoculate you with this, with a Pox to you." Many proper Bostonians agreed with the sentiments expressed by the mad bomber and rejected Mather's strange ideas, whether they came from African slaves, heathen Turks, or the Royal Society. Of all the physicians Mather appealed to, only Zabdiel Boylston was willing to test the efficacy of inoculation. On June 26, 1721, Boylston tried the experiment on his own 6-year-old son, a 2-year-old boy, and a 36-year-old slave. The operation was successful. After performing more than 200 inoculations, Boylston concluded that this was the most beneficial and effective medical innovation ever discovered. Nevertheless, as word of his experiments spread, Boston became a true "hell on earth" for Mather and Boylston. Boston residents were shocked and alarmed by these unprecedented experiments; physicians denounced Mather and Boylston for imposing a dangerous and untried procedure on the community. Boston officials prohibited further inoculations.

Some ministers denounced inoculation as a challenge to God's plan, an invitation to vice and immorality, and an attempt to turn man to human rather than Divine guidance, but Mather and other ministers were the most zealous advocates of inoculation. William Douglass, Boston's best educated physician, opposed inoculation as a strange and suspect practice, and expressed amazement at the way in which clergymen reconciled inoculation with the doctrine of predestination. Sounding more like a theologian than a physician, he claimed that it was a sin to deliberately infect healthy people with a dangerous disease that they might not have contracted otherwise.

In reflecting on the turmoil in Boston, Mather asked the people of New England to think about how many lives could have been saved if the physicians had not "poisoned and bewitched" them against smallpox inoculation. Although Mather admitted that some people died after the operation, he reminded his critics that some people died after having a tooth pulled, while others casually risked their lives by dosing themselves with emetics and cathartics, or by smoking tobacco. William Cooper, associate pastor of the Brattle Street Church, simply said that it was proper to accept God's guidance and thank him for providing the means of averting a calamity.

As the epidemic died down, the fear and hostility aroused by Boylston's experiments also ebbed away. People began to ask whether inoculation really worked. Even a crude analysis of Boylston's statistical evidence provided strong support for the value of inoculation. During the epidemic of 1721, 844 had died of smallpox. Therefore, the mortality rate for naturally acquired smallpox had been about 14%. Of 247 people inoculated, only six had died. Of course, such crude calculations do not take into account many important complications, such as the problem of assessing the risk of acquiring smallpox naturally, nor the possibility that some of those inoculated had already contracted the disease, or were improperly inoculated and later acquired the natural disease. Today a vaccine with a 2.4% fatality rate would be unacceptable, but when compared to naturally acquired smallpox, the benefits of inoculation exceeded the risks.

Inoculation had important ramifications for medical practitioners and public health officials willing to accept the responsibilities inherent in this unprecedented promise of control over epidemic disease. As Benjamin Franklin so poignantly explained, weighing the risks and benefits of inoculation became an awesome responsibility for parents. In 1736, Franklin printed a notice in the *Pennsylvania Gazette* denying rumors that his son Francis had died of inoculated smallpox. Franklin was afraid that the false reports would keep other parents from protecting their children. The child acquired natural smallpox while suffering from a "Flux" that had forced Franklin to postpone the operation. In his *Autobiography*, Franklin reflected on the bitter regrets he still harbored about failing to protect Francis. Knowing that some parents refused to inoculate their children because of fear that they would never forgive themselves if the child died after the operation, he urged them to consider that uninoculated children faced the greater risk of naturally acquired smallpox. As epidemics of smallpox continued to plague New England communities, the isolation and recovery period required for safe inoculation tended to limit the practice to wealthy families. An inoculated person with a mild case of smallpox was obviously a danger to others. During the Revolutionary War, the British were accused of conducting "germ warfare" by inoculating agents and sending them about the country to spread the infection. With smallpox a constant threat to the army, General George Washington ordered secret mass inoculation of American soldiers in order to prepare an effective military force. Through such measures, smallpox gradually ceased to be "the terror of America."

Perhaps the greatest medical achievement of the Age of Enlightenment was recognition of the possibility of preventing epidemic smallpox. This achievement might be traced to the enthusiastic search for natural curiosities from around the world that was such a prominent feature of eighteenth-century intellectual life. In England, the Royal Society provided the primary forum for the discussion of such novelties, and its journal provided a vehicle for the dissemination of curious information. A perfect example of an inquiry into strange and exotic customs appeared in the Royal Society's *Philosophical Transaction* of 1714; it was Emanuel Timoni's "Account, or history, of the procuring of the smallpox by incision, or inoculation, as it has for some time been practised at Constantinople." Timoni's credentials were quite respectable; he was a graduate of Padua and a Fellow of the Royal Society. At about the same time, another description of inoculation was submitted to the Society by Jacob Pylarini. According to Timoni and Pylarini, the inoculator took pus from a favorable smallpox case by opening a pustule with a needle. The needle was placed in a clean glass vessel which was carried about in the inoculator's armpit or bosom to keep it warm. Several small wounds were made in a healthy subject's skin and a little blood was allowed to flow. The smallpox matter was mixed with the blood and the incision was covered with half a walnut shell. A magical or religious touch could be added by inoculating at several sites to form a cross.

Seven years after the appearance of these papers, a series of experimental trials were conducted, under royal sponsorship and with the cooperation of the Royal Society and College of Physicians, to evaluate the safety of inoculation. Six felons, who had volunteered to participate in exchange for pardons (if they survived), were inoculated by Maitland on August 9, 1721, in the presence of at least 25 witnesses. On September 6, the experiment was judged a success and the prisoners were released. As a further test, the orphans of St. James's parish were inoculated. These experiments were closely studied by the Prince and Princess of Wales (later King George II and Queen Caroline). The favorable reports led the Princess to submit two of her daughters to inoculation. Inevitably, there were some highly publicized failures which were exploited in the war of sermons and pamphlets disputing the religious, social, and medical implications of inoculation.

Advocates of inoculation believed that protecting individuals from smallpox was only the beginning. Matthieu Maty (1718–1776), who championed inoculation in England, France, and Holland, predicted that within 100 years people might totally forget smallpox and all its dangers. By the second half of the eighteenth century, inoculation was a generally accepted medical practice. Based on information reported by inoculators for the years 1723 to 1727, James Jurin calculated a death rate from inoculated smallpox of about one in 48 to 60 cases, in contrast to one death per every six cases of natural smallpox. Individual inoculators reported morality rates ranging from 1 in 30 to 1 in 8000; the mortality rate probably averaged about 1 in 200. Because inoculation was most commonly demanded during epidemic years, some of the deaths attributed to inoculation were probably the result of naturally acquired smallpox. Although inoculation probably had a limited impact on the overall incidence of smallpox, inoculation paved the way for the rapid acceptance of Jennerian vaccination.

EDWARD JENNER, COWPOX, AND VACCINATION

Edward Jenner (1749–1823), son of a vicar, was 13 years old when he was apprenticed to a physician. He obtained a respectable medical degree from St. Andrews, but preferred the life of country doctor to a fashionable London practice. Although he was often described as modest in both professional ambitions and intelligence, his mind was lively enough to maintain a life-long friendship with the distinguished anatomist John Hunter (1728–1793). Thanks to a study of the rather nasty habits of the cuckoo and Hunter's sponsorship, Jenner became a member of the Royal Society. In their correspondence, Hunter and Jenner exchanged information about natural history and medicine. Thus when Jenner became intrigued by local folk beliefs about smallpox and cowpox, he asked Hunter for his opinion of the hypothesis that inoculation with cowpox might eliminate the danger of smallpox. Hunter offered the advice that guided his own work: don't speculate, do the experiment.

In 1793, the Royal Society rejected Jenner's paper "Inquiry into the Natural History of a Disease known in Gloucestershire by the name of the 'Cowpox.'" Five years later, Jenner published *An Inquiry into the Causes and Effects of the Variolae Vaccinae, a Disease Discovered in Some of the Western Counties of England, particularly Gloucestershire, and Known by the Name of the Cow Pox.* In view of the medical profession's tendency to resist new ideas and methods, the fact that Jennerian vaccination had spread throughout Europe and the Americas by 1800 is as remarkable as the rewards and honors heaped upon the modest country doctor who championed the new technique. In the *Inquiry*, Jenner suggested that a disease of horses, called "the grease," was modified by passage through the cow and caused a disease in humans that was so similar to smallpox that it might be the primordial source of the disease. Because both men and women in Gloucestershire milked dairy cows, a man who had taken care of horses could transfer the grease to cows where it appeared as cowpox. Infected milkmaids noted lesions on their hands, along with symptoms of generalized illness. While the cowpox was a minor inconvenience, those who had the infection seemed to be immune to natural and inoculated smallpox.

Eighteenth-century standards of proof, medical ethics, informed consent, and clinical trials were, of course, very different from those of modern medicine. Jenner's evidence would probably intrigue, but certainly not convince, a modern scientist. In addition to compiling case histories, Jenner performed a few experiments on the transmission and effect of cowpox. For example, on May 14, 1796, Jenner inoculated 8-year old James Phipps with cowpox lymph taken from the hand of a milkmaid named Sara Nelmes. About a week later the boy complained of mild generalized discomfort, but within a few days he had completely recovered. When he was tested by inoculation with pus taken from a patient with smallpox, no reaction occurred. To distinguish between the old practice of *inoculation* with smallpox matter and his new method, Jenner coined the term *vaccination* (Latin *vaccinus*, relating to the cow). For the sake of convenience, and to distance his procedure from unwelcome associations

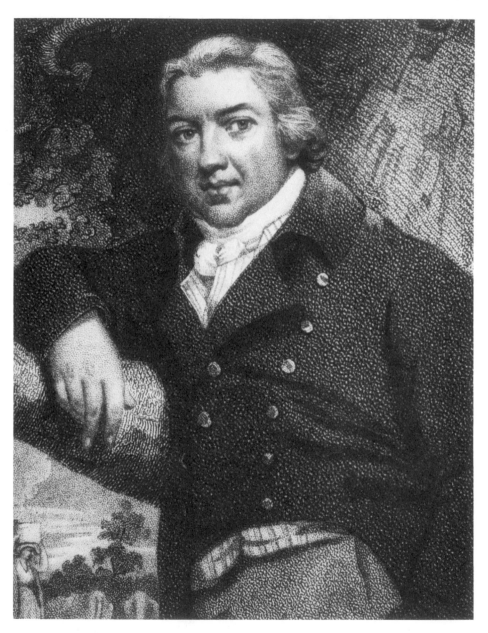

Edward Jenner

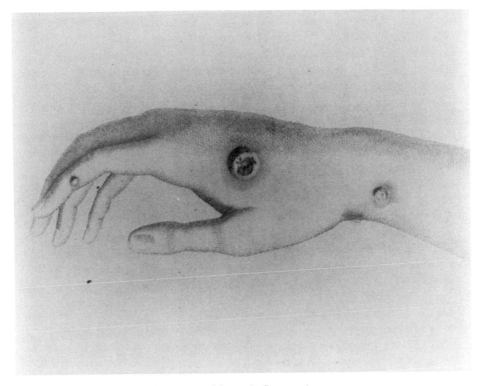

The source of Jenner's first vaccine

with "brute animals," Jenner proved that immunity could be transmitted directly from person to person.

Some of Jenner's contemporaries denounced him as a fraud and a quack and raged against the use of vile animal matter in human beings, while others called vaccination the greatest discovery in the history of medicine. Physicians, surgeons, apothecaries, clergymen, and assorted opportunists vied for control of vaccination. But maintaining control and conducting careful trails was all but impossible because recipients of the vaccine could use their own vesicles to vaccinate family and friends. Critics warned that transmitting disease from a "brute creature" to human beings was a loathsome, immoral, and dangerous act. However, experience substantiated Jenner's major contention: vaccination was simple, safe, inexpensive, and effective, and vaccination rapidly displaced inoculation. Within one brief decade enterprising practitioners had carried vaccination all around the world. Threads impregnated with cowpox lymph were generally the medium of transmission, but on long voyages vaccine was kept alive by a series of person-to-person transfers. At times the supply of unvaccinated orphans was so depleted that the chain of transmission was threatened.

In America, the case for vaccination was energetically promoted by Benjamin Waterhouse (1754–1846). Waterhouse was not the first person to perform vaccination in North America, but he was the first vaccinator to capture the attention of the public and the medical profession. Like many ambitious American doctors, Waterhouse studied medicine in Europe. His reward was a professorship of Theory and Practice of Physic at Harvard. Early in 1799 Waterhouse received a copy of Jenner's *Inquiry* from a friend. A few months later, under the heading "Something Curious in the Medical Line," Waterhouse published a brief note on vaccination in Boston's *Columbian Centinel*. After several frustrating attempts to obtain active vaccine, Waterhouse secured a sample and in July 1800 began experimenting on his children and servants. Waterhouse sent some of his vaccine to Thomas Jefferson, who vaccinated his entire household. In 1806 Jefferson predicted in a letter to Jenner; "Future generations will know by history only that the loathsome smallpox existed and by you has been extirpated." Although his prediction would not come true until the 1970s, Jefferson helped set the process in motion through his example and support.

Debates about the safety and efficacy of preventive vaccines have raged ever since the first experiments on smallpox inoculation and vaccination, experiments done long before the establishment of the sciences of microbiology and immunology. Many arguments about vaccination were more emotional than scientific: any interference with nature or the will of God was immoral; deliberately introducing disease matter into a healthy person is obscene; inoculations may appear to be beneficial, but the risks must ultimately outweigh the benefits. Other critics objected to the enactment of laws that infringed on personal liberty. For example, the British philosopher Herbert Spencer wrote: "Compulsory vaccination I detest, and voluntary vaccination I disapprove." On the other hand, Johann Peter Frank had no doubt that vaccination was the most important medical discovery ever made and that if all states adopted compulsory vaccination, smallpox would soon disappear.

Early attempts to measure the impact of preventive immunizations lacked the rigorous controls that modern scientists demand. Indeed, clinical trails performed in hospitals were often little better than purely anecdotal evidence. When a disease is widespread, it is difficult to compare experimental and control groups because some people in both groups may have had the disease or, in the case of smallpox, may have contracted the disease just before the beginning of the experiment. Despite uncertainty and protests, variolation was declared illegal and vaccination was made compulsory in the United Kingdom in the 1850s. The death rate from smallpox fell from the eighteenth-century level of 3000–4000 per million to 90 per million after 1872 when enforcement of the vaccination laws became more common. Nevertheless, Alfred Russel Wallace, English naturalist and co-discoverer of evolution by natural selection, denounced vaccination as one of the major failures of the nineteenth century. According to Wallace, the public health authorities were not only guilty of incompetence and dishonesty in their use of statistics, but had conspired with the medical establishment to cover up numerous deaths caused by vaccination. Reflecting the views of many Englishmen, Wallace asserted that those who promulgated and enforced the vaccination statutes were guilty of a crime against liberty, health, and humanity.

Many Americans must have agreed with Wallace, because in the 1910s epidemiologists were still complaining that the United States was the least vaccinated civilized country in the world. Individual states were almost as likely to pass laws prohibiting compulsory vaccination as laws mandating vaccination. A survey conducted in 1928–1931 found that more than 40% of United States residents had never been vaccinated. Enforcement of vaccination laws improved dramatically after World War II, and the risk of contracting smallpox within the United States eventually became so small that in 1971 the Public Health Service recommended ending routine vaccination. At that point, the United States had been smallpox-free for over 20 years, but six to eight children were dying each year from vaccination-related complications. Hostility to compulsory immunization never entirely disappeared; in the 1980s, opponents of immunization even claimed that vaccinia virus was responsible for the AIDS epidemic.

Vaccinia virus made the eradication of smallpox possible, but the origin of vaccinia remains as great a puzzle as the nature of the relationships among smallpox, cowpox, and vaccinia viruses. As demonstrated in the 1930s, vaccinia is different from cowpox; indeed, vaccinia can be defined as a species of laboratory virus which has no natural reservoir. Smallpox, cowpox, and vaccinia viruses are all members of the genus *Orthopoxvirus*, but they are distinct species and cannot be "transformed" into each other. Horsepox was extinct by the time immunological identification of particular strains was possible. Because cowpox and horsepox were rare and sporadic, virologists think that the ancestral pox was normally found in some wild species and was only occasionally transmitted to horses and cattle. Since the 1960s vaccines have been produced from three basic vaccinia strains maintained in England, America, and Russia. But the early trials of vaccination seem to have involved an uncontrollable mixture of viruses, with natural smallpox ever present, as inoculators took their material indiscriminately from cows and people, from primary pustules and secondary pustules of uncertain origin. Jenner claimed that vaccination, if properly done, produced life-long immunity, but immunity from vaccination, inoculation, and natural smallpox falls off with time and is variable in any population. Thus it is not surprising that different results were found among different populations, especially during epidemics.

After World War II, smallpox was no longer considered endemic in Britain or the United States. Nevertheless, imported cases continued to touch off minor epidemics and major panics. Because the disease was so rarely seen in England, Europe, and the United States, smallpox patients often infected hospital personnel and visitors before the proper diagnosis was made. Once a smallpox outbreak was identified, some cities launched heroic vaccination campaigns. During smallpox panics in the 1940s, newspaper and radio messages exhorted young and old: "Be Sure, Be Safe, Get

Vaccinated!'' In New York City, Mayor O'Dwyer set a good example by having himself vaccinated in the presence of reporters and photographers five times in 6 years. Although vaccination was supposedly required before admission to the city school system, public health officials estimated that at the outset of the 1947 outbreak only about 2 million of New York's nearly 8 million residents had any immunity to smallpox. Under the threat of an epidemic, 5 million New Yorkers were vaccinated within 2 weeks. This world record was achieved with the help of some 400 volunteers out of the city's 13,000 private physicians. The vast majority refused to help.

THE GLOBAL ERADICATION OF SMALLPOX

By the 1960s, for most residents of the wealthy industrialized nations, the odds of suffering ill effects from vaccination became greater than the chance of encountering smallpox. However, given the extensive and rapid movement of people in the Jet Age, as long as smallpox existed anywhere in the world, the danger of outbreaks triggered

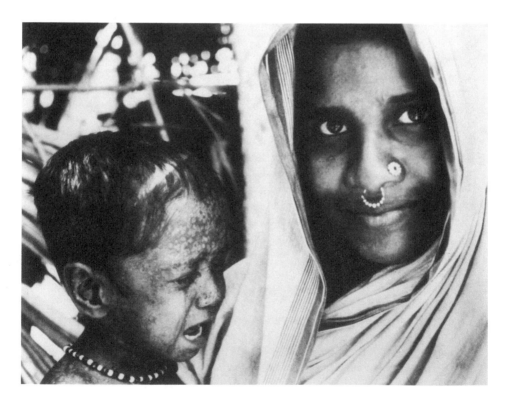

Smallpox in Bangladesh: the last of smallpox on the Asian subcontinent (courtesy of the World Health Organization)

by imported smallpox could not be ignored. For the United States, Great Britain, and the Soviet Union, the world-wide eradication of smallpox offered a humane and economical solution to the vaccination dilemma. Increasing certainty that there was no animal reservoir or human carrier state for smallpox made global eradication a practicable goal. The Smallpox Eradication Program was adopted by the World Health Organization in 1958, but the intensive campaign for global eradication was not launched until 1967 when smallpox was endemic in 33 countries and another 11 were experiencing only "imported" cases. Despite the availability of large stocks of donated vaccine, few public health specialists were optimistic about the possibility of eradicating smallpox from the world's poorest nations, with their negligible medical resources and overwhelming burden of poverty and disease. Surprisingly, within 4 years eradication programs in West and Central Africa were successful. During this phase of the global campaign, public health workers learned to modify their strategy in ways appropriate to special challenges. Originally, the smallpox eradication strategy called for mass vaccination using jet immunization guns that could deliver hundreds of doses per hour. Epidemiologists considered it necessary to target 80 to 100% of the population for vaccination. However, maintaining vaccine in hot, humid climates became a problem, as did maintenance of injector guns. Simpler equipment, like the bifurcated needle, proved to be more efficient. As a result of shortages of personnel and equipment in eastern Nigeria, public health workers discovered almost by accident that a strategy called "surveillance-containment" effectively broke the chain of transmission. By concentrating limited resources on the most infected areas, the new strategy proved effective even when only 50% of the population had been vaccinated. In October 1977, Ali Maow Maalin of Somalia became the last person outside a laboratory setting to contract smallpox. The case might have spelled disaster for the containment program; Maalin worked as a cook in a busy city hospital and his disease was first diagnosed as malaria and later as chickenpox. During the most contagious stage, Maalin had more than 160 contacts, but no other cases were found.

Although humanitarian motives were not absent from the decision to declare war against smallpox, there is no doubt that economic factors loomed large in the choice of this target. For developing nations, malaria and other tropical diseases caused more serious problems than smallpox. Most victims of smallpox die or recover within a matter of weeks, and in areas where the disease was endemic it was usually just one of many childhood illnesses. In contrast, malaria is a debilitating recurrent illness that reduces productivity, resistance to other infections, and the live birth rate. Global eradication of smallpox cost billions of dollars, but elimination of the disease will save at least one billion dollars per year that smallpox-free nations were spending to deal with the threat of imported disease. The December 1979 Final Report of the Global Commission for the Certification of Smallpox Eradication solemnly declared that: "The world and all its peoples have won freedom from smallpox." In describing the 10-year campaign led by the World Health Organization, Donald A. Henderson proposed the next logical step: what had been learned in the smallpox campaign should form the basis of global immunization programs for controlling diphtheria, whooping cough, tetanus, measles, poliomyelitis, and tuberculosis. Such global campaigns could transform the mission of health services "from curative medicine for the rich to preventive medicine for all."

Now that global eradication of smallpox has been achieved, the only reservoirs of smallpox virus are those remaining in research laboratories. The danger of maintaining such laboratory stocks was emphasized in 1978 when Janet Parker, a photographer who worked in the Birmingham University Medical School, died of smallpox. The virus seems to have entered rooms on the floor above the virus research laboratory through air ducts. Parker was hospitalized and diagnosed 13 days after becoming ill; she died 2 weeks later. The accident also led to the death of Henry Bedson, director of the virus research laboratory. After confirming the source of the virus involved, Bedson wrote a note admitting that safety precautions had been ignored and he committed suicide. Bedson's laboratory was due to close at the end of 1978 because inspectors considered it too old and unsafe to be used for smallpox research. With the threat of naturally occurring smallpox eliminated, fears have grown that the virus could be used as an agent of biological warfare. Smallpox has been called the ideal agent for germ warfare because the virus is stable, easy to grow, easily dispersed as an aerosol, and causes a terrifying, highly contagious disease.

SUGGESTED READINGS

Ackerknecht, Erwin (1967). *Medicine at the Paris Hospital 1794–1848*. Baltimore. MD: Johns Hopkins Press.

Altman, Lawrence K. (1987). *Who Goes First? The Story of Self-Experimentation in Medicine*. New York: Random House.

Altschule, Mark D. (1989). *Essays on the Rise and Decline of Bedside Medicine*. Philadelphia, PA: Lea & Febiger.

Ashburn, Percy Moreau (1947). *The Ranks of Death: A Medical History of the Conquest of America*. Ed. Frank D. Asburn. New York: Coward-McCann. Cambridge, England.

Bacon, Francis (1909). *The New Atlantis*. ed. by G. C. Moore Smith. Cambridge University Press.

Baxby, Derrick (1981). *Jenner's Smallpox Vaccine. The Riddle of Vaccinia Virus and Its Origins*. London: Heinemann Educational Books.

Beeuwkes, A. M., Todhunter, E. N., and Weigley, compilers (1967). *Essays on the History of Nutrition and Dietetics*. Chicago: American Dietetic Association.

Blake, John B. (1957). *Benjamin Waterhouse and the Introduction of Vaccination. A Reappraisal*. Philadelphia: University Pennsylvania Press.

Bowers, John Z. (1981). The Odyssey of Smallpox Vaccination. *BHM* 55:17–33.

Bruce-Chwatt, L. J. (1987). Malaria—From Laveran's Discovery to DNA Probes: New Trends in Diagnosis of Malaria. *Lancet* 2:1509–1511.

Burnet, Sir Macfarlane, and White, David O. (1972). *Natural History of Infectious Disease*, 4th ed. New York: Cambridge University Press.

Bynum, W. F., and Nutton, V., eds. (1981). *Theories of Fever From Antiquity to the Enlightment*. *Medical History*, Supplement No. 1. London: Wellcome Institute for the History of Medicine.

Bynum, W. F., and Porter, Roy, eds. (1988). *Brunonianism in Britain and Europe. Medical History,* Supplement No. 8. London: Wellcome Institute for the History of Medicine.

Carpenter, Kenneth J. (1986). *The History of Scurvy and Vitamin C*. New York: Cambridge University Press.

Chick, Harriette, Hume, Margaret, and Macfarlane, Marjorie (1971). *War on Diseases: A History of the Lister Institute*. London: Deutsch.

Comrie, John D. (1922). *Selected Works of Thomas Sydenham, M.D., with a Short Biography and Explanatory Notes*. New York: William Wood

Copeman, W. S. C. (1964). *A Short History of the Gout and the Rheumatic Diseases*. Berkeley, CA: University of California Press.

Creighton, Charles (1887). *The Natural History of Cowpox and Vaccinial Syphilis*. London: Cassell.

Creighton, Charles (1889). *Jenner and Vaccination*. London: Sonnenschein.

Crookshank, Edgar M. (1889). *History and Pathology of Vaccination*. 2 vols. London: H. K. Lewis.

Crosby, Alfred W. (1972). *The Columbian Exchange. Biological and Cultural Consequences of 1492*. Westport, CT: Greenwood Press.

Cunningham, Andrew, and French, Roger, eds. (1990). *the Medical Enlightenment of the Eighteenth Century*. New York: Cambridge University Press.

Cunningham, Andrew (1989). Thomas Sydenham: Epidemics, experiment and the 'Good Old Cause.' In French, Roger, and Wear, Andrew, eds. *The Medical Revolution of the Seventeenth Century*. New York: Cambridge University Press.

Curtin, Philip D. (1989). *Death by Migration. Europe's Encounter with the Tropical World in the Nineteenth Century*. New York: Cambridge University Press.

Dewhurst, Kenneth, ed. (1966). *Dr. Thomas Sydenham (1624–1689): His Life and Original Writings*. Berkeley, CA: University of California Press.

Dixon, Cyril W. (1962). *Smallpox*. London: J. & A. Churchill.

Downie, A.W. (1970). Smallpox. In *Infectious Agents and Host Reaction*, ed. S. Mudd. Philadelphia, PA: W. B. Saunders, pp. 487–518.

Duffy, John (1953). *Epidemics in Colonia America*. Baton Rouge, LA: Louisiana State University Press.

Edelstein, Stuart J. (1986). *The Sickled Cell: From Myths to Molecules*. Cambridge, MA: Harvard University Press.

Etheridge, Elizabeth W. (1972). *The Butterfly Caste. A Social History of Pellagra in the South*. Westport, CT: Greenwood.

Fenner, F., Henderson, D. A., Arita, I., Jezek, Z., and Ladi, I. D. (1988). *Smallpox and Its Eradication*. Geneva: WHO.

Frank, Johann Peter (1976). *A System of Complete Medical Police*. Selection from Johann Peter Frank. Edited with an Introduction by Erna Lesky. (1976). Baltimore, MD: Johns Hopkins University Press.

Goldblith, Samuel A., and Joslyn, M. A. (1964). *Milestones in Nutrition. An Anthology of Food Sciences*. 2 vols. Westport, CT: Avi Publ. Co.

Halsband, Robert (1967). *The Life of Mary Wortley Montague*. Oxford, England: Clarendon Press.

Headrick, Daniel R. (1981). *The Tools of Empire: Technology and European Imperialism in the Nineteenth Century*. New York: Oxford University Press.

Henderson, Donald A. (1976). The Eradication of Smallpox. *Sci. Amer.* 235(4):25–33.

Hirsch, August (1883–86). *Handbook of Geographical and Historical Pathology*. (Trans. by Charles Creighton from the 2nd German ed.) 3 volumes. London: New Sydenham Society.

Hopkins, Donald R. (1983). *Princes and Peasants. Smallpox in History*. Chicago: University of Chicago Press.

Hopkins, Sir Frederick Gowland (1936). *Discovery and Significance of Vitamins*. Smithsonian Inst. Annual Report, Washington, DC., 1935.

Janssens, Uta (1981). Matthieu Maty and the Adoption of Inoculation for Smallpox in Holland. *BHM* 55:246–256.

Jenner, Edward (1923). An Inquiry into the Natural History of a Disease Known as the Cowpox. *Lancet* 1:137–141.

Johns, Timothy (1990). *With Bitter Herbs They Shall Eat It. Chemical Ecology and the Origins of Human Diet and Medicine*. Tucson, AZ: University of Arizona Press.

King, Lester S. (1971). *The Medical World of the Eighteenth Century*. New York: Kreiger.

Kiple, Kenneth F. (1981). *Another Dimension to the Black Diaspora: Diet, Disease, and Racism*. New York: Cambridge University Press.

Langer, William L. (1975). American Foods and Europe's Population Growth, 1750–1850. *J. Social History* 8: 51–66.

Langer, William L. (1976). Immunization Against Smallpox before Jenner. *Sci. Amer.* 234: 112–117.

Lilienfeld, Abraham M., ed. (1980). *Times, Places, and Persons. Aspects of the History of Epidemiology*. Baltimore, MD: Johns Hopkins University Press.

Lind, James (1953). *Treatise on Scurvy*. A bicentenary volume containing a reprint of the first edition of "A Treasite of the Scurvy" by James Lind with additional notes. Ed. by C.P. Stewart and D. Guthrie. Edinburgh, Scotland: University Edinburgh Press.

Lindeboom, G. A. (1968). *Herman Boerhaave, The Man and His Work*. London: Methuen.

Lloyd, Christopher, ed. (1965). *The Health of Seamen: Selections from the Works of Dr. James Lind, Sir Gilbert Blane and Dr. Thomas Trotter*. London: Navy Records Society.

Lusk, G. (1928). *The Elements of the Science of Nutrition*. 4th ed. Philadelphia, PA: W. B. Saunders.

Macleod, Roy and Lewis, Milton, eds. (1988). *Disease, Medicine, and Empire. Perspectives on Western Medicine and the Experience of European Expansion*. London: Routledge.

Mather, Cotton (1972). *The Angel of Bethesda. An Essay on the Common Maladies of Mankind*. Reproduction of the 1724 manuscript. Ed. by G.W. Jones. Barre, MA: American Antiquarian Society.

McCollum, E. V. (1957). *A History of Nutrition: the Sequence of Ideas in Nutrition Investigations*. Boston: Houghton Mifflin.

McKeown, Thomas (1976). *The Modern Rise of Population*. New York: Academic Press.

Miller, Genevieve (1957). *The Adoption of Inoculation for Smallpox in England and France*. Philadelphia, PA: University of Pennsylvania Press.

Miller, L. H., Howard, R. J., Carter, R., Good, M. F., Nussenzweig, Victor, and Nussenzweig, Ruth S. (1986). Research Toward Malaria Vaccines. *Science* 234:1349–1356.

Morgagni, G. B. (1769). *The Seats and Causes of diseases*. 3 vols. English trans. by B. Alexander. London, 1769. (Facsimile reprint, Mount Kisco, New York: Futura, 1980.)

Morgagni, Giambattista (1984). *The Clinical Consultations of Giambattista Morgagni*: The Edition of Enrico Benassi (1935). Trans. and intro. Saul Jarcho. Charlottesville: University of Virginia Press.

Moss, Ralph W. (1987). *Free Radical. Albert Szent-Györgyi and the Battle Over Vitamin C*. New York: Paragon House Publishers.

Pauling, Linus (1971). *Vitamin C and the Common Cold*. New York: Bantam.

Pauling, Linus (1986). *How to Live Longer and Feel Better*. New York: Avon Books.

Pepper, William (1910). *The Medical Side of Benjamin Franklin*. New York: Argosy-Antiquarian Ltd., repr. 1970.

Perkus, Marion E., Piccini, A., Lipinkas, B.R., and Paoletti, E. (1985). Recombinant Vaccinia Virus: Immunization Against Multiple Pathogens. *Science* 229: 981–984.

Porter, Dorothy, and Porter, Roy (1988). *Patient's Progress. Sickness, Health, and Medical Care in England, 1650–1850*. Berkeley, CA: University of California Press.

Rather, L.J. (1965). *Mind and Body in Eighteenth Century Medicine. A Study Based on Jerome Gaub's 'De regimine mentis'*. Berkeley, CA: University of California Press.

Razzell, Peter (1977). *Edward Jenner's Cowpox Vaccine: The History of a Medical Myth*. Sussex, England: Caliban Books.

Reiser, Stanley Joel (1978). *Medicine and the Reign of Technology*. Cambridge, England: Cambridge University Press.

Riese, Walther (1953). *Conception of Disease: Its History, Its Versions, and Its Nature*. New York: Philosophical Library.

Roe, Daphne, A. (1973). *A Plague of Corn: The Social History of Pellagra*. Ithaca, NY: Cornell University Press.

Rosen, George (1974). *From Medical Police to Social Medicine: Essays on the History of Health Care*. New York: Science History Publications.

Salaman, Redcliffe, (1985). *The History and Social Influence of the Potato*. Ed. by J.G. Hawkes. New York: Cambrige University Press.

Schwartz, Hillel (1986). *Never Satisfied. A Cultural History of Diets, Fantasies and Fat*. New York: The Free Press.

Shiltz, Randy (1988). *And the Band Played On. People, Politics and the AIDS Epidemic*. New York: St. Martin's Press.

Shurkin, Joel N. (1979). *The Invisible Fire. The Story of Mankind's Triumph Over the Ancient Scourge of Smallpox*. New York: Putnam.

Smith, Alice Henderson (1919). A historical inquiry into the efficacy of lime juice for the prevention and cure of scurvy. *J. Army Med. Corps* 32:93–116, 188–208.

Starfield, Barbara et al. (1986). *The Effectiveness of Medical Care: Validating Clinical Wisdom*. Baltimore, MD: Johns Hopkins University Press.

Stearn, E. W., and Stearn, A. E. (1945). *The Effect of Smallpox on the Destiny of the Amerindian*. Boston: Bruce-Hamphries.

Stone, Irwin (1972). *The Healing Factor: Vitamin C Against Disease*. New York: Grosset and Dunlap.

Sydenham, Thomas (1848–50). *The Works of Thomas Sydenham, M.D.* 2 vols. Trans. by R.G. Latham (including a "Life of Thomas Sydenham"). London: The Sydenham Society.

Vogel, Morris J. and Rosenberg, Charles, eds. (1979). *The Therapeutic Revolution: Essays in the Social History of American Medicine.* Philadelphia, PA: University of Pennsylvania Press.

Wade, N. (1978). New Smallpox Outbreak Leads Scientist to Suicide. *Science* 201:1108.

Wade, Nicholas (1978). Biological Warfare Fears May Impede Last Goal of Smallpox Eradicators. *Science* 201:329–330.

Wedeen, Richard P. (1984). *Poison in the Pot. The Legacy of Lead.* Carbondale, IL: Southern Illinois University Press.

Whelan, E. M., and Stare, F. J. (1983). *The 100% Natural, Purely Organic, Cholesterol-Free, Megavitamin, Low-Carbohydrate Nutrition Hoax.* New York: Atheneum.

Whorton, James C. (1982). *Crusaders for Fitness: The History of American Health Reformers.* Princeton, NJ: Princeton University Press.

Winslow, Ola E. (1974). *A Destroying Angel: The Conquest of Smallpox in Colonial Boston.* Boston: Houghton Mifflin.

World Health Organization (1980). *The Global Eradication of Smallpox.* Final Report of the Global Commission for the Certification of Smallpox Eradication, Geneva, December, 1979. Geneva: WHO.

10

CHILDBED FEVER, MIDWIFERY, AND OBSTETRICS

The eighteenth century is of particular interest to philosophers, political scientists, demographers, and historians of medicine. Eighteenth-century philophers and scientists called their century the age of enlightenment, revolutions, philosophy, reason, and natural law. On a less exalted plane, it should be noted that during the second half of the eighteenth century, the population of Europe began a steep increase, unprecedented in extent, duration, and permanence. For the history of women and medicine, it is also a time of special interest. This is the time that puerperal or childbed fever first seems to have emerged as an epidemic disease, and it is the time during which medical men began to make significant inroads into the traditionally female domain of childbirth. As we have seen, eighteenth-century thinkers and physicians, such as Johann Peter Frank, believed that the greatest wealth of the state should be measured in terms of the number, health, and productivity of its subjects. The state could not afford to lose its peasants, workers, sailors, and soldiers to disease; moreover, it could not afford to lose its potential mothers. In an ideal state, women would be encouraged and enabled to carry out their duty to the state of producing new workers by the activities of the Medical Police and the Supreme Medical Board. Among the foremost duties of the Supreme Medical Board would be the collection of annual lists of birth and deaths from each town or village, in each district and province, and the careful analysis of the causes of excessive mortality, especially that of pregnant women, women in childbirth, postpartum women, and children.

It has been a tenet of historical demography and of many feminist writers that there must have been a causal relationship between the rise of epidemic puerperal fever and the development of a new medically oriented obstetrics, characterized by the "man-midwife" and the lying-in ward of the urban hospital. (The term "lying-in" refers to the confinement of women in the period before, during, and after childbirth. Postpartum refers to the period after birth.) Puerperal fever, or childbed fever, is generally and nonspecifically defined as a form of postpartum sepsis with rising fever that sets in after the first 24 hours following delivery, but before the 11th postpartum day. Although the term implies a causal link to the experience of childbirth, the definition provides no specific information about the etiology of the disease. Not all postpartum fevers and infections should be called puerperal fever; this makes the task of tracing the history of the disease and its possible causal connection to changes in patterns of fertility, use of lying-in hospitals, the rise of gynecology and obstetrics as areas of specialization within the medical profession, and the utilization of traditional female birth attendants and midwives very difficult.

In addition to its place within the larger history of women and medicine and the professionalization of the healing arts, the battle against puerperal fever can be seen as part of the story of the development of antiseptic surgery, because puerperal fever is essentially equivalent to wound infection. Even in the 1930s, before the introduction of sulfonilamide, puerperal fever remained the most important illness confronting the obstetrician; in the maternity wards of even the best American teaching hospitals, it was not unusual for at least 20% of the women to develop fevers after giving birth and for several women to die of puerperal infection every year. Once the fever set in there was little the doctor could do to help. One regimen adopted with great enthusiasm involved the copious administration of mercurochrome via vaginal instillation during labor and intravenously in infected patients. Probably the only effect was to turn both patient and bed sheets a bright red. Other useless cures included intramuscular injections of sterile cow's milk, blood transfusions, hysterectomy, and intravenous injections of alcohol.

Case histories in the Hippocratic texts indicate that puerperal infection was rare, but not unknown in ancient Greece. The transformation of a rare, private tragedy into a well-known, frequent, and much feared epidemic disease of lying-in hospitals seems to have occurred in the eighteenth century. Epidemics occurred at the Hôtel Dieu in Paris and in the newly established lying-in hospitals in the British Isles. Epidemic puerperal fever was first recognized as a specific disease in the eighteenth century and became the subject of special medical treatises. John Burton (1697–1771) and John Leake (1729–1792) were among the first to suggest that puerperal fever was contagious. However, Alexander Gordon of Aberdeen (1752–1799) and Charles White of Manchester (1728–1813) realized that doctors could carry the fever from patient to patient. White boasted that he had never lost a patient to puerperal fever, while colleagues who performed autopsies often lost several patients in succession.

OLIVER WENDELL HOLMES

In 1843, the American poet and physician Oliver Wendell Holmes (1809–1894) read a paper to the Boston Society for Medical Improvement entitled "The Contagiousness of Puerperal Fever." The audience response ranged from indifference to hostility, although the paper is now generally regarded as a clear, convincing, and logical argument concerning the transmission and prevention of puerperal fever. Holmes, the father of the famous jurist Oliver Wendell Holmes, Jr. had spent several years "yawning over law books" before taking up the study of medicine. After completing his medical training in Europe, Holmes combined private practice with various academic positions, including professorships at Dartmouth and Harvard. However, he first gained national attention with the publication of "Old Ironsides," the poem that gave him a taste for the "intoxicating pleasure of authorship."

A report on a fatal case of childbed fever presented at a meeting of the Boston Society for Medical Improvement piqued Holmes's curiosity about the disease. The physician who conducted the autopsy died of "pathologist's pyemia" (septicemia) within a week. Before his own demise he attended several women in labor; all of these patients were stricken with puerperal fever. Such a pattern suggested to Holmes that puerperal fever was a form of contagion which could be transmitted from one patient to another by the attending physician. To test this hypothesis, Holmes needed the kind of data that doctors were understandably reluctant to share—a record of patients who had died under their care, perhaps because of their care. Nevertheless, Holmes gathered evidence which should have been more than sufficient to convince a "Committee of Husbands" to demand that a practitioner be dismissed "after five or six funerals had marked the path of his daily visits."

America's foremost authorities on obstetrics consistently rejected the doctrine of the contagiousness of puerperal fever. Holmes' critics defended the "value and dignity" of the medical profession and denied the possibility that a physician could become a "minister of evil" carrying disease to his patients. Rather than acknowledge a personal role in the transmission of this disease, they attributed puerperal fever to chance or to God. But, because the disease followed particular practitioners and spared women attended by other practitioners, Holmes argued that it must be transmitted by contagion rather than miasma. (The term "contagion" refers to the agent of an infectious disease transmitted by touch or direct contact; the term "miasma" refers to poisonous vapors which were thought to arise from decomposing matter to infect the air and cause disease.) In other words, Holmes contended, the disease was connected with a particular *person,* who obviously had a vested interest in "denying and disbelieving the facts." Enraged by the intransigence of his colleagues, Holmes denounced them as self-righteous, ignorant men guilty of "professional homicide" and thundered a warning that for their voluntary blindness, interested oversight, and culpable negligence these pestilence-carriers of the lying-in chamber "must look to God for pardon, for man will never forgive him."

For many and complex reasons, given the longstanding debate about the nature of the transmission of disease, physicians denied the possibility that puerperal fever was contagious. Still, it is difficult to ignore Holmes's charge that at least a part of the learned debates could be reduced to a self-serving refusal to believe that a gentleman with apparently clean hands could be the agent of death. Steeped in these attitudes, doctors were a source of grave danger to their patients. This point is well illustrated by Dr. Warrington's account of how he had performed five deliveries shortly after conducting an autopsy of a puerperal fever case in which he had scooped out the contents of the abdominal cavity with his bare hands. All five women were stricken with puerperal fever. Another example reported by Holmes concerns an opponent of the doctrine of contagion who participated in the autopsy of a patient who had died of puerperal fever. For the edification of his students, Dr. Campbell "carried the pelvic viscera in his pocket to the class-room." That evening, without changing his clothes, he attended a woman in labor. This patient died. The next day he delivered another patient with the obstetrical forceps. This patient also died, as did many others during the next few weeks. A few months later, Dr. Campbell participated in another autopsy of a victim of puerperal fever after which he was called to attend two patients before he found time to properly wash his hands or change his clothes. Both of these patients died of puerperal fever.

Having presented his case for the contagiousness of puerperal fever, Holmes outlined methods of prevention. He thought it best that obstetricians avoid active participation in all post-mortems. If a physician had been an observer at an autopsy he should wash thoroughly, change every item of clothing, and allow 24 hours to pass before attending women in labor. A physician who had two cases of puerperal fever among his patients should give up obstetrics for at least one month and try to rid himself of the contagion. Finally, when a "private pestilence" appeared in the practice of one physician, it should be seen as a crime rather than a misfortune. Professional interests must then give way to the physician's duty to society. Even admirers of Holmes's ability to present a logical case in luminous prose have been dubious of his claim to the discovery of the cause and prevention of puerperal fever, on the grounds that Holmes was unable to compel the medical community to accept his doctrine. Others dismissed him as merely a worthy poet who had restated observations already made by Gordon and White. Holmes fought the battle against puerperal fever with no weapons other than logic and his eloquent pen, but no one ever accused his Hungarian counterpart, Ignaz Philipp Semmelweis, of excessive eloquence. Semmelweis, a man apparently lacking in even a rudimentary sense of tact and diplomacy, fought childbed fever with the blunt club of statistical and empirical evidence.

IGNAZ PHILIPP SEMMELWEIS

The life of Ignaz Philipp Semmelweis encompasses elements of heroism and tragedy more appropriate to treatment by a novelist than a historian. Born in Budapest in 1818,

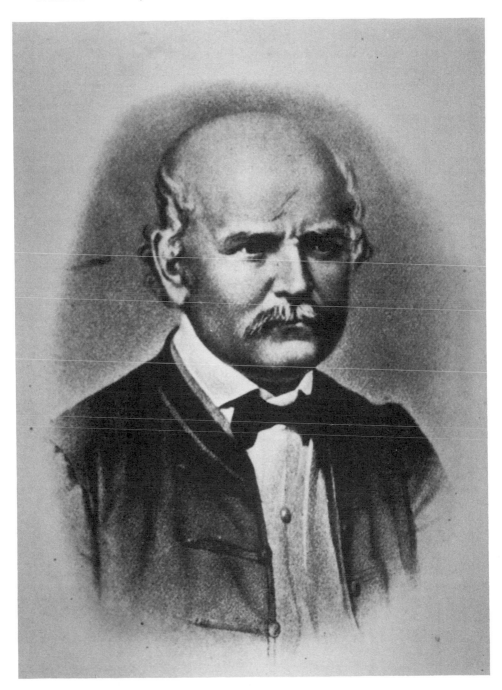

Ignaz Philipp Semmelweis

Ignaz Philipp Semmelweis was sent to Vienna to study law, but he soon transferred to the school of medicine. The University of Vienna, especially the medical school, at this time was aptly described as a hotbed of revolutionary activity, where senior, well-entrenched professors with close ties to conservative government officials were being confronted by younger faculty members with opposing views of politics, society, and scientific research. Semmelweis came under the influence of three of the leaders of the new approach to pathological and clinical investigation: Karl von Rokitansky, Josef Skoda, and Ferdinand von Hebra. Rokitansky, professor of pathological anatomy, had personally conducted some 30,000 autopsies. His prodigious efforts to bring order and system to the classification of disease through the study of internal pathological lesions led the great Rudolf Virchow to call him the "Linnaeus of pathological anatomy." After obtaining his medical degree, Semmelweis became assistant to Johann Klein, house officer of the First Obstetrical Clinic at the Vienna General Hospital.

The Vienna General Hospital had been quite large even in the eighteenth century when Johann Peter Frank described it as having many advantages over other contemporary hospitals in terms of space and suitable divisions for the isolation of certain contagious diseases. But even the Vienna Hospital did not have all the special departments Frank recommended; it did have a lunatic tower, a lazaret, small rooms for paying customers and pregnant women, and large sick rooms, with 20 or more beds. The purposes of the well-equipped hospital, according to Frank were: (a) curing poor, sick people; (b) perfecting medical science; and (c) educating good practitioners. Eighteenth- and nineteenth-century hospitals were generally far from ideal. Most faced major problems of overcrowding and lack of special facilities and resources. Contagious diseases become a major threat in a general hospital because of crowding and the difficulty of maintaining cleanliness and healthy air. Such conditions were especially dangerous to women in childbed. To protect new mothers from acquiring contagious diseases in the hospital, Frank stipulated that the lying-in ward should be quite separate from the general hospital. The lying-in ward should have three departments: one for pregnant women so that they could save their strength "for the coming ordeal"; the second should be dedicated to women giving birth; the third should be reserved for postpartum women. Postpartum women should be kept in small rooms with only two or three beds. Women who needed surgical intervention in birth should not be kept in the common labor room because the sight and sounds of such "artificial births" would have a bad effect on women in labor. The lying-in ward did not need rooms for the sick because postpartum women who became ill should be transferred to the general hospital. Unfortunately, hospital managers paid little attention to such costly recommendations.

In the 1840s, the Vienna Hospital provided medical researchers with a plethora of "clinical material"—patients forced by poverty, if not expectation of a cure, to use the hospital. Researchers and students could anticipate about 3000 childbirth cases and some 1600 autopsies. Thus, Vienna was a magnet for foreign medical students.

The founder of the Vienna obstetrical department, Lucas Boër (1788–1822), established the enviable record of a 1.25% maternal mortality rate among over 71,000 patients. Boër confined medical students to use of the phantom (a mannequin with uterus and birth canal), but his successor, Johann Klein, let students take an active role in examinations and deliveries. Moreover, Klein enthusiastically endorsed the idea that the dead should serve educational purposes. Therefore, the cadavers of women and infants who died in the hospital were used for demonstrations of the birth process. Klein's methods gave medical students better clinical experience, but maternal mortality soared to 10%.

During a period of expansion and reorganization, Klein divided the obstetrical service into two separate divisions: one was supervised by midwives training midwifery students. In the other division, medical students practiced under the supervision of physicians. Women in the second division were sometimes examined by five or more different students, who moved freely between the wards and the adjoining dissection room. From 1841 to 1846 the maternal mortality rate averaged 10%; during epidemic years, 20–50% of the maternity patients died of the fever. A 2–3% mortality rate generally prevailed in the midwives' section.

Unlike Dr. Klein, who was quite indifferent to the high death rate of women in his hospital, Semmelweis became obsessed by the suffering of his patients. Each day he examined every patient in his ward, demonstrated the proper methods for examining patients in labor, and performed operations. Before beginning work in the wards, Semmelweis conscientiously dissected the bodies of puerperal fever victims. During the first month of his assistantship, July 1846, the mortality from puerperal fever was 13.1%; in August it had risen to 18.05%. Ironically, it was not his systematic study of mortality rates, observations of patients, or diligent work in the dissection room that gave Semmelweis his flash of insight into the cause of the fever; it was the death of his friend Jakob Kolletschka (1804–1847), professor of forensic medicine. In 1847, while Semmelweis was on vacation, Kolletschka died of pathologist's pyemia from a minor wound incurred during an autopsy. Pyemia was a well known risk to anatomists. A small wound incurred during dissection might go unnoticed until redness, throbbing pain, and red streaks up along the arm announced the presence of a potentially fatal infection. When Semmelweis studied the autopsy report, he realized that the findings were nearly identical to those characteristic of death from puerperal fever. Kolletschka's massive infection had obviously been triggered by the introduction of ''cadaveric matter'' into a small wound caused by a dissection knife. Therefore, he concluded, *cadaveric matter must also be the cause of puerperal fever*. Few maternity patients underwent any surgical interventions, but after childbirth women were especially vulnerable to infection because, in addition to the trauma of passage of the infant through the birth canal, a large internal wound was created by the detachment of the placenta from the wall of the uterus. Just as the dissecting knife introduced cadaveric matter into the anatomist's bloodstream, the contaminated hand of the examining physicians carried cadaveric matter from the autopsy room to the laboring woman. As demonstrated by the persistence of "cadaveric odor," washing with soap and water did not entirely remove the contamination carried from the death house.

The insight gained from Kolletschka's tragic death was the foundation upon which Semmelweis constructed what he called his "doctrine:" puerperal fever was identical to wound infection and was caused by the introduction of cadaveric matter into the body. In opposition to almost all medical authorities, Semmelweis asserted that only his doctrine was consistent with the statistics and facts observed at the Vienna Lying-in Hospital. His major argument was that none of the prevailing theories could explain away the threefold difference in mortality rates between the First Division, staffed by medical students, and the Second Division, staffed by midwives. Actually, this threefold difference was an understatement because, whenever possible, women with the fever were transferred to wards in the General Hospital and their deaths were not included in the reports of the First Division. Very few patients in the Second Division were transferred to other wards unless they had a contagious disease like smallpox.

According to official medical dogma, childbed fever was caused by "atmospheric-cosmic-tellurgic influences" or an "epidemic constitution" that peculiarly affected puerperal women because of internal predisposing conditions, such as milk-fever, or a peculiarity of the blood associated with childbirth and lactation. Many complicating factors were suggested to explain away the differences between Division I and Division II. Some physicians blamed overcrowding for the high mortality in Division I, but Division II was actually more crowded. Semmelweis drew attention to another interesting correlation: in the midwives' ward long labors were not more fatal than short labors, but in Division I, women with long labors were especially prone to the fever. Women brought into the hospital after "street-births" seemed to be immune to the fever. (Hospital charity was formally extended to women and their infants in return for their use as "teaching material," but the hospital accepted women after "street-births" if the patient could convince the authorities that she had intended to be delivered in the hospital but was unable to get there in time. To avoid being used for "public instruction," some women employed a midwife before coming to the hospital.)

Hospital administrators blamed high mortality rates on the miserable condition of the poor, desperate, unmarried women who delivered in the hospital. While such a theory might explain the difference between charity patients in hospitals and private patients giving birth at home, it could not explain the difference between Division I and II. Another explanation attributed differential mortality to the shame women experienced when attended by male physicians. Ironically, delicate upper-class ladies were able to employ physicians, rather than midwives, without dying of shame. The fear inspired by the bad reputation of Division I was also cited as a possible factor in the genesis of disease. Semmelweis proved that statistical differences in mortality rates preceded the recognition that they existed. Moreover, he dismissed the idea that fear could produce the anatomical findings characteristic of both puerperal fever and pathologist's pyemia as patently ridiculous. The authorities attempted to blame the high mortality rate on injuries caused by physical examinations conducted by the foreign medical students who were accused of being particularly rough and coarse in their treatment of patients. Semmelweis protested that compared to the birth of a baby, manual examination, even by an uncouth medical student, hardly constituted a major trauma. Nevertheless, limiting the number of foreign medical students and the number of manual examinations per patient did produce a temporary decline in maternal mortality rates. The "doctrine" explained all these observations: The attempt to improve medical education by giving students clinical experience and anatomical instruction had produced ideal conditions for the transmission of puerperal fever. The foreign medical students, who had come to Vienna at great trouble and expense, were especially eager to use the cadavers and the "clinical material" available only in the great teaching hospitals of European cities.

To eliminate cadaveric particles, Semmelweis insisted that all students and physicians scrub their hands with chlorinated lime. As a consequence, the mortality rate in his Division dropped to about 3%. Contrary to popular belief, handwashing was not an unknown custom among nineteenth-century doctors. But the soap and water wash that might bring the hands to a state of socially acceptable cleanliness did not remove all the dangerous cadaveric matter. In 1848, the first full year of chlorine scrubbing, the mortality rate in Semmelweis's division fell to 1.27%. Nevertheless, the simple precautions Semmelweis suggested were not thought appropriate for a charity hospital. Professor Klein, who remained a bitter enemy of Semmelweis and his doctrine, accused his assistant of insubordination and other crimes.

For Semmelweis the discovery of the cause and prevention of puerperal fever was complete by the autumn of 1847; all further observations, including some experiments on laboratory animals, simply confirmed and extended the doctrine. The discovery of the cause and prevention of puerperal fever brought him a terrible burden of guilt. Driven by concern for his patients and the desire to understand the disease, Semmelweis had pursued pathological studies more diligently than any of his colleagues. Therefore, every day when he entered the clinic after his work in the autopsy room, he had carried with him the deadly cadaveric particles that caused the fever.

Unfortunately, even among his friends the doctrine was generally misunderstood as a simplistic attempt to link childbed fever to "cadaveric matter." Thus, some rather half-hearted attempts to test or duplicate Semmelweis's success by scrubbing after autopsy, or forbidding practicing obstetricians from conducting autopsies, were failures because of lack of attention to more subtle factors, such as disinfection of instruments, linens, dressings, and the isolation of patients with infections. Indeed, after Semmelweis had explained his doctrine to one foreign obstetrician, the Englishman replied that all this was nothing new. All English doctors washed their hands when they left the hospital.

Although Semmelweis had provided a practical system of antisepsis that could have prevented both puerperal fever and postsurgical infection, it would be wrong to assume that his discovery changed medical practice. Just as the term "classic" is generally applied to a book that nobody reads, the term "landmark" is applied to an insight that was largely ignored. To say that Semmelweis's discovery was a "breakthrough" would imply that after it was made, hospitals were significantly safer places for women. In reality, Semmelweis lost his sanity and his life in the battle against puerperal fever and prevailing medical opinion. Unwilling to compromise with corrupt and ignorant authorities, and lacking any talent for diplomacy, oratory, or literary exposition, Semmelweis destroyed his own career and made few converts to his doctrine. He also displayed a perverse sense of timing by establishing his doctrine just as a wave of revolutions swept through Europe; 1848 was a year quite appropriate for making a revolutionary discovery, but not a convenient time for a foreigner in Vienna to achieve the official recognition that could win the support of the medical establishment.

The resistance and apathy that greeted Semmelweis's doctrine and methods were due in part to medicine's conservative traditions, but his reluctance to publish his extensive observations also played a role. Declaring himself pathologically averse to writing, Semmelweis left the task of publicizing the doctrine to colleagues who overemphasized the problem of cadaveric matter. Since some hospitals boasted a 26% maternal mortality rate despite the absence of routine autopsies, the doctrine seemed irrelevant to their problems. Moreover, chloride of lime seemed too simple an answer to epidemics spawned by the ineluctable cosmic forces which had always absolved the doctor of responsibility for the fate of his patients. Without hope of professional advancement in Vienna, Semmelweis abruptly left the city and returned to Budapest. Not surprisingly, misfortune followed him—poverty, professional rejection, and two broken limbs within a year. The only ray of hope to fall into Semmelweis's life was his marriage to Marie Weidenhofer, a woman 20 years his junior. Their first child died within 48 hours of hydrocephalus; the second died when 4 months old of peritonitis, but two daughters and a son survived.

In 1861 Semmelweis finally overcame his aversion to writing, and published *The Etiology, Concept, and Prophylaxis of Childbed Fever*. Many physicians who knew of the "doctrine" from vague, secondhand accounts assumed that it had been discredited since 1848. Critics dismissed his book as the obsolete ravings of the "Pester Narr" (the fool from Budapest). Having finally accepted the burden of authorship, Semmelweis dispatched an avalanche of vitriolic pamphlets and open letters accusing his critics of having massacred mothers and infants. Citing the names of his enemies, he denounced them "before God and the world" as medical Neros, guilty of willful homicides. His depression deepened as he brooded upon the deaths that could have been prevented had his doctrine been accepted in 1848. His condition continued to deteriorate until his wife agreed to send him to a mental asylum where he died 2 weeks later from an infected wound.

Despite demonstrations of the value of the doctrine in the hospitals of Budapest and Vienna, few physicians were interested in the work of Semmelweis. Rudolf Virchow (1821–1902), the German "Pope of Pathology," initially rejected the doctrine in favor of the theory that pregnant women were predisposed to inflammations; not until 1864 did Virchow accept the concept of the contagiousness of puerperal fever. By 1880, as part of the Listerian system, rather than the work of Semmelweis, the doctrine was more or less incorporated into obstetrical practice throughout Europe. Shortly after the death of Semmelweis, Joseph Lister (1827–1912) began to publish a series of papers describing his antiseptic system. Although Lister later acknowledged Semmelweis as his "clinical precursor," Lister's immediate inspiration was Louis Pasteur's work on the diseases of wine and beer, not puerperal fever. Despite the work of Pasteur and Lister, the concept of a special "epidemic constitution" of parturient women was still blamed for puerperal fever well into the 1870s when Louis Pasteur announced his discovery of the probable cause of puerperal fever. Actually, the role of germ theory in the transformation of obstetrics and surgical practice is problematic. Oliver Wendell Holmes did not think that acceptance of germ theory was a prerequisite to the acceptance of the doctrine of the contagiousness of puerperal fever. Indeed, in the 1880s, he reminded his colleagues that he had given his warning and advice long before the advocates of germ theory had marshaled their "little army of microbes" in support of his doctrine of the contagiousness of childbed fever.

MIDWIVES VS. MEDICAL MEN

Of course puerperal fever was not always an epidemic disease and childbirth did not always fall within the province of the medical man. While women were almost universally excluded from the medical profession, the practice of midwifery was once exclusively theirs. Until very recent times, childbirth was considered a natural, rather than a medical event. When labor began, a woman sent for female friends, relatives, and the midwife. This "social childbirth" provided a support system in which women comforted the laboring woman, shared experience and advice, provided witnesses against accusations of infanticide, and helped the new mother through the lying-in period.

Throughout much of European history, religious authorities had exerted considerable influence over the selection of midwives; character and piety were essential criteria for obtaining approval. Midwives were forbidden to perform abortions or conceal a birth; they were expected to make the mothers of illegitimate infants reveal the name of the father. If the child seemed likely to die before proper baptism, a qualified midwife could perform an emergency baptism. Should the mother die in labor, the midwife might attempt baptism in utero or cesarean section. Witch-hunters considered midwives the most pernicious of all witches. Midwives were accused of

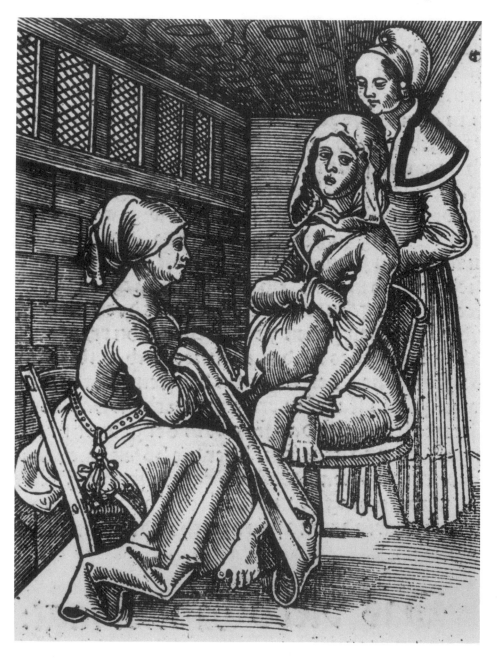

Midwives attending a delivery

inducing miscarriages and offering newborn infants to Satan. The products of miscarriages and abortions, stillborn infants, the umbilical cord, and the afterbirth (placenta) played a notorious role in the pharmacology of witchcraft. Given the midwife's low status and wretched fees, the temptation to engage in magic, sell forbidden materials, or accept bribes for family planning through infanticide, must have been overwhelming. Because of the biblical curse on Eve, midwives were forbidden to use drugs or magical practices to ease the pain of childbirth. Nevertheless, midwives trafficked in charms, amulets, and drugs said to relieve pain and facilitate labor. When discovered, the patient and the midwife might face heavy penalties.

As women became increasingly disadvantaged in terms of legal opportunities to study and practice medicine, those women who had served as healers were extirpated from historical memory. One example of this process is the treatment of Trotula, or Trota, of Salerno, in histories of medicine. There has been considerable disagreement as to whether Trotula was a professor at the University of Salerno and the author of major treatises on obstetrics and gynecology, or a mythical and somewhat ludicrous figure sometimes referred to as "Dame Trots." According to true believers, Trotula was a member of the faculty of the medical school of Salerno during the twelfth century, a period during which women were allowed to study and teach at this remarkable school. Two important obstetrical treatises, known as the *Trotula minor* and the *Trotula major*, are attributed to Trotula, but it appears more likely that she was actually the author of a general work on medicine. Simplified translations of the gynecological texts attributed to Trotula were treasured by generations of women. The *English Trotula* contains complex and bizarre remedies, advice about conception, pregnancy, and childbirth, and methods guaranteed to cure "wind in the uterus" and other female problems. The author suggested that skeptical readers test prescriptions on a rooster.

By the middle of the fifteenth century, secular authorities were beginning to displace the church in regulating the practice of midwifery. When labor did not proceed normally, the midwife, who was prohibited by law from using surgical instruments, was required to send for a doctor. Although the penalty for disobedience might be death, midwives apparently adapted common tools to suit their needs, as indicated by accusations that midwives used hooks, needles, spoons, and knives in difficult deliveries. Most midwives were illiterate, or too poor to buy books; only those working in large cities could expect to earn a decent income. Nevertheless, many medical men objected to the publication of midwifery texts in the vernacular. The earliest printed textbook for midwives, Eucharius Rosslin's *Garden of Roses for Pregnant Women and Midwives*, was first published in 1513; it was still in use in the 1730s.

A few women were able to emerge from the unlettered and unknown legions of marginal practitioners and issue strong calls for improvements in the training and status of midwives. In France, Louise Bourgeois (1563–1636) gained fame as midwife to the French Court. After retiring from active practice, Bourgeois spent her remaining years writing about the art of midwifery. Elizabeth Cellier, a seventeenth-century English midwife, was unquestionably a "fearless, ingenious, and energetic woman," but nineteenth-century male obstetricians considered her efforts to raise the status of midwives "unscrupulous." In a petition submitted to King James II in 1687, Cellier alleged that perhaps two-thirds of all infant and maternal mortality was due to a lack of skill among those who practiced midwifery. Cellier hoped the king would support a Royal Hospital managed by a corporation of well-trained midwives, but the College of Physicians easily suppressed this scheme.

MALE MIDWIFERY, OR THE EVOLUTION OF OBSTETRICS AND GYNECOLOGY

Soranus of Ephesus (98–138) was the first of the great Greek medical writers to be recognized as an authority on obstetrics and gynecology. The midwife described in the *Gynecology* was female, literate, familiar with medical theory, free from superstition, strong, sober, respectable, and dexterous. Obviously, Soranus expected the midwife to do much more than simply catch the baby. Although physicians from Hippocrates to William Harvey were interested in obstetrics and gynecology, they took it for granted that the practice of midwifery belonged to women. Even in the seventeenth century, the man-midwife was a controversial, menacing, but somewhat ridiculous figure. The doctor was only called for in cases of difficult or obstructed labor. Since "ocular inspection" was not allowed, the man-midwife operated blindly on a patient covered with sheets in a darkened room. Ancient misconceptions about the female reproductive system were closely linked to medical theories about conception, gestation, sex determination, and childbirth. Of special significance in the management of birth was the idea that the fetus, rather than the mother, was the active participant in this process. Since the laboring woman was regarded as the obstacle, the physician's task was to employ whatever tools were necessary to help the poor little prisoner in its struggle to escape from the womb. Nevertheless, as medical men challenged the midwives for control of childbirth during the eighteenth and nineteenth centuries, their claims were heavily based on their alleged possession of superior knowledge of female reproductive anatomy and physiology. Of course, much had been learned about the human reproductive system since the ancient Greeks described the uterus as a mobile, restless, two-chambered organ with an innate hunger for child-bearing. Still, there was considerable controversy over the morphology of the uterus, the function of the cervix, and the mechanism of labor in the early twentieth century.

A good example of the way in which authors create rather than recreate the past can be found in two books written by James Hobson Aveling (1828–1892), Physician to the Chelsea Hospital for Women and Examiner of Midwives for the Obstetrical

Society of London. Dr. Aveling's hagiography, *The Chamberlens and the Midwifery Forceps*, was written to demonstrate the great contributions of medical men to midwifery. In contrast, the stated purpose of his *English Midwives: Their History and Prospects*, was to call attention to female midwives and show the misery and damage that had resulted from their ignorance. In trying to explain just how low the midwife's status was, Aveling noted that she might even be called to aid cows that could not calve. However, in rural areas, where a cow might be considered more valuable than a wife, such a request was probably not taken as an insult.

Aveling claimed that the great William Harvey had rescued English midwifery from its place as the most despised part of the medical profession. It would be more accurate to say that it was a monopoly on the obstetrical forceps and large claims as to specialized professional knowledge that were responsible for male domination of the field rather than Harvey's remarkable studies of embryology. The origins of the obstetrical forceps are obscure, although the instrument seems simple enough in form and function. All that is known with certainty is that the "hands of iron" evolved from instruments of death. Before surgeons adopted the obstetrical forceps they could do little more than kill and extract an impacted fetus with knives, hooks, perforators, and lithotomy forceps, or attempt cesarean section on a moribund woman in hopes of delivering a live infant. By about 1720, medical men had several versions of the obstetrical forceps, with which they could deliver a live, if rather squashed baby. But the instrument had been invented at least 100 years before by a member of the Chamberlen family.

Just which of the Chamberlens invented the obstetrical forceps is uncertain, because of the family's obsessive secrecy and strange penchant for naming almost all sons Peter or Hugh. Between 1600 and 1728, four generations of Chamberlens enjoyed a lucrative midwifery practice because of their special instrument. The Chamberlens boasted that their skills in managing difficult labors far exceeded those of any member of the Royal College of Physicians. Not surprisingly, a state of war existed between brothers Peter the Elder and Peter the Younger and the College. Even after Peter the Younger's son "Dr. Peter" became a member of the College of Physicians, the battle continued. Dr. Peter's son Hugh was the first to write about the family secret. In 1673, Hugh referred to the great fear women had of seeing the doctor enter the lying-in chamber. Women believed that when "the man" came, mother or child would die. But, Hugh revealed, this need not be the case because the Chamberlens had, "by God's Blessing" and their own genius and industry, discovered a way of safely delivering the infants of women in difficult cases where any other practitioner "must endanger, if not destroy one or both with Hooks." Apologizing for not sharing the secret of his success, Hugh explained that he could not do so without financial injury to his family.

The secret of the Chamberlen forceps was finally revealed in 1818 when a cache of obstetrical instruments was discovered in a hidden compartment in a house once owned by the Chamberlens. The original obstetrical forceps had separable, curved, and fenestrated blades. After the blades had been inserted into the birth canal, one at a time, they were positioned around the head of the infant. The crossed branches were then joined and fastened with a rivet or thong. Aveling made the startling claim that among the forceps discovered in Dr. Peter's house was "doubtless the first midwifery forceps constructed by the Chamberlens, and from which sprung all the various forms now in use." How these instruments could have *sprung* from such a well-kept secret is something of a mystery. In any case, by the mid-eighteenth century several versions of the obstetrical forceps had been independently invented. Over the years, many variations on the basic instrument were introduced—some trivial, some futile, and some dangerous. Perforators and hooks on the handles of the instrument were employed when a forceps delivery was unsuccessful.

An early warning of the threat medical men would pose to midwives and their patients was issued by the English midwife, Jane Sharp, author of *The Compleat Midwife's Companion* (1671). Sharp argued that female midwives were sanctioned by the Bible, whereas male midwives were not, and that women should place greater reliance on God than on the College of Physicians. Although Sharp acknowledged that infant and maternal mortality rates were distressingly high, she refused to let midwives bear all the blame. Emphasizing the poverty and misery endured by the majority of women, she insisted that poor women needed meat more than they needed the services of physicians and surgeons. Poorly trained midwives and surgeons contributed to infant and maternal mortality, but malnutrition, crowded and unsanitary housing, contaminated food and water, bad air, and occupational hazards deserved equal honors, as demonstrated by the work of the leaders of the nineteenth-century sanitary reform movement. Although infant mortality averaged about 150/1000 live births for England as a whole, in working-class areas the rate was much higher. Where mothers were employed and drugs were used as "babysitters," infant mortality rates soared to 200–260/1000. Druggists sold hundreds of pounds of opium per year in the form of pills, elixirs, and soothing cordials. While mothers worked in fields or factories, their tranquilized babies were left at home to die of drugs, dysentery, and malnutrition.

Eighteenth-century moralists and journalists found the man-midwife controversy a wonderful source of salacious and titillating stories. Social critics warned that French dances, French novels, and male midwifery would lead to the complete corruption of female virtue, social chaos, and the end of civilization. The man-midwife was also the object of scorn within the medical profession, where all forms of specialization were regarded with suspicion. The College of Physicians was reluctant to allow obstetricians the rights and privileges of membership, because midwifery was a manual operation, foreign to the ways of learned gentlemen who should not stoop to participating in the "humiliating events of parturition." But to keep the spoils within the family, leaders of the College of Surgeons suggested that midwifery should be conducted by the wives, widows, and daughters of surgeons and apothecaries.

Critics charged the man-midwife with deliberately exaggerating the dangers of childbirth in order to turn a natural event into a surgical process for self-serving motives. Doctors were also accused of misusing instruments to save time and justify large fees. According to one English midwife, the man-midwife hid his mistakes in a cloud of scientific jargon so that confused patients thanked the man who had killed the infant and maimed the mother. Obstetricians cynically shared tricks for impressing the patient and avoiding blame. For example, if the doctor left during the early stages of labor, he should poke the patient intravaginally and tell her he was doing something to help the progress of labor. Thus, even if he was not present when the child was born, he could claim the credit if all went well, and blame the nurse for any problems. Some doctors admitted that factors other than the sex of the birth attendant might determine the outcome of labor. Dr. Charles White noted that sick, half-starved, impoverished, rural women served only by the worst sort of midwives might actually have a lower rate of maternal mortality than city women delivered in lying-in hospitals, or wealthy women attended by male doctors. In contrast, Dr. Samuel Merriman, Physician to the Middlesex Hospital, argued that women were totally unable to master scientific knowledge or use medical instruments. Since problems could develop suddenly, even in apparently normal labors, all cases should be attended by male practitioners.

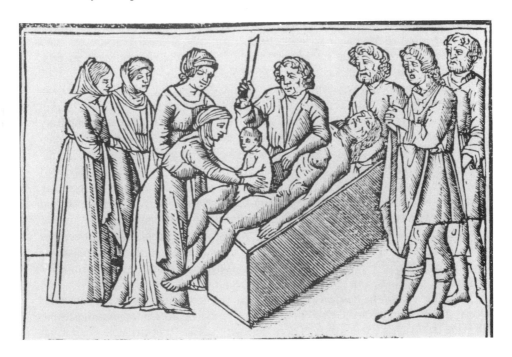

Cesarean section

Many doctors were willing to accept a class of midwives who would relieve them of unprofitable cases, but they would not tolerate women who might offer real competition. Members of the Obstetrical Society saw a clear division between the role of the midwife and that of the obstetrician. Midwives were proper for poor women, because they were stronger than rich women and, therefore, less in need of sophisticated medical assistance at childbirth. Midwives should be restricted to "the hard, tedious, ill-paid work appropriate for women" while medical men maintained a "manly and dignified position" in service to wealthy clients. Midwives were supposed to call for a doctor in case of abnormal labor, but doctors might refuse to take on a case begun by a midwife. Even in notorious cases at the beginning of the twentieth century where deaths had occurred because of the lack of surgical intervention, many doctors argued that such cases would teach the improvident to mend their ways, save their money, and call a doctor first. When potential patients realized that doctors would not to "cover" for midwives, these pesky competitors would disappear.

The outcome of the rivalry between midwives and medical men was obvious by the end of the nineteenth century; the smell of total victory was already obvious in Aveling's claim that the sordid history of the ignorant and incompetent midwife was drawing to a close. Nevertheless, the triumph of the medical man in the nineteenth century is an enigma. Certainly, "science" had not yet entered the lying-in chamber. The transition from midwifery to obstetrics occurred at a time when intervention was often performed by rough, inexperienced, surgically oriented practitioners, still concerned with strength and speed, uninhibited by considerations of asepsis. Moreover, the transition occurred in a period obsessed with "female modesty." The proper Victorian lady was expected to prefer death to a discussion of gynecological problems with a male physician.

Paradoxically, the most prudish societies of all were those which most completely accepted the new male-dominated obstetrics. It has been argued that the medicalization of birth reflected a deepened concern for the welfare of women. Alternatively, the paradox can be explained as a reflection of hostility towards women which generated a desire to punish them for their sexuality by the ultimate degradation: taking away their female support system and substituting the control of the male doctor who would transform the dangerous, unpredictable process of childbirth into a routine surgical operation. The argument that birth was a "pathological process," and that perhaps nature deliberately intended for women to be "used up in the process of reproduction, in a manner analogous to that of salmon," suggests a deep-seated contempt for women, or at least a lack of sympathy.

As the role of the hospital expanded in the eighteenth and nineteenth centuries, physicians in the great cities of Europe were able to gain the clinical experience that made it possible for the "hands of iron" to emerge as the "imperishable symbol and weapon" with which the battle between traditional female-centered births and the medicalization of birth would be fought. With the introduction of obstetrical anesthesia in the 1850s, the physician could add the promise of pain-free labor to his monopoly on obstetrical instruments. Forceps and anesthesia could make childbirth faster and less painful, but the resultant burden of injury and infection was a heavy price to pay. Critics warned that when the mother was under anesthesia the forceps were used brusquely and unnecessarily, causing profound damage to mother and infant. Often the damage was done simply because the doctor had not troubled himself to be sure that maternal tissues were not trapped within the locking mechanism of the forceps. On the other hand, doctors who took the precaution of passing a finger around the lock—a finger ungloved and probably unwashed—also endangered the patient. Although the poor and desperate women who served as ''clinical material'' in the hospitals of the nineteenth century had little choice in birth attendants, wealthy women increasingly chose physician-attended home delivery in the hope of safer and less painful deliveries.

During the mid-twentieth century childbirth moved out of the sphere of women's domestic culture and into the hospital. The trend towards hospital delivery had been accelerating since the 1920s. Before 1938, in the United States, half of all babies were still born at home; by 1955, about 95% of all births took place in hospitals where the laboring woman found herself ''alone among strangers.'' This transition has been called the most significant change in the history of childbirth, but it occurred *before* the medicalized hospital birth had actually become statistically safer than home births. Nevertheless, women chose hospital delivery with the expectation that the hospital offered experitise, new technology, freedom from pain, and increased safety for both mother and infant.

Ever since medical men gained a monopoly over the ''hands of iron'' and the ''potions of oblivion,'' the midwife has been an endangered species. Unlike chiropractors, optometrists, podiatrists, and dentists, the midwife never had a chance at the title ''doctor.'' In the 1960s and 1970s interest in ''natural'' approaches to health care and the Women's Rights Movement led to calls for a return to ''woman-centered childbirth,'' but the trend towards medicalization of birth had become so powerful that in the 1980s more than 25% of babies born in some American hospitals were brought into the world by cesarean section. In this context, the history of puerperal fever and midwifery is clearly only part of a complex transformation with respect to medical institutions, professional roles, social expectations, and concepts of the nature of woman. The man-midwife entered the female-dominated world of ''social childbirth'' as a surgeon, transformed childbirth into a surgical event in the physician-dominated world of the hospital, and created a new professional role for fellow practitioners as obstetricians and gynecologists.

SUGGESTED READINGS

Antler, Joyce, and Fox, Daniel M. (1976). The movement toward a safe maternity: physician accountability in New York City, 1915–1940. *BHM* 50: 569–595.

Arms, Suzanne (1984). *Immaculate Deception. A New Look at Women and Childbirth.* Westport, CT: Greenwood Press.

Arney, William R. (1983). *Power and the Profession of Obstetrics.* Chicago: University of Chicago Press.

Aveling, James Hobson (1882). *The Chamberlens and the Midwifery Forceps; Memorials of the Family and an Essay on the Invention of the Instrument.* London: Churchill.

Aveling, James Hobson (1872). *English Midwives: Their History and Prospects.* London: Churchill.

Barker-Benfield, G. J. (1976). *The Horrors of the Half-Known Life: Male Attitudes Toward Women and Sexuality in Nineteenth Century America.* New York: Harper & Row.

Benton, John (1985). Trotula, Women's Problems, and the Professionalization of Medicine in the Middle Ages. *Bulletin of the History of Medicine* 59: 30–53.

Bodemer, Charles W. (1973). Historical interpretations of the human uterus and cervix uteri. In *The Biology of the Cervix*, R. J. Blandau and K. Moghissi, eds., Chicago: University of Chicago Press.

Céline, Louis-Ferdinand (Dr. Destouches) (1937). *Mea Culpa and the Life and Work of Semmelweis.* Trans. by R. A. Parker. Boston: Little, Brown and Co.

Das, K. N. (1929). *Obstetric Forceps: Its History and Evolution.* St. Louis, MO: C. V. Mosby.

Declercq, Eugene, and Lacroix, Richard (1985). The Immigrant Midwives of Lawrence: The Conflict Between Law and Culture in Early Twentieth-Century Massachusetts. *BHM* 59:232–246.

DeLacy, Margaret (1989). Puerperal Fever in Eighteenth-Century Britain. *BHM* 63: 521–556.

Dennison, Jean (1977). *Midwives and Medical Men: A History of Interprofessional Rivalries and Women's Rights.* New York: Schocken.

Diulio, Rosemary Cline (1988). *Childbirth. An Annotated Bibliography and Guide.* New York: Garland.

Donegan, Jane B. (1978). *Women and Men Midwives: Medicine, Morality, and Misogyny in Early America.* Westport, CT: Greenwood Press.

Edwards, Margo, and Waldorf, Mary (1984). *Reclaiming Birth: History and Heroines of American Childbirth Reform.* New York: The Crossing Press.

Ehrenreich, Barbara, and English, Deidre (1973). *Witches, Midwives, and Nurses. A History of Women Healers.* New York: Feminist Press.

Enkin, Murray, Keirse, Marc J. N. C., and Chalmers, Iain (1989). *A Guide to Effective Care in Pregnancy and Childbirth.* New York: Oxford University Press.

Fisher, Sue (1986). *In the Patient's Best Interest: Women and the Politics of Medical Decision-Making.* New Brunswick, NJ: Rutgers University Press.

Forbes, Thomas R. (1966). *The Midwife and the Witch.* New Haven, CT: Yale University Press.

Gortvay, György, and Zoltan, Imre (1968). *Semmelweis: His Life and Work.* Trans. by E. Rona. Budapest: Akademiai Kiado.

Haller, John S., and Haller, Robin M. (1974). *The Physician and Sexuality in Victorian America.* Urbana, IL: University of Illinois Press.

Harris, Seale (1950). *Woman's Surgeon; The Story of J. Marion Sims.* New York: Macmillan.

Hartman, Mary, and Banner, Lois W., eds. (1974). *Clio's Consciousness Raised: New Perspectives on the History of Women*. New York: Harper and Row.

Holmes, Oliver Wendell (1892). *Holmes' Works*. Vol. IX. Medical Essays, 1842–1882. Boston: Houghton, Mifflin and Co.

Korbin, Frances E. (1966). The American Midwife Controversy: A Crisis of Professionalization. *BHM* 40:350–363.

Laufe, Leonard (1968). *Obstetric Forceps*. New York: Harper & Row.

Leavitt, Judith W. (1986). *Brought to Bed: Childbearing in America, 1750–1950*. New York: Oxford University Press.

Leavitt, Judith W. (1983). "Science" Enters the Birthing Room: Obstetrics in America Since the Eighteenth Century. *Jounal of American History* 70: 281–304.

Lesky, Erna (1976). *The Vienna Medical School of the Nineteenth Century*. Baltimore, MD: Johns Hopkins University Press.

Litoff, Judy Barrett (1978). *American Midwives 1860 to the Present*. Westport, CT: Greenwood Press.

McKeown, Thomas, and Brown, R. G. (1969). Medical Evidence Related to English Population Changes in the Eighteenth Century. In David V. Glass and D. E. C. Eversley, eds. *Population in History: Essays in Historical Demography*. London: Edward Arnold.

Moscucci, Ornella (1990). *The Science of Woman. Gynecology and Gender in England 1800–1929*. New York: Cambridge University Press.

Murphy, Frank P. (1946). Ignaz Philipp Semmelweis (1818–65): An Annotated Bibliography. *BHM* 20:653–707.

Nuland, Sherwin B. (1979). The Enigma of Semmelweis—An Interpretation. *JHMAS* 10: 255–272.

Oakley, Ann (1984). *The Captured Womb: A History of the Medical Care of Pregnant Women*. Oxford: Basil Blackwell.

Radcliffe, Walter (1967). *Milestones in Midwifery*. Bristol, England: Wright.

Rosser, Sue V., ed. (1988). *Feminism Within the Science and Health Care Professions: Overcoming Resistance*. New York: Pergamon Press.

Rosser, Sue V. (1987). *Teaching Science and Health from a Feminist Perspective*. New York: Pergamon Press.

Rothman, Barbara Katz (1982). *In Labor: Women and Power in the Birthplace*. New York: W. W. Norton.

Rowland, Beryl, ed. (1981). *Medieval Woman's Guide to Health: The First English Gynecological Handbook*. Middle English Text, with Intro. and modern English trans. Kent, OH: Kent State University Press.

Schnorrenberg, Barbara Brandon (1981). Is Childbirth Any Place for a Woman? The Decline of Midwifery in 18th Century England. *Studies in Eighteenth Century Culture* 10: 393–408.

Semmelweis, Ignaz (1983). *The Etiology, Concept, and Prophylaxis of Childbed Fever*. Trans., ed., introductory essay by K. Codell Carter. Madison, WI: University of Wisconsin Press.

Shorter, Edward (1982). *A History of Women's Bodies*. New York: Basic Books.

Shryock, Richard H. (1967). *Medical Licensing in America, 1650–1965*. Baltimore, MD: Johns Hopkins University Press.

Sinclair, William J. (1909). *Semmelweis, His Life and Doctrine*. Manchester, England: Manchester University Press.

Slaughter, Frank G. (1950). *Immortal Magyar. Semmelweis, Conqueror of Childbed Fever*. New York: Henry Schuman.

Smith, F. B. (1979). *The People's Health 1830–1910*. New York: Holmes & Meier.

Soranus, (1956). *Soranus' Gynecology*. Trans. by O. Temkin. Baltimore, MD: Johns Hopkins University Press.

Stotland, Nada Logan (1988). *Social Change and Women's Reproductive Health Care: A Guide for Physicians and Their Patients*. Westport, CT: Greenwood Press.

Towler, Jean, and Bramall, Joan (1986). *Midwives in History and Society*. New York: Routledge, Chapman & Hall.

Walsh, Mary Roth (1977). *Doctors Wanted: No Women Need Apply*. New Haven, CT: Yale University Press.

Wertz, Richard W., and Wertz, Dorothy C. (1977). *Lying-in. A History of Childbirth in America: Its Technologies and Social Relations*. New York: Free Press.

White, Charles (1773). *A Treatise on the Management of Pregnant and Lying-in Women and the Means of Curing, More Especially of Preventing the Principal Disorders to Which They Are Liable*. Repr., Canton, MA: Science History Publications, 1986.

Yong, Diony, ed. (1983). *Obstetrical Intervention and Technology in the 1980s*. New York: Haworth Press.

Young, J. H. (1944). *Cesarean Section, the History and Development of the Operation from Earliest Times*. London: H.K. Lewis.

THE ART AND SCIENCE OF SURGERY

odern surgery has evolved from one of the most despised branches of medicine
into one of the most respected, most powerful, and best compensated areas of
medical specialization. The transformation seems to have occurred with remarkable
speed once surgeons were given the tools to overcome two of the greatest obstacles
to major operative procedures: pain and infection. General anesthesia was introduced
in the 1840s and antisepsis in the 1870s. A closer examination of the evolution of
surgery, however, suggests a more complex explanation for the remarkable
transformation that occurred in the nineteenth century. First of all, surgeons could
point to a long history of successes, if not in major operative procedures, then, at least,
in the treatment of wounds, ulcers, skin diseases, fractures, dislocations, and so forth.
In comparison to the treatment of internal diseases by physicians, the surgeons who
treated traumatic injuries, urinary disorders, and venereal diseases had good reason
to boast of the efficacy of their methods. Indeed, it can be argued that as surgeons
used their claims of expertise and knowledge to close the gap between medicine and
surgery, they established the basis for the professionalization and modernization of
a powerful, unified, and inclusive medical profession.

Taking a broader view of surgery, the remarkable progress made between about
1700 and 1830 can be largely attributed to the work of inventive and courageous
surgeons, better education and practical training, and above all, to advances in
anatomy and physiology. Even when allegiance to humoral pathology was all-
pervasive, the surgical point of view had to focus more narrowly and pragmatically

on a localized lesion. As the study of correlations between the course of disease in the living and pathological lesions in the dead gained support, physicians increasingly accepted the validity of a localized pathology. Surgery gained much from the researches of physicians, but also contributed an empirical, anatomically based point of view which was to have important ramifications for medicine as a whole.

ANESTHESIA

During the eighteenth century, progress in anatomical investigation and the acceptance of a localized, lesion-based, or solidistic approach to pathology provided an intellectual framework for advances in surgery. However, from the patient's point of view, pain was a powerful reason for avoiding even the most desperately needed operation. Despite the fact that narcotics have been used in rituals and recreation for thousands of years, Oliver Wendell Holmes reflected conventional medical wisdom when he said that nature offered only three natural anesthetics: sleep, fainting, and death. Experimentation with mind- and mood-altering substances is older than agriculture, but the potions prepared for ceremonial, religious, or social purposes were rarely used for the relief of surgical pain. Perhaps the powerful religious associations of intoxicants militated against their use as secular anesthetics. On the other hand, the magical agents used in ceremonies culminating in ecstasy and self-mutilation might have worked primarily through the power of suggestion. If the potion did not work, the user was to blame for lack of faith.

Thus, it is unreasonable to assume that the preparations used to induce ceremonial intoxication would satisfy the criteria for anesthetic agents considered essential by nineteenth-century surgeons: relief of pain must be *inevitable, complete*, and *safe*. Drugs that are appropriate for ceremonial purposes might cause unpredictable and dangerous effects in a person undergoing surgery. As twentieth-century statistics for deaths due to drug overdoses indicate, people are willing to take risks with "recreational drugs" that they would not find acceptable in medical procedures. In the religious context, death was in the hands of the gods; in the operating room, the responsibility belonged to the surgeon.

If anesthetics are "tamed inebrients," then alcohol should have been the drug of choice for surgery. Alcoholic preparations have been used as the "potion of the condemned" and in preparation for ceremonial tribal rites, such as circumcision and scarification. Unfortunately, the large doses of alcohol needed to induce stupefaction are likely to cause nausea, vomiting, and death instead of sleep. Healers could also try to induce what might be called a state of psychological anesthesia by means of mesmerism, hypnotism, shamanistic rituals, prayers, and the symbolic transference of pain to an animal or inanimate item. Such methods might not be inevitable and complete, but a mixture of hope and faith is likely to be safer than complex mixtures of drugs and alcohol. Various forms of self-hypnosis were used in India, but these

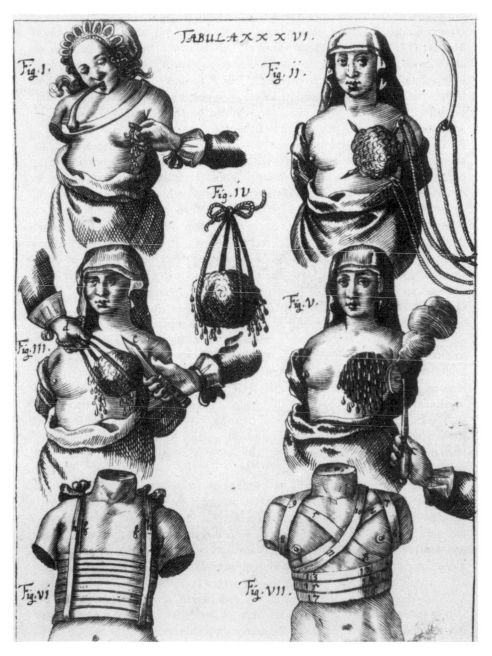

Mastectomy procedures depicted in a 1666 text by Johann Schultes (1595–1645)

practices require high levels of training, concentration, and self-discipline. The best known European version of psychological anesthesia was developed by Anton Mesmer (1734–1815). Although Mesmer's methods were criticized by physicians and exposed as fraudulent by skeptical scientists, "sensitive" patients were easily put into a somnambulistic state by Mesmer's "animal magnetism." Mesmerism and hypnotism have been so closely associated with quackery that impartial evaluation is difficult. The term "hypnotism" was coined by James Braid (1795–1860) to separate the scientific study of "nervous sleep" from spiritualism and quackery. Braid argued that mesmerism was a subjective condition that depended on the suggestibility of the patient. Nevertheless, it could produce a state of somnambulism deep enough to overcome the pain of surgical operations. To demonstrate the power of this technique, the French "midwifery mesmerist" Charles Lafontaine mesmerized women in a lying-in hospital and a lion at the zoo.

By the time European physicians began to take hypnotism seriously, the triumph of inhalation anesthesia was virtually complete. Somewhat out of phase with the tides of history, John Elliotson (1791–1868), lecturer on medicine at the University of London, founded a hospital for studies of mesmerism. He reported that even amputations at the thigh could be carried out under hypnotism. Dr. James Esdaile (1808–1859), who became interested in mesmerism while working in India, claimed to have had a mortality rate of only 5 1/2% in 261 operations performed under mesmerism. Unfortunately, when he returned to Scotland in 1851, he found that mesmerism did not work as well as it had in India. Eventually, hypnotism proved to be more significant in the development of psychoanalysis than in surgical anesthesia. The Parisian neurologist Jean Martin Charcot (1825–1893) used hypnotism in his clinical studies of hysteria, but considered the hypnotic state pathological in itself. Recent studies of the neuroendocrinology of pain may help explain the mechanism of hypnotism. Surprisingly, although hypnotism has generally been denigrated as "mere suggestion," it is more likely to ameliorate "real" pain than "imaginary" pain.

A direct, but crude way of inducing a state of insensitivity was to knock the patient unconscious with a blow to the jaw. This technique is not very specific or complete, but the surgeon might be able to extract a bullet before his patient recovered from the shock. Distraction could also be achieved by rubbing the patient with counterirritants such as stinging nettles. Pressure applied to nerves or arteries can induce insensitivity to pain, as well as asphyxia and death. Even phlebotomy could act as a pain-killer when it was carried out aggressively enough to induce fainting. Such bleedings were used in preparation for childbirth, reducing dislocations, and setting fractures. Traditional methods were too unpredictable to fit the criteria for modern surgical anesthesia. Thus, the search for a safe and effective agent takes us back to the world of drug lore and chemical experimentation.

Mythology and folklore are rich in allusions to wondrous potions such as the one used by Helen of Troy to quench pain and strife. Unfortunately, the ingredients in

the perfect pain killers of antiquity are quite mysterious. Real sleep potions contained
so many dangerous ingredients that it was safer to inhale them than to ingest them.
With inhalation, the amount of the active ingredient need not be calculated too
precisely, because the inhalant could be withdrawn as soon as the patient was
sufficiently affected. In contrast, an overdose of drugs swallowed or injected could
not be removed. The medieval prototype of the ''sleep apple'' that appears in the story
of Snow White usually contained opium, mandrake, henbane, hemlock, wine, and
musk. The user was expected to inhale the fumes of the apple rather than eat it. The
''soporific sponges'' recommended by medieval surgeons contained similar mixtures. By the sixteenth century, surgeons were describing old favorites like mandrake
as poisonous drugs that lulled the senses and made men cowards. In Shakespeare's
Antony and Cleopatra, Cleopatra safely used mandrake to sleep away the hours before
Antony's return, but surgeons found that drugged patients who slept like the dead
during surgery often failed to awaken afterwards. Shakespeare alludes to various
soporific agents, such as poppy, mandragora, and ''drowsy syrups,'' but these agents
were unreliable at best. Nevertheless, opium retained its favored status long after
mandrake was discarded. Eminent physicians like Thomas Sydenham and John
Hunter saw opium as a powerful drug and proof of God's mercy. As the eighteenth-
century surgeon John Hunter told a colleague seeking advice about treating a patient
with a painful malignant cancer, the only choice was ''Opium, Opium, Opium!''

In large doses, opium generally causes somnolence and depression, but excitation,
vomiting, headaches, and constipation are not uncommon side-effects. Opium was
used in cough medicines, sleeping potions, and soothing elixirs for crying babies.
Some critics recognized the dangers of drug dependence, but opium remained widely
available into the twentieth century. Soporifics and narcotics were also prepared from
marijuana, hellebore, belladonna, henbane, jimsonweed, and enough miscellaneous
greens to make a very exotic salad. Henbane was known as the poor man's opium.
Sixteenth-century herbals recommended it for insomnia, toothache, and pain.
Poisonous substances are present throughout the tissues of the ubiquitous jimsonweed, but the powerful alkaloids atropine and scopolamine are concentrated in the
seeds. Reports of atropine-like poisoning in persons who have eaten the seeds, often
washed down with alcohol, are not uncommon. Long used as a hypnotic and sedative,
scopolamine became popular with twentieth-century obstetricians who claimed that
the ''twilight sleep'' induced by the drug allowed scientific management of ''painless
childbirth.'' Scopolamine has even been marketed for relief of sea sickness, despite
the fact that it can produce dangerous hallucinations. Hemlock was the active
ingredient in the infamous ''drink of death'' given to the condemned Socrates.
Although clearly a dangerous drug, hemlock was sometimes used in anesthetic
concoctions. The drug depresses the motor centers before the sensory centers are
affected; this is good for the surgeon, but bad for the patient. Curare, an arrow poison
used by South American Indians, was brought to the attention of European scientists
by Alexander von Humboldt (1769–1859), who came close to killing himself in the

course of this research. Curare does not relieve pain, but it is useful in surgery because it prevents movement and provides profound muscle relaxation.

Despite the wealth of soporific agents available in nature's medical garden, the remarkable products of the eighteenth-century chemical revolution eventually eclipsed the ancient anodynes. Joseph Priestley (1733–1804), British theologian, educator, writer, and political theorist, is best known as the discoverer of oxygen, but as Sir Humphry Davy (1778–1829) said of this indefatigable chemist, "no single person ever discovered so many new and curious substances." Most curious of all was the gas known as nitrous oxide, or "laughing gas." As he was in the habit of testing the effect of new gases on himself, Priestley might have discovered the anesthetic properties of laughing gas if his research had not been interrupted by the political and religious conflicts that forced him to emigrate to America in 1794.

The genius that characterized the birth of pneumatic chemistry soon gave way to confusion and quackery. Conscientious experimentalists could not compete with charlatans promising miraculous cures for asthma, catarrh, consumption, and cancer through the inhalation of oxygen, hydrogen, and other "factitious airs." However, some physicians attempted to find legitimate medical uses for the new gases. Fascinated by pneumatic chemistry, Thomas Beddoes (1760–1808) persuaded his friends Thomas Wedgwood (1771–1805) and James Watt (1736–1819) to help him establish the Pneumatic Institute, a hospital in which the inhalation of factitious airs was used in the treatment of lung disease. Many scientists, including the great Humphry Davy (1778–1829), were intrigued by his work. While suffering from toothache in 1795, Davy began inhaling nitrous oxide. In addition to feeling giddy, relaxed, and cheerful, Davy noted that the pain caused by his wisdom teeth had almost disappeared. Soon after the exhilaration wore off the pain returned, worse than ever. Nevertheless, Davy suggested that nitrous oxide might be useful during surgical operations. Davy's associate Michael Faraday (1791–1867) discovered the soporific effect of ether vapor during experiments on various gases. In comparing the effects of ether and nitrous oxide, Faraday found that both chemicals produced similar responses. Most subjects found inhalation of ether or nitrous oxide very pleasant, but occasionally participants experienced frightening and bizarre effects, such as loss of sensations, prolonged lethargy, hallucinations, and fainting. Conservative physicians used such reports to prove that the inhalation of gases was dangerous, uncertain, and likely to produce scandalous behaviors. Even the valiant attempts of Henry Hill Hickman (1801–1830) to validate the safety and efficacy of inhalation anesthesia failed to arouse the interest of the medical profession. Unlike many pioneers of anesthesia, Hickman did not simply sniff at various chemicals. Dogs and mice placed in a sealed glass vessel were subjected to various test gases until they were in a state of "suspended animation." In this state, animals were insensitive to pain, but were at risk of circulatory collapse during surgery. Hickman attempted to call attention to surgical anesthesia, but no one in England seemed interested. Overwhelmed with a sense of failure, Hickman killed himself.

LAUGHING GAS, ETHER, AND SURGICAL ANESTHESIA

The story of the successful development of surgical anesthesia in the 1840s involves a most unlikely cast of characters more suited to farce than historical drama. Moreover, the action took place not in the prestigious medical schools and hospitals of Europe, but at the periphery of the medical and scientific world. The characters featured in the play were peripatetic professors, show-business chemists, and dentists, who at the time were regarded as closer to quacks than to doctors.

The story is so complicated that a brief introduction to the cast of characters is necessary before we explore the events in detail. Horace Wells and William Thomas Green Morton were dentists who had shared a successful partnership before Wells recognized the anesthetic properties of nitrous oxide and Morton demonstrated the value of ether. Charles T. Jackson, chemist and physician, later claimed to have discovered ether anesthesia and to have instructed Morton in its use. While the priority battle raged in New England, Georgia physician Crawford Williamson Long announced that he had operated under ether anesthesia before Morton.

During the nineteenth century, "medicine shows" and "philosophical lectures" by self-appointed "professors" brought edification and entertainment to the citizens of cities and towns throughout America. "Professors of chemistry" enlivened lectures on the amazing properties of newly discovered gases by breathing fire with hydrogen and encouraging volunteers to make fools of themselves after inhaling

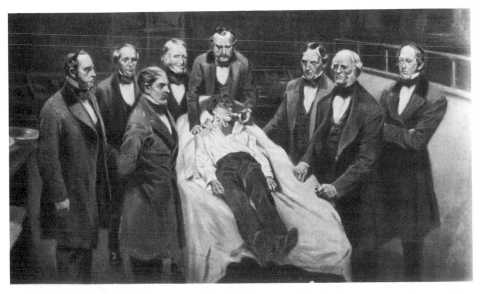

Surgical anesthesia at Massachusetts General Hospital, 1846

nitrous oxide. Students of dentistry, medicine, and chemistry did not have to wait for the itinerant professors, but could enjoy "laughing gas parties" and "ether frolics" whenever they wished. Indeed, the "champagne effect" of these substances was so well known that when Jackson attempted to claim priority, Morton's defenders noted that one could hardly find a school or community in America where the boys and girls had not inhaled ether.

Dentists were probably more highly motivated than any other practitioners to discover novel and powerful anesthetics. Until the excruciating pain of a rotting tooth exceeded the anticipated agony of extraction, the victim of toothache was unlikely to submit to the services of a dentist. Throughout history dentists claimed to possess potions that would save the tooth or eliminate pain. Ancient tooth-dressings included everything from honey and opium to sour apples and powdered beetles. Among the most peculiar treatments for toothache we must include kissing a donkey, biting off the head of a mouse, inserting a live louse in the tooth, and applications of powdered crow dung.

As nineteenth-century American dentists introduced improved dental appliances and instruments, their professional advances were limited by the fears of prospective patients and the disdain of the medical profession. These obstacles were especially resented by men like Horace Wells (1815–1848) and his partner William Morton (1819–1868). Wells and Morton had developed improved sets of false teeth and dental solder, but potential customers were unwilling to accept their "money-back-if-not-satisfied" deal because it required extraction of all remaining teeth and roots. Thus, Wells and Morton were keenly interested in any agent that could achieve painless dentistry. On December 10, 1844, Wells attended a lecture by Dr. Gardner Quincy Colton, during which the remarkable properties of nitrous oxide were demonstrated. Wells was struck by the fact that a volunteer remained in a state of euphoria while under the influence of laughing gas even though he fell off the stage and injured his leg. Wells asked Colton to bring laughing gas to his office for an experiment. The next morning, Colton administered the gas to Wells, and John M. Riggs, a dental student, extracted a tooth. When Wells regained consciousness, he was elated to realize that he had not experienced the slightest sensation during the operation. By mid-January of 1845 Wells had used nitrous oxide on over a dozen patients. At Morton's request, Dr. John Collins Warren (1778–1856), Professor of Anatomy at Harvard Medical School, allowed Wells to address a class in surgery. However, Dr. Warren's skeptical attitude towards painless dentistry was evident in his introductory remarks. "There's a gentleman here," Warren warned his students, "who pretends he has something which will destroy pain in surgical operations." When the medical student who "volunteered" to have a tooth extracted groaned during the operation, Wells and Morton were ridiculed and humiliated by the hostile audience. Ironically, the patient later admitted that he had felt no pain. In evaluating the anesthesia controversy Dr. Henry J. Bigelow argued that Wells had not satisfied the criteria for surgical anesthesia which must be complete, inevitable, and safe. Behaviors elicited by nitrous oxide inhalation were unpredictable and suggestion played an important role in determining the effect of the gas. Those who inhaled for amusement became exhilarated; those well prepared for surgery became drowsy and lost consciousness.

Morton later complained that he was the only one involved in the discovery of anesthesia who had suffered a "pecuniary loss," but Wells paid for his part in the controversy with his sanity and his life. Failing to find professional recognition, Wells resorted to sniffing ether and chloroform to cope with depression. In January 1848, Wells was arrested for allegedly accosting a young woman and throwing something (acid, ether, or chloroform) at her. Two days later, Wells was found dead in his cell along with an empty vial of chloroform, a penknife, a razor, and a suicide note. Only a short time after Wells's dismal performance reassured the Boston Brahmins that a mere dentist could not teach them the secret of painless surgery, Morton convinced the same elite physicians that inhalation anesthesia was "no humbug."

Like nitrous oxide, ether had long been used for recreational purposes. Moreover, during its 300-year history several investigators came tantalizingly close to discovering its anesthetic properties. The honor of being first to synthesize ether has been attributed to several Renaissance alchemists, but the nature of these alchemical preparations is obscure. The starting materials (sulfuric acid and alcohol) would have been widely available, but careful temperature regulation is needed to enhance the production of ethyl ether as opposed to other possible reaction products. Certainly, if ether had been synthesized, it would have been impure, and, as William T. G. Morton discovered, purity was critical when ether was used as an anesthetic agent. Even though ether had been used as a sedative in the treatment of tuberculosis, asthma, and whooping cough, its anesthetic potential was rarely exploited. Extrapolating from the pleasant experience of an "ether frolic" to dental and surgical operations was not a self-evident step before practitioners deliberately set forth on a quest for inhalation anesthetics.

According to family tradition, Morton graduated from the Baltimore College of Dental Surgery in 1842. There is, however, no proof that Morton ever matriculated at any dental school. Dentistry was hardly considered a profession at that time, but attempts to improve the training and status of dentists had been made as early as 1839 when the *American Journal of Dental Science* was established. The American Society of Dental Surgeons held its first meeting in August, 1840, 6 months after Baltimore College, the first of its kind in America, was chartered. Both Wells and Morton seem to have been skillful and inventive dentists who specialized in "mechanical dentistry," or "plate work." Because of the suffering of his patients and their tendency to prefer death to dentistry, Morton was obsessed with finding a way to mitigate the pain of dental operations. Like surgeons, dentists could offer their patients only unreliable soporifics. Moreover, the nausea caused by alcohol and laudanum was especially dangerous during dental procedures because vomiting could lead to suffocation and death.

Despite the financial success of the Wells-Morton partnership, Morton became one of Dr. Charles Thomas Jackson's (1805–1880) private pupils in order to make the transition from dentistry to medicine. In a discussion of toothache, Jackson recommended using ether in the form of "tooth-ache drops." But when Morton performed tooth extractions on Jackson's wife and aunt, the physician merely encouraged the ladies to be brave. Therefore, during the priority battle over the discovery of anesthesia, Morton argued that his former mentor had never thought of going beyond the application of liquid ether *"in the same manner that laudanum and other narcotics have always been applied to sensitive teeth."* Always on the lookout for pain-relieving agents, Morton was intrigued by Jackson's "tooth-ache drops" and consulted the literature concerning the use of ether as antispasmodic, anodyne, and narcotic. Noting that when ether was applied to a rotten tooth the gums became numb, Morton wondered whether ether could numb the whole body. Taking elaborate precautions to ensure secrecy, he tested the effects of ether inhalation on various animals. Disconcerted by the variability of the results, Morton sought Jackson's advice and learned that the ether sold by pharmacists was rarely pure enough for special uses.

On September 30, 1846, Morton saturated a handkerchief with ether, looked at his watch, and inhaled deeply. He regained consciousness about 8 minutes later with no ill effects other than mild exhilaration, followed by headache. That evening Morton tested his discovery while extracting a patient's firmly rooted bicuspid. After the painless operation, the happy patient gave Morton a written testimonial. Convinced of the validity of his discovery, Morton again approached Dr. Warren to ask for an opportunity to demonstrate his method of producing insensibility to pain. Thinking that inhaling ether through some special apparatus might produce more reliable results, Morton sought the assistance of a well-known scientific instrument-maker. Although Morton could have gotten the equipment from Jackson, he did not wish to alert the chemist to his discovery.

By October 16, 1846, the day of the hospital demonstration, Morton was in a state of terrible anxiety and his inhalation apparatus was still unfinished. The patient was already strapped to the table in preparation for his ordeal when Morton rushed in with his new inhaler and "Letheon gas." Amazed by the patient's complete quiet and tranquility during the extirpation of a large tumor from his mouth and tongue, Dr. Warren announced: "Gentlemen, this is no humbug." Witnesses later recalled this demonstration of ether anesthesia as "the most sublime scene ever witnessed in the operating-room." This operation would end the era of the surgeon as "armed savage" and allow a remarkable series of improvements in the art of surgery. It also precipitated a vicious priority battle. According to Morton, the first intimation of the trouble to come was a visit from Dr. Jackson on October 23, 1846. Jackson had heard that Morton intended to take out a patent for ether anesthesia and expected to make a good deal of money. Dentists routinely patented their inventions, but physicians supposedly answered to a higher code of ethics. However, Jackson demanded fees for professional advice, his name on the patent, and 10% of the net profits. Shortly after presenting his demands to Morton, Jackson sent a sealed report to the Academy of Sciences of France in which he claimed that he had discovered ether anesthesia and instructed a certain dentist to use ether when extracting teeth. Jackson's sealed report was his insurance policy; if ether proved to be dangerous his report could be destroyed, but if it was successful, he intended to use it to claim priority. As soon as the success of ether anesthesia seemed assured, Jackson presented himself as its sole discoverer and denounced Morton as a ''stooge'' acting under his direction. When Jackson spoke to the Massachusetts Medical Society, most of his audience accepted the claims of the eminent physician, chemist, and geologist against the ''quack dentist.'' Not every one was convinced and Jackson was asked whether he would have accepted the blame if Morton's patient had died.

The Massachusetts Medical Society's rules of ethics did not allow the use of ''secret remedies''; therefore, when Morton offered his services for another operation, hospital surgeons refused to employ him until he revealed the identity of Letheon. They also assured him that the patient would die if her leg was not amputated, and would probably die of shock if the operation was conducted without anesthesia. It was not easy for Morton to envision the greater good of humanity while his dreams of fame and fortune evaporated even more quickly than ether itself. Opportunities to profit from his discovery continuously eluded him. In July of 1868 Morton went to New York City in a state of extreme agitation caused by the conflict with Jackson and died of a cerebral hemorrhage shortly after consulting his lawyer. An inscription on Morton's tomb, composed by Dr. Bigelow, honors him as the inventor of anesthetic inhalation. Jackson survived Morton by 12 years, but he did not enjoy a peaceful old age. According to a story probably too good to be true, in July of 1873, after considerable drinking, Jackson wandered into the Mount Auburn Cemetery and was overcome by a frenzy while reading the inscription on Morton's tomb. Declared hopelessly insane, Jackson was confined to a mental asylum for the rest of his miserable life.

While Wells, Morton, and Jackson were disputing the discovery of inhalation anesthesia, Crawford W. Long (1815–1878) emerged from his obscure existence in rural Georgia with testimonials documenting his own priority claim. Like Wells, Long came to an appreciation of the medical potential of a drug from casual observations of its recreational uses. When a traveling chemist sparked local interest in laughing gas, Long suggested that ether would be just as exhilarating. According to Long, sniffing ether became a popular form of entertainment at social gatherings. After these ''ether frolics,'' participants sometimes discovered bruises and other injuries acquired while ''under the influence.'' Long realized that ether might be used to induce insensitivity to pain during surgery, but he had more opportunities to stage ether frolics than surgical operations. In March 1842 Long persuaded James M. Venable to have a tumor on his neck surgically removed. Knowing that Venable was afraid of the knife, but fond of ether, Long suggested that he sniff ether prior to the operation. It was not until 1849 that Long published an account of his discovery in the *Southern Medical and Surgical Journal*. Technically, Long established his priority, but as Sir William Osler said: "In science the credit goes to the man who convinces the world, not to the man to whom the idea first occurs."

Despite warnings from the Philadelphia *Medical Examiner* that the physicians of Boston would soon constitute one fraternity with the quacks, ether anesthesia quickly spread to Paris and London. Although anesthesia was certainly an important factor in the surgical revolution, more subtle and complex factors were also involved. Indeed, given the increased use of the knife that accompanied the decline of humoralism and the rise of morbid anatomy during the period from about 1700 to the 1830s, quite possibly the rapid acceptance of anesthesia was the outcome of the rise of surgery rather than the reverse. In any case, with the rapid dissemination of surgical anesthesia advances in the art were inevitable; so too were accidents and deaths.

The changing nature of surgical practice must have been painful indeed to those who had established their reputation through speed and strength and now saw surgeons developing a deliberate and subtle touch. Practitioners who had struggled to attain the professional detachment (or callousness) needed to operate in the pre-anesthetic era had taken great pride in the achievement. Like the librarian who objects to people taking books from neatly ordered shelves, the master surgeon resented the trick that obviated the need for his painstakingly acquired skills. Anesthesia so transformed the art of surgery that Henry J. Bigelow urged reform of the curriculum at Harvard Medical School to inculcate humanity and sensitivity back into medical students. Within 2 years of Morton's first public demonstration of Letheon, ether, nitrous oxide, chloroform, and other anesthetics were widely used in dentistry, obstetrics, and surgery. Anesthetics were also used by physicians for convulsions, asthma, whooping cough, menstrual cramps, neuralgia, insomnia, and insanity. While some practitioners denounced anesthesia as a dangerous and blasphemous novelty and others adopted it without reservations, most cautiously accepted it as a mixed blessing which had to be used selectively. The risks and benefits of anesthesia had to be evaluated by a new "utilitarian calculus" which considered age, sex, race, ethnicity, the seriousness of the operation, and other subtle factors. Some surgeons justified anesthesia by arguing that pain itself was evil because it caused shock, depleted precious stores of vital energy, and damaged the body. Moreover, anesthesia encouraged patients to accept operations and allowed surgeons to refine their skills. Advocates of universal anesthetization accused doctors of exaggerating individual idiosyncrasies in order to maintain exclusive control over anesthesia. The American Medical Association's Committee on Medical Science warned that chloroform and ether should only be used by physicians; with respect to anesthesia, even dentists should defer to physicians. To put this concern in context, note that doctors also warned patients that bathing could prove fatal unless prescribed by a physician instead of a hydropath ("water-cure" healer).

Many nineteenth-century critics of anesthesia sincerely believed that pain was God's punishment for human failures and wickedness. William Henry Atkinson, M.D., first president of the American Dental Association, contended that anesthesia was a Satanic plot to deprive men of the capacity to reason and endure the pain that God intended them to experience. Certainly doctors were influenced by religious dogma, but professional norms also conditioned them to be suspicious of an innovation that challenged centuries of medical experience in which insensitivity to pain (as in coma, shock, or brain damage) was a harbinger of death. Pain, life, and healing had always been inextricably linked. Opponents of the new surgery pounced upon reports of deaths after anesthesia, ignoring the fact that it was not uncommon for patients to die after operations performed without anesthesia. Many critics feared that anesthetics gave doctors excessive power over patients. Anesthetics might be used to subdue and tranquilize uncooperative patients into unnecessary, experimental operations. It was even possible that the relief of pain was an illusion; the patient might actually suffer pain but be rendered incapable of expressing or recalling the experience. Anesthesia might poison the blood, retard healing, cause hemorrhages, convulsions, miscarriage, asphyxia, pneumonia, paralysis, insanity, and death. Although some of these fears were obviously exaggerated, further experience proved that anesthetics, like any potent drug, could cause serious side effects. Even under optimum, fully modern conditions, the dangers of anesthesia should not be underestimated. In many cases, general anesthesia may be the most dangerous part of an operation.

Inspired by his successful use of ether, James Young Simpson (1811–1870), Professor of Midwifery at Edinburgh and one of Scotland's leading surgeons and obstetricians, initiated a search for an anesthetic without ether's disadvantages. Using himself and his friends as guinea pigs, Simpson began a systematic, but dangerous search for a volatile agent with an agreeable odor. Having sniffed his way through samples of acetone, benzene, benzoin, and many other reagents, Simpson tested chloroform. This dense, colorless liquid produced a sense of euphoria as well as loss of consciousness. Within a week, Simpson's patients were enjoying the benefits of chloroform analgesia. Chloroform was easier to administer than ether, but it also seemed to be more dangerous. Indeed, it was fortunate that the *principle* of surgical anesthesia had been established with ether, because the relatively high mortality rate with chloroform would have inhibited development of this branch of the healing art.

The safety of anesthesia was not the only point of contention, as demonstrated by the ferocity of the attack on the use of anesthetics in obstetrics. Clergymen, doctors, and assorted amateur moralists argued that pain had a God-given, and therefore holy role to play in the lives of men, and especially in the lives of women. Midwives had been put to death for the blasphemous, sinful, unnatural crime of attempting to alleviate the pains of childbirth. Clergymen denounced Simpson and commanded women to endure the pains of childbirth with patience and fortitude. Did the Bible not say that Eve was condemned to bring forth children in sorrow? Obstetricians warned women that labor contractions were identical to labor pains; therefore, without pain there would be no contractions and normal delivery could not occur. Suffering was inherent in female physiology, and labor pains enhanced woman's capacity for tenderness, femininity, and maternal feelings. Saddened by the controversy, Simpson met his critics on theological as well as scientific grounds. Using the Bible to substantiate his work, Simpson asserted that the curse in Genesis had been revoked by a passage in Deuteronomy that promised: "The Lord will bless the fruit of the womb and the land." Moreover, the word translated as "sorrow" in the case of Eve's punishment was really the word for "labor" which referred to both farming and childbirth. Furthermore, God established the principle of anesthesia when he caused a deep sleep to fall upon Adam before operating on his rib. When Dr. John Snow (1813–1858) administered chloroform to Queen Victoria in 1853 during the birth of her eighth child, the issue of whether a proper lady would accept anesthesia was settled. Unlike his American counterparts, Simpson died rich in honors and respect. He was knighted, appointed Physician in Scotland to the Queen, awarded an honorary doctorate by Oxford University, received the Freedom of the City of Edinburgh, and after his untimely death at age 59, academic and commercial activities in Scotland were suspended to accommodate one of the largest funerals ever to honor a Scottish doctor.

LOCAL ANESTHESIA

With proper management, inhalation anesthesia was generally safe, complete, and inevitable. However, complete insensibility is not suitable for all operations. Although some of the drugs and instruments involved in the development of local, regional, and spinal anesthesia predate Morton's demonstration, the development of special techniques for their use in surgery began in earnest after the acceptance of inhalation anesthesia. In 1803, Friedrich Wilhelm Sertürner (1783–1841) isolated crystals of a powerful analgesic agent from crude opium. Sertürner named the chemical *morphine*, after Morpheus, the Greek god of dreams. Morphine paste could be introduced locally with the point of a lancet, or a solution of morphine could be instilled into a wound. In the 1850s Charles Gabriel Pravaz (1791–1853), a French surgeon, and Alexander Wood (1817–1884) of Edinburgh independently invented the modern type of hollow metal needle. (The device known as a hypodermic syringe in the United States and England is called a Pravaz syringe on the Continent.) Injections of morphine were generally used for the relief of local pain, but some surgeons administered morphine in preparation for surgery under general anesthesia in the belief that it prevented shock, delirium, nausea, and lessened the amount of inhalant needed.

The ancient Incas had successfully exploited the anesthetic qualities of the coca leaf as well as its mood-altering properties, and their Peruvian descendants continued to use coca leaves to drive away pain, hunger, nausea, fatigue, and sorrow. While Europeans quickly took up the native American custom of smoking tobacco, they ignored coca until nineteenth-century chemists isolated cocaine from coca leaves. After reading a report on the physiological effects of cocaine, Sigmund Freud (1856–1939) decided that the drug might serve as a remedy for mental and physical diseases. Using himself as guinea pig, Freud discovered that cocaine banished his depression and increased his energy. Freud urged his friend Carl Koller (1857–1944), a physician who specialized in eye disorders, to try cocaine for the relief of eye diseases such as trachoma and iritis. When a solution of cocaine was instilled into the eye of a frog, Koller could touch the cornea without eliciting any reaction. Following successful tests on rabbits and humans, Koller announced his discovery at the 1884 Opthalmological Congress in Heidelberg. By the end of the nineteenth century, many popular ointments, snuffs, suppositories, cigarettes, and beverages contained cocaine. The best known is Coca-Cola, a patent medicine introduced in 1886 as a therapeutic agent, sovereign remedy, and general tonic. In addition to extract of coca leaves, Coca-Cola contained an extract of the kola nut, which is high in caffeine. By 1906 when the Pure Food and Drug Law was passed in the United States, the makers of Coca-Cola were using decocainized coca leaves, but the caffein remained.

William S. Halsted (1852–1922), one of New York's leading surgeons, realized that Koller had barely begun to exploit the possible range of cocaine anesthesia. Impressed with the drug's effects, Halsted performed a series of tests on himself, his medical students, and experimental animals. Because cocaine constricts blood vessels, it seemed to be the ideal local anesthetic for surgery in highly vascularized areas. Halsted developed a technique he called ''conduction anesthesia''—a means of specifically anesthetizing various parts of the body by injecting cocaine solutions into the appropriate nerves. When using cocaine, Halsted and his assistants enjoyed feelings of increased energy and creativity, as well as freedom from pain and fatigue. But Halsted soon noticed that some of his students were becoming irresponsible, and that when he stopped taking cocaine he experienced vertigo, cramps, anxiety, insomnia, and hallucinations. (A century later descriptions of cocaine abuse included intense anxiety, depression, psychosis, and seizures followed by respiratory or cardiac arrest.) Some of Halsted's addicted students wound up in the slums of New York, while Halsted was sent to an asylum for the mentally ill. He was quite a different person when he emerged a year later, now addicted to morphine. Encouraged and supported by his colleages William Osler and William Henry Welch, Halsted continued his distinguished career as the first professor of surgery at Johns Hopkins. With increasing use of cocaine anesthesia, reports of serious side effects and deaths soon appeared.

PAIN AND THE SEARCH FOR ENDOGENOUS OPIATES

It is impossible to divorce the story of anesthesia from the study of the mechanism of pain. While scientific understanding of the mechanism of pain is far from complete, the problem can now be reformulated in terms of the discovery that the body makes its own morphine-like analgesics. In 1972, Dr. Avram Goldstein, a neurobiologist at Stanford University, suggested that the search for natural substances with the pain-relieving characteristics of opium and morphine should be fruitful. Just as enzymes and substrates fit together like locks and keys, so too might natural opiates interact with receptors in nerve cells. One year later, researchers at three independent laboratories demonstrated the existence of opiate receptors (Solomon Snyder and Candace Pert of Johns Hopkins; Eric Simon of New York University School of Medicine; Lars Terenius of Uppsala University, Sweden). Given the fact that opium is not a natural constituent of the nervous system, investigators reasoned that the opiate receptors must play a role in the control of pain via some endogenous narcotic. Substances that mimic the action of morphine were found in brain, pituitary gland, and other tissues. Because these agents function as endogenous morphine-like substances, they have been called "endorphins." Neurobiologists and pharmacologists now foresee the possibility of finding ways to control the production of endorphins and developing safe endorphin-like drugs.

HOSPITALISM

The impact of anesthesia on the frequency of operations has been a matter of debate, but careful analyses of patterns of surgery in nineteenth-century hospitals indicate that anesthesia did expand the amount of surgery performed. In part, the rise in surgical cases was an outgrowth of urbanization and industrialization, but the increase in gynecological surgery, especially ovariotomy, was especially dramatic. Many gynecological operations were done to "cure" nonspecific "female complaints" and emotional problems. Those who harbored suspicions that surgeons acted to satisfy their own "savage desire for cutting" were convinced that surgeons operated on moribund accident victims not because they expected to save them, but because they were viewed as "teaching material" or experimental specimens. A striking upsurge in novel operations did occur in the post-anesthesia, pre-antiseptic period, but there is some evidence that the notorious rise in post-surgical infections associated with this era had more to do with changing patterns of poverty, urbanization, and industrialization than anesthesia. The deplorable conditions of the hospitals, the misery of the typical hospital patient, and the growing evils of poverty and industrialization provide an explanatory framework for the prevalence of hospital infections in the second half of the nineteenth century.

Ideally, surgery should be judged in terms of the survival and rehabilitation of the patient, but the drama of the operation tends to overwhelm the mundane details of post-surgical management. In the pre-anesthetic era, the dazzling strength, speed, and daring of the master surgeon were displayed to good advantage in a limited range of operations. The legendary surgeon who amputated a leg at the thigh, along with two fingers of his assistant, and both testes of an observer represented the epitome of this genre of surgery. Better authenticated heroes of this era were men like William

Cheselden (1688–1752) who could perform an operation for bladder stones in less than 1 minute, and James Syme (1799–1870), who amputated at the hip joint in little more than 60 seconds. Surgeons were as obsessed with setting speed records as modern athletes, but their goal was the reduction of the stress, pain, and shock endured by the patient. In this context, surgical anesthesia might be seen as a prerequisite for the standardized antiseptic ritual, because it would have been virtually impossible for the lightning-quick surgeon to carry out such procedures while coping with a screaming, struggling patient. When the art of anesthesia had been mastered, the surgeon was no longer damned as the "armed savage," but, in the crowded, filthy wards of the typical nineteenth-century hospital, wound infection was transformed from a sporadic event into an epidemic condition which could be referred to as hospitalism. Although honest surgeons were forced to admit that the patient on the operating table in a hospital was more likely to die than a soldier on the battlefield, the poor prognosis did not inhibit rising interest in surgical intervention.

The cause of wound infection was not clearly understood until the elaboration of germ theory, but "uncleanliness" had been a major suspect since the time of Hippocrates. Hippocratic physicians knew that it was preferable for a wound to heal by first intention, i.e., without suppuration (pus formation). The surgeon hoped that if a wound was washed with wine, vinegar, freshly voided urine, or boiled water, cleansed of foreign objects, and covered with a simple dressing, healing would proceed without complications. However, wound infection was such a common occurrence that by the medieval period, surgeons had developed elaborate methods to provoke suppuration. The theoretical rationalization for these procedures is known as the "doctrine of laudable pus." According to this offshoot of humoral pathology, recovery from disease or injury required casting off putrid humors from the interior of the body. The appearance of nice creamy white pus in a wound was, therefore, a natural and necessary phase of healing.

The relationship between changing surgical practice and mortality rates is obscured by the simultaneous shift to hospital-based medical practice. However, statistics such as the 74% mortality rate among Parisian hospital patients who had undergone amputation at the thigh in the 1870s seem to speak for themselves. Knowing how often successful operations were followed by fatal infections, doctors were among those who refused to submit to the knife. For example, when the great French surgeon, diagnostician, and anatomist Guillaume Dupuytren (1777–1835) faced death, he rejected the possibility of an operation, saying he would rather die by God's hand than by that of the surgeon.

Physicians and surgeons knew all too well that a pin prick opened a doorway to death. The doctor was no more immune to the danger than his patient; as we have seen previously, minor wounds incurred during dissections could lead to death from a massive systemic infection known as pathologist's pyemia. With but slight exaggeration, doctors warned that it was safer to submit to surgery in a stable, where veterinary surgery was routinely and successfully performed, than in a hospital. When miasmata generated by ineluctable cosmic tellurgic influences permeated the hospital, patients in the wards inevitably succumbed to hospital gangrene, erysipelas, puerperal fever, pyemia, and septicemia. Physicians endlessly debated about the nature of these forces and disease entities, but all of these hospital fevers can be subsumed by the term hospitalism. When epidemic fevers were particularly virulent, the only way to prevent the spread of infection was to burn down the institution.

Ironically, the evolution of the hospital into a center for medical education and research may have been a major factor in the appalling mortality rates of the large teaching hospitals. Changes in the hospital's social role may also have contributed to the pandemic of hospitalism. By the nineteenth century, the reputation of many of these institutions was so low that no horror story seemed impossible. Impoverished slum dwellers were convinced that hospital patients were doomed to death and dissection to satisfy the morbid curiosity of doctors. Among the more bizarre rumors that circulated in France was that of the dissection room where human fat was collected to light the lamps of the Faculty of Medicine. Descriptions of major hospitals invariably refer to the overcrowding, stench, and filth of the wards. Surgeons complained that the nurses were rarely sober enough to work; patients complained that they were being starved to death. Hospital floors were covered with expectorations, excrement, urine, blood, and pus. Operations were often performed in the center of such wards rather than a separate operating room. The same wash basin, water, and sponge were used to treat a whole row of patients. Pus-saturated dressings were collected in the common "pus-pail." On a more positive note, the great quantity and diversity of patients provided invaluable clinical experience for young surgeons, physicians, and pathologists. Indeed, the appalling conditions of the large urban hospitals of Europe provided the environment in which a new form of medical science, based on physical examination, pathological anatomy, and medical statistics, could emerge. (Indeed, these are the conditions that allowed Friedrich Miescher (1844–1895) to use pus cells for work that led to the discovery of the nucleic acids.)

Hospitals began as places of refuge and charity, to care for the sick and comfort of the dying. Changing medical theory, training, practice, and intense interest in pathological anatomy, as well as socioeconomic factors, created new roles for this institution. But the hospital remained embedded in a matrix of poverty in which the virtues of economy and efficiency were more important than cleanliness. Philanthropists, administrators, and physicians, as members of the "better classes," expected their "lower class" patients to be conditioned to crowding, discomfort, and filth; excessive cleanliness might even shock and distress such people. Surgeons began operations without any special preparation, although a brief hand wash was considered appropriate when leaving the dissecting room. During operations, surgeons protected their clothes with an apron or towel, or wore an old coat already covered with blood and pus. Patients were "worked up" for surgery by the removal of outer clothing and a swish of a well-used sponge. Observers were often invited to probe and examine interesting wounds. Habits acquired in the pre-anesthetic era were not easily broken; the pace of surgery was less frantic, but certainly not leisurely. A surgeon took pride in his ingenious methods for saving time, such as holding a knife in his mouth while operating. Using the same coat for all operations was convenient, because needles, sutures, and instruments could be kept handy in the lapel, buttonhole, and pockets.

It would be wrong to extrapolate from the epidemics of infection that swept through nineteenth-century hospitals to the problem of surgical infection in other ages. Indeed, it has been suggested that fluctuations in hospital mortality rates reflected the level of distress in the community. Famine, scurvy, and disease would certainly affect resistance to infection. This hypothesis is consistent with the observation that veterinary surgery was relatively free of the problem of wound infection, although it was carried out under rather primitive conditions with little concern for asepsis. Hospitalism might, thus, have been a unique nineteenth-century plague, perhaps caused by the effects of the Industrial Revolution, rather than a reflection of surgical practice from Hippocrates to Lister.

JOSEPH LISTER AND THE ANTISEPTIC SYSTEM

Nineteenth-century hospital surgery is so inextricably associated with epidemic hospitalism that modern surgery seems to be a direct product of Joseph Lister's (1827–1912) introduction of his antiseptic system. The factors involved in the evolution of modern surgery were certainly more complex, but the importance of Lister's appreciation of germ theory and his obsession with preventing infection by attention to both the surgical operation and the quality of post-surgical care should not be underestimated. Too sensitive to have become a surgeon in the pre-anesthetic era, under the tutelage of the great Scottish surgeon James Syme (1799–1870), Lister learned to love the most "bloody and butcherly department of the healing art." Happily married to his mentor's daughter, Lister established his repuation as a surgeon, scientist, and teacher. By the time Lister retired in 1892 his methods were finally winning due recognition. He was the first British surgeon to be elevated to the peerage, an original member of the Order of Merit, and the recipient of numerous other honors.

Unlike Semmelweis, Lister was an experimental scientist who shared Louis Pasteur's insights into the relationship between theory and practice. Like most of his contemporaries, Lister initially believed that infection might be caused by the entry of noxious air into a wound. However, when his attention was drawn to Louis Pasteur's research on the diseases of wine and beer, Lister reached an understanding of the applicability of germ theory to surgical infection. Although few physicians were willing to believe that what occurred in the chemist's test tubes was relevant to medicine, Lister began a study of inflammation in which he used various animal models. Insights gained through these experiments and in hospital wards provided the basis for the development of the antiseptic system.

In attacking the problem of hospital infections, Lister deliberately chose compound fractures for his critical tests, because ''disastrous consequences'' were frequent with open or compound fracture (a fracture in which the broken ends of the bone protrude through the skin), in contrast to the uncomplicated healing characteristic of simple fracture (a fracture in which the skin remains unbroken), although the trauma involved and the possibility of deformity were similar. Infection often claimed more than 60% of patients with compound fractures. Surgeons traditionally probed and enlarged the opening of the wound, but the prognosis was so poor that immediate amputation was considered a reasonable course of treatment. Nevertheless, as we have seen in the case of Ambroise Paré, amputation and/or death were not inevitable consequences of compound fracture. According to experienced surgeons, any blockhead could perform an amputation after such an injury, but great skill was needed to cure compound fractures without operation.

The search for antiseptics and disinfectants has been part of folk-medicine and surgery throughout history. As Florence Nightingale (1820–1910), pioneer of modern nursing and sanitary reform often said, most of these agents were useless,

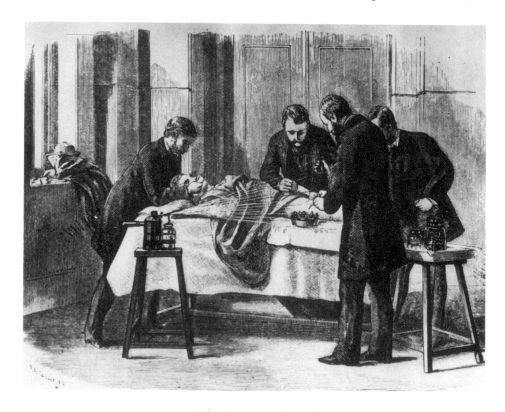

Antiseptic surgery in 1882

except when they overwhelmed the nose and forced people to open the windows. Carbolic acid was one of many chemicals used in the nineteenth century as a general disinfectant for cesspools, outhouses, stables, and drains. After reading about the beneficial effects the town of Carlisle enjoyed after adding carbolic acid to its sewage works, Lister tested it in animal and human experiments. Several cases ended in failure, but suggested ways in which Lister could improve his technique. In 1865, an 11-year-old boy with a compound fracture of the leg was admitted to the Glasgow Royal Infirmary. The limb was splinted and the wound was washed and dressed with carbolic acid. Within 6 weeks the bones were well united and the sore had healed without suppuration. Further refinements of the antiseptic system led to successful treatments for a variety of life-threatening conditions. Moreover, when the antiseptic system was fully incorporated into the hospital routine, the overall rate of hospitalism declined dramatically.

Lister always attributed his success to his appreciation of Pasteur's argument that the "septic property of the atmosphere" was due to germs suspended in the air and deposited on surfaces. To attack the germs in the air directly, Lister experimented with devices that sprayed carbolic acid into the air of the operating room. His favorite pump—known as the mule—dispensed a fine mist which his patients and assistants found extremely irritating. Eventually, Lister acknowledged that he had overemphasized the problem of airborne germs and, focusing his attention on improvements in disinfection of hands, instruments, and wound dressings, he abandoned the spray.

ANTISEPSIS AND ASEPSIS

By the end of the nineteenth century, many surgeons had joined microbiologists in using improved methods of sterilization and were full participants in the debates concerning the relative merits of heat versus chemical sterilization, and antiseptic versus aseptic methods. The goal of *antisepsis* is to kill the germs in and around a wound by means of germicidal agents. The goal of *asepsis* is to prevent the introduction of germs into the surgical site. Because almost all wounds contain some bacteria, the concept of *aseptic wounds* is essentially an oxymoronic microbiological myth. On the other hand, antiseptics alone cannot guarantee uncomplicated healing; the immunological status of the patient is an important factor. Lister tended to remain attached to his own antiseptic methods and, despite his admiration for Louis Pasteur, insisted on keeping his instruments in carbolic acid, even after Pasteur and Charles Chamberland demonstrated that heat sterilization was superior to chemical disinfection of surgical instruments. Chamberland's autoclave, a device for sterilization by moist heat under pressure, was in general use in bacteriology laboratories by 1883. Indeed, the relationship between Listerian antisepsis and the acceptance of asepsis by nineteenth-century surgeons involves a complex web of motives, prejudices, and theories. What has been called the "full aseptic ritual" never became part of Lister's routine. Indeed, Lister had little enthusiasm for some of the later additions to the surgical ritual, such as white gowns, masks, and gloves. After adopting the aseptic ritual, some of Lister's associates recalled that Lister, operating in his old coat under a cloud of carbolic acid spray, had had just as much success with much less fuss.

As surgeons adopted asepsis and antisepsis with increasing rigor, operations that had once been the miraculous achievements of truly gifted or unusually lucky performers became a matter of routine. However, the conversion of surgeons to the gospel of antisepsis and asepsis was not rapid or universal, nor were all hospitals capable of providing a supportive staff and environment. Even at the turn of the century indifference towards aseptic procedures was not uncommon. Advocates of asepsis adopted the habit of answering the question "What is new in surgery?" with the declaration: "Today we wash our hands *before* operations!"

Surprisingly, one of the last of the critical factors considered in the battle against infection was the surgeon's hand. William Stewart Halsted, a pioneer of local anesthesia, was also a leader in the battle for aseptic surgery. Pasteur said that if he had been a surgeon he would not only use perfectly clean instruments and heat-sterilized water and bandages, he would willingly submit his hands to a rapid flaming after washing them with the greatest care. It is difficult to imagine surgeons agreeing to a routine "flaming" of their hands, but the antiseptic solutions used for scrubbing were almost as unpleasant. When Halsted came to terms with the fact that the human hand could not be sterilized, he decided that it should be covered by flexible gloves, resistant to harsh disinfectants. Initially, Halsted asked the Goodyear Rubber Company to make two pairs of rubber gloves for Miss Caroline Hampton, head nurse in the surgical division, who was very sensitive to disinfectants. The experiment was successful, except for the fact that Johns Hopkins lost an efficient nurse when Miss Hampton married Halsted. In the 1890s the use of flexible rubber gloves was added to the surgical ritual at Johns Hopkins. Doctors had previously used gloves to protect themselves from patients, especially those who might be syphilitic, but surgical gloves were an innovation designed to protect the patient from the surgeon.

The remainder of Halsted's life was devoted to the improvement of surgical technique. He attempted to instill in his associates an understanding of antiseptic and aseptic principles and an operating style that minimized injury and insult to the tissues. Recalling the surgical technique taught at Johns Hopkins in the 1890s, Dr. William G. MacCallum remembered it as "rigorous and even painful to the staff if not to the patient." For the sake of asepsis, some surgeons even trimmed their magnificent beards and mustaches and refrained from talking to observers and yelling at their assistants. Another safety measure was the complete removal of spectators from the operating room. Some hospitals installed special mirrors or glass domes so that observers could watch without contaminating the operating room. When properly applied, antisepsis, asepsis, and anesthesia transformed the operating room from a doorway to death into an arena of quiet routine.

To explore the achievements of the many famous surgeons of the post-Listerian period would be an impossible task, and rather like compiling a catalogue of all the parts of the body. It is more important to recognize the fact that the surgical revolution involved much more than the obvious technical triumphs of anesthesia and asepsis. More subtle, but fundamental factors involved changes in the status and training of the surgeon which made it possible for practitioners of a once lowly craft to integrate advances in pathological anatomy, medical instrumentation, and the life sciences into the science and art of surgery. Since the late nineteenth century, progress in controlling the three major obstacles to successful surgery—pain, infection, and bleeding—has been remarkable. Understanding of the immunological basis of blood-group substances and practical methods for the storage and transfusion of blood and blood products have made survival possible even when accidents or operations cause catastrophic blood loss. Knowledge of the most hidden parts of the body has grown via the classical pathway of anatomical study and through the introduction of new instruments and techniques for visualizing, exploring, and sampling body parts and products. The surgeon is no longer engaged in single-handed combat, but is part of a team of specialists in anesthesia, pathology, radiology, bacteriology, immunology, etc. Surgical triumphs had become so routine by the 1960s that gaining an international reputation, or at least a cover story in *Time* magazine, required nothing less than a return to the stuff of myth: the transplantation of human hearts.

Not all of the factors that determine the success of surgery are, strictly speaking, a part of medical science. Some of the major post-operative threats to the patient are so humble that it would have been an insult to the dignity of the medical profession to take notice of them. For example, hospital bandages were generally made of rags which had gone through a laundry process that scarcely inconvenienced their microbial inhabitants. Rags were a major item of international trade and a good vehicle for the exchange of disease. No matter how skillful the surgeon, if the patient was later bandaged with contaminated dressings, and put into soiled bedding, infection and death could claim another victim.

FROM HOSPITALISM TO NOSOCOMIAL INFECTIONS

Surgeons no longer fear the old hospital fevers, but few patients realize that *nosocomial infections* are still a very significant threat. Probably few patients know that nosocomial infection simply means hospital-acquired infection. Although it is difficult to assess the morbidity and mortality directly due to nosocomial infections, according to the National Nosocomial Infections Surveillance System (NNISS), the overall infection rate is highest in large teaching hospitals and lowest in nonteaching hospitals. In all hospitals, the incidence of such infections is highest in the surgery department, followed by the medicine and gynecology wards. Semmelweis and Lister would be dismayed to find that the most common and most preventable cause of nosocomial infections is a general neglect of hand washing by hospital doctors and staff members.

One hundred years after the development of the Listerian system the Study on the Efficacy of Nosocomial Infection Control, a retrospective study involving a representative sample of American hospitals, found that 5–6% of hospitalized patients developed a nosocomial infection. Moreover, investigators suggested that the true incidence of nosocomial infections was actually much higher. If all nosocomial infections were accurately reported, they would probably rank as the tenth leading cause of death in the United States.

Although there is no doubt that nosocomial infections add to morbidity and mortality rates and increase the costs of hospital care, it is still very difficult to determine the actual risk assumed when a patient enters a hospital. The proportion of extremely sick and vulnerable patients found in today's hospitals—transplant patients, premature infants, elderly patients with multiple disorders, cancer patients, burn victims, AIDS patients—has dramatically increased. Such patients would not have lived long enough to contract hospital infections in the not so distant past.

SUGGESTED READINGS

Bigelow, Henry J. (1900). *Surgical Anaesthesia; Addresses and Other Papers*. Boston: Little, Brown and Co.

Boland, Frank K. (1950). *The First Anesthesia; The Story of Crawford Long*. Athens, GA: University of Georgia Press.

Cartwright, F. F. (1952). *The English Pioneers of Anaesthesia: Beddoes, Davy, and Hickman*. Bristol, England: Wright.

Cartwright, Frederick Fox (1967). *The Development of Modern Surgery from 1830*. London: Arthur Barker.

Cherry, Laurence (1985). A Hospital Is No Place for a Sick Person to Be. *Discover*, October 1985, pp. 96-101.

Cheyne, W. Watson (1925). *Lister and His Achievement*. London: Longmans, Green.

Churchill, Edward D. (1964). Healing by First Intention and with Supuration: Studies in the History of Wound Healing. *JHMAS* 19:193-214.

Churchill, Edward D. (1965). The Pandemic of Wound Infection in Hospitals: Studies in the History of Wound Healing. *JHMAS* 20:390-404.

Cole, Frank (1965). *Milestones in Anesthesia: Readings in the Development of Surgical Anesthesia, 1665-1940*. Lincoln, NE: University of Nebraska Press.

Crowe, S.J. (1957). *Halsted of John Hopkins. The Man and His Men*. Springfield, IL: Charles C. Thomas.

Davis, Audrey B. (1982). The Development of Anesthesia. *Amer. Sci.* 70:522-528.

Davis, Audrey B. (1984). Silent Sleep: An Essay Review. *BHM* 58:111-139.

Davy, Humphrey (1800). *Researches, Chemical and Philosophical, Chiefly Concerning Nitrous Oxide or Dephlogisticated Nitrous Air, and its Respiration*. London: J. Johnson. Repr. London: Butterworths, 1972.

Duffy, John (1944). Anglo-American Reaction to Obstetrical Anesthesia. *BHM* 38:32-44.

Edmondston, William E. (1986). *The Induction of Hypnosis*. New York: Wiley.

Ellis, Edgar S. (1946). *Ancient Anodynes: Primitive Anaesthesia and Allied Conditions*. London: Heinemann.

Faulconer, Albert, and Keys, Thomas Edward, eds. (1965). *Foundations of Anesthesiology.* 2 vols. Springfield, IL: Charles C. Thomas.

Fisher, Richard B. (1977). *Joseph Lister, 1827-1912.* London: Macdonald and Jane's.

Flood, Ann Barry, and Scott, W. Richard with Brown, Byron W. et al. (1987). *Hospital Structure and Performance.* Baltimore, MD: Johns Hopkins University Press.

Godlee, Sir Rochard John (1924). *Lord Lister.* 3rd ed. rev. Oxford, England: Clarendon Press.

Hamilton, David (1982). The Nineteenth-Century Surgical Revolution--Antisepsis or Better Nutrition? *BHM* 56:30-40.

Harvey, Samuel C. (1929). *The History of Hemostasis.* New York: Hoeber.

Horan, Teresa C., et al. (1986). Nosocomial Infection Surveillance, 1984. CDC Surveillance Summaries. *MMWR* 35, No. 1SS: 17SS-29SS.

Hurwitz, Alfred, and Degenshein, George A. (1958). *Milestones in Modern Surgery.* New York: Hoeber-Harper.

Keys, Thomas E. (1963). *The History of Surgical Anesthesia.* New York: Dover.

Leake, Chauncy D. (1947). *Letheon: The Cadenced Story of Anesthesia.* Austin, TX: Univeristy of Texas Press.

Lister, Joseph (1909). *Collected Papers of Joseph, Baron Lister.* 2 vols. Oxford, England: Clarendon Press.

Ludovici, L. J. (1961). *The Discovery of Anaesthesia.* New York: Thomas Y. Crowell.

MacCallum, William George (1930). *William Stewart Halsted, Surgeon.* Baltimore, MD: Johns Hopkins Press.

Majno, Guido (1975). *The Healing Hand. Man and Wound in the Ancient World.* Cambridge, MA: Harvard University Press.

McDonell, Katherine Mandusic, ed. (1988). *The Journals of William A. Lindsay. An Ordinary Nineteenth-Century Physician's Surgical Cases.* Indianapolis, IN: Indiana Historical Society.

Melzak, Ronald (1973). *The Puzzle of Pain.* New York: Basic Books.

Metchnikoff, Elie (1939). *The Founders of Modern Medicine. Pasteur. Koch. Lister.* New York: Walden Publications.

Miller, Timothy S. (1985). *The Birth of the Hospital in the Byzantine Empire.* The Henry E. Sigerist Supplements to the BHM, New Series, no. 10.

Morton, W. T. G. (1946). *W.T.G. Morton's Memoir on Sulphuric Ether 1847.* Foreword by John F. Fulton. New York: Schuman.

Nightingale, Florence (1859). *Notes on Hospitals.* London: John W. Parker & Son.

Olsen, D. B., Kim, S. W., Stephen, R. L., Brophy, J. J., Normann, R. A., and Detmer, D. E., eds. (1987). *Symposium on Artificial Organs, Biomedical Engineering and Transplantation.* New York: VCH Publishers.

Pattison, F. L. M. (1987). *Granville Sharp Pattison Anatomist and Antagonist, 1791-1851.* Tuscaloosa, AL: University of Alabama Press.

Pernick, Martin S. (1985). *A Calculus of Suffering: Pain, Professionalism, and Anesthesia in 19th-Century America.* New York: Columbia University Press.

Peterson, J. Jeanne (1978). *The Medical Profession in Mid-Victorian London.* Berkeley, CA: University of California Press.

Randers-Peterson, Justine (1960). *The Surgeon's Glove.* Springfield, IL: Charles C. Thomas.

Ravitch, Mark M. (1982). *A Century of Surgery. 1880-1980.* 2 vols. Philadelphia, PA: J.B. Lippincott Co.

Rodgers, R., and Cooper, S., eds. (1988). *Endorphins, Opiates and Behavioural Processes.* New York: Wiley.

Scrimshaw, Nevin S., Taylor, Carl E., and Gordon, John E. (1968). *Interactions of Nutrition and Infection.* Geneva: World Health Organization.

Smith, Theodore C., Cooperman, Lee H., and Wollman, Harry, (1980). History and Principles of Anesthesiology. In *The Pharmacological Basis of Therapeutics*, 6th ed. Alfred Goodman Gilman, Louis S. Goodman, and Alfred Gilman, eds. New York: Macmillan.

Sykes, William Stanley (1982). *Essays on the First Hundred Years of Anaesthesia.* 3 vols. Chicago, IL: American Society of Anesthesiologists, 3 vols.

Temkin, Owsei (1951). The role of surgery in the rise of modern medical thought. *BHM* 25:248-259.

Thomas, Vivien T. (1985). *Pioneering Research in Surgical Shock and Cardiovascular Surgery. Vivien Thomas and His Work with Alfred Blalock.* Philadelphia, PA: University of Pennsylvania Press.

Thompson, John D., and Goldin, Grace (1975). *The Hospital: A Social and Architectural History.* New Haven, CT: Yale University Press.

Volpitto, Perry P., and Vandam, Leroy D. eds. (1982). *The Genesis of Contemporary American Anesthesiology.* Springfield, IL: Charles C. Thomas.

Wallace, Abraham (1928). *Reminiscences of Lister.* Manchester, England: Two Worlds.

Wallace, Antony F. (1982). *The Progress of Plastic Surgery: An Introductory History.* Oxford, England: William A. Meeuws.

Wangensteen, Owen H., and Wangensteen, Sarah D. (1978). *The Rise of Surgery. From Empiric Craft to Scientific Discipline.* Minneapolis, MN: University of Minnesota Press.

Welch, Claude E., ed. (1966). *Advances in Surgery.* Chicago, IL: Year Book Medical Publishers.

Whipple, Allen O. (1963). *The Story of Wound Healing and Wound Repair.* Springfield, IL: Charles C. Thomas.

Willis, W. D., Jr. (1985). *The Pain System. The Neural Basis of Nociceptive Transmission in the Mammalian Nervous System.* Basel: Karger.

Zimmerman, Leo M., and Veith, Ilza (1967). *Great Ideas in the History of Surgery.* 2nd ed. New York: Dover.

THE GERM THEORY OF DISEASE: MEDICAL MICROBIOLOGY

D espite the antiquity of the concepts of contagion and germs or seeds of disease, microbiology was not established as a scientific discipline until the end of the nineteenth century. In the process, scientists and medical reformers often cast their arguments in terms of an opposition between *contagion theory* and *miasma theory*. While the miasma theory of disease was the primary stimulus to the public health campaigns of the nineteenth century, closer inspection of the evolution and usage of these terms in earlier periods suggests that they were not necessarily seen as mutually exclusive. Sharp distinctions between contagion and miasma models might be considered rather misleading and anachronistic when applied to the period between Fracastoro's publication of *On Contagion* in 1546 and the triumph of microbiology at the end of the nineteenth century. That is, Renaissance authors and those who followed them often switched back and forth between the two terms; when contagion was defined loosely enough to include harmful material that was indirectly, as well as directly transmitted, it was not incompatible with equally vague definitions of miasma as disease-inducing noxious, contaminated air. Thus, when nineteenth-century bacteriologists expressed their interest in Fracastoro as the precursor of germ theory, they were probably interpreting his views in a manner very different from the way in which Fracastoro and other Renaissance physicians saw them. It should be noted that the microscope, the instrument so intimately linked to microbiology, had been invented at the end of the sixteenth century. During the seventeenth century, microscopists established the existence of tiny "animalcules," infusoria, the capillary network, and certain kinds of cells. Antoni van Leeuwenhoek (1632–1723), one of the most ingenious microscopists of that period, described molds, protozoa, bacteria, sperm cells, and other assorted "little animals." The work of the pioneering microscopists of the seventeenth century was the best to be done until the middle of the nineteenth century, when various technical problems with the lens systems and sample preparation were finally solved.

In medical research the period from the 1850s to the 1880s was a time of great excitement and confusion. In order to simplify our survey of the development of medical microbiology, we will focus on the work of Louis Pasteur and Robert Koch, the scientists who have come to exemplify the establishment of the theoretical and methodological basis for the new science of microbiology. In terms of their practical legacy, Pasteur established the fundamentals of disinfection, sterilization, immunization, and procedures for the development of vaccines.

CONTAGION AND MICROPARASITES AS CAUSES OF DISEASE

The idea that disease, impurity, or corruption can be transmitted by contact is an ancient folk belief, but it was generally ignored in Hippocratic doctrine. *On Contagion* (1546) by Girolamo Fracastoro is generally regarded as the earliest exposition of germ theory, but it was Giovanni Cosimo Bonomo (d. 1697) who provided the first convincing demonstration that a contagious human disease was caused by a minute parasite close to the threshold of invisibility. Bonomo proved that scabies, commonly known as "the itch," was caused by a tortoise-like mite just barely visible to the naked eye. The mites could be transferred directly from person to person or by means of bedding or clothing used by "itchy" persons. The itch mite, however, was regarded as an interesting curiosity rather than an example that might apply to other diseases. Even after the popularization of the microscope in the 1660s, most physicians and naturalists regarded the notion of "disease-causing animalcules" as little better than ancient superstitions about elf-shot, worms, and flying venom. Moreover, there was little evidence available to decide between the hypothesis that the minute entities observed by microscopists were the *product* of disease, putrefaction, and fermentation and the alternative hypothesis that they were the *cause* of these phenomena.

Further evidence for contagion theory appeared in studies of silkworm diseases. Agostino Bassi (1773–1857) found that he could transfer the disease called muscardine to healthy silkworms by inoculating them with material taken from worms that had died of the disease. According to Bassi, muscardine was caused by a minute living plant or parasitic fungus. Bassi suggested that other contagious diseases might be caused by similar parasites. The fungus that causes muscardine was later named *Botrytis bassiana* in honor of Agostino Bassi. Johann Lucas Schönlein's (1793–1864) search for the cause of ringworm was influenced by Bassi's work on muscardine. In 1839 Schönlein, a professor of medicine at Zurich, reported finding a fungus in the pustules of ringworm. Unlike the prolix Bassi, Schönlein set forth his case for a causal relationship between parasite and disease in barely 200 words.

When Jacob Henle (1809–1895), Professor of Anatomy at Zurich, published *On Miasmata and Contagia* in 1840, several examples of microparasites as putative agents of disease had been added to scabies and muscardine. Critically evaluating the experimental evidence, Henle discussed the nature of the proofs that would be required to establish a causal relationship between microbes and disease. While it is possible to link Fracastoro's account of contagion and miasma to Henle's hypothesis, the context in which they worked and the centuries that separated them infused very different meanings into their use of the terms miasma and contagion.

According to Henle, physicians blamed disease on miasma, which they defined as something that mixed with and poisoned the air, but, he argued, no one had ever demonstrated the existence of miasma with scientific instruments. Miasma was only presumed to exist, by exclusion, because no other cause could be demonstrated. According to Henle's hypothesis, *contagia animata* (living organisms) caused contagious diseases because whatever the morbid matter of disease might be, it obviously had the power to increase in the afflicted individual. Given the fact that the pus from pox pustules could be used to infect a multitude of people, the contagion must be an animate entity that multiplies within the body of the sick organism. Chemicals, organic or not, remain fixed in amount; only living things have the power of multiplying themselves.

One could most logically explain the natural history of epidemics by assuming that an agent excreted by sick individuals was the cause. If this agent was excreted by the lungs, it might easily pass to others through the air; if excreted by the intestines, it would enter sewers and wells. Acknowledging the lack of rigorous evidence for the germ theory of disease, Henle argued that science could not wait for unequivocal proofs because scientists could only conduct research in "the light of a reasonable theory." Although Henle's theory was generally ignored by his contemporaries, after the establishment of microbiology, his essay on contagion was awarded the status of a landmark.

LOUIS PASTEUR

Microbe hunting was not uncommon in the first half of the nineteenth century, and Louis Pasteur (1822–1895) was not the first to argue that infectious diseases were caused by germs, but his work was of paramount importance in demonstrating the relevance of germ theory to infectious disease, surgery, hospital management, agriculture, and industry. Pasteur's work illuminated virtually every branch of nineteenth-century microbiology, from chemistry to fermentation, from spontaneous generation to the germ theory of disease, from the preparation of protective vaccines to immunology and virology. Generally, Pasteur was involved in several research problems simultaneously. The interaction between his many interests makes it impossible to discuss his work as a neat chronological progression, but this complexity reflects his belief that "the sciences gain by mutual support." His career can also

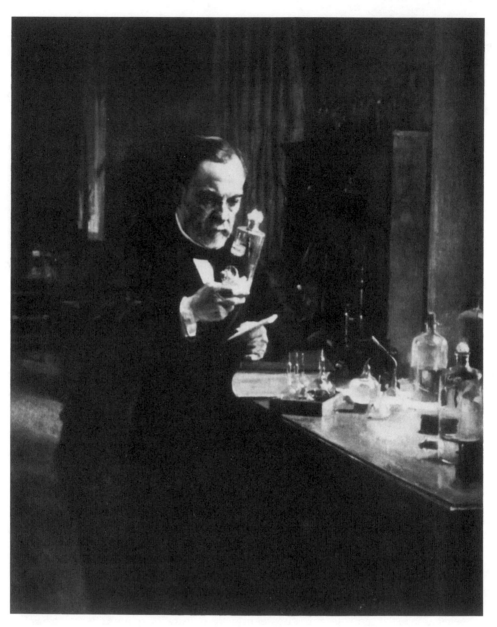

Louis Pasteur

serve as a case study for the interplay between researches devoted to practical problems and so-called pure or basic scientific knowledge.

As a youth, Pasteur was a diligent student and talented artist. He abandoned art in order to devote all his energies to science, but his high school work in chemistry was rated only mediocre. (Stories about such ludicrous errors in judgment by teachers of the gifted and talented seem to be a required part of the hagiography of great scientists, perhaps to give hope to underachieving students and make teachers more humble.) Pasteur went on to study chemistry and physics with distinction, but the most important lesson he learned from his studies at the elite École Normale Supérieure of Paris was a willingness to apply the experimental approaches he had learned in chemistry to a broad range of problems in biology and medicine, areas in which he had no specific training. The research problems and methods that Pasteur assimilated as a doctoral student led down many paths. However, nine specific aspects of his work were carved into the marble walls of the chapel at the Pasteur Institute in Paris where he was buried: molecular dissymmetry, fermentations, studies of so-called spontaneous generation, studies of wine, diseases of silkworms, studies of beer, contagious diseases, protective vaccines, and prevention of rabies. Although Pasteur was more interested in broad philosophical questions and basic scientific issues than specific medical problems, in terms of the history of medicine, he is primarily remembered for the practical aspects of his work that are most directly related to infectious diseases.

Studies of crystal structure, stereoisomerism, and molecular dissymmetry seem remote from medical microbiology, but this work provided the unifying thread that guided Pasteur through the labyrinth of research. Pasteur discovered that certain organic molecules can exist as mirror images, that is, in right-handed and left-handed versions. As he pursued this remarkable trait from the behavior of crystals to that of microorganisms, Pasteur came to see molecular dissymmetry as a fundamental criterion which distinguished the chemical processes of vital phenomena from those of the inanimate world.

Among the aphorisms of Louis Pasteur, the most quoted have to do with the importance of theory and the role of chance in discovery. He insisted that the theoretical was as important as the practical, although he accepted the idea that, for the good of the state, scientific education should be made relevant to industrial and commercial needs. "Without theory," Pasteur argued, "practice is but routine born of habit." When asked the use of a purely scientific discovery, Pasteur liked to answer: "What is the use of a new-born child?" By chance, Pasteur discovered that mold growing on his solutions of organic acids fermented the right-handed form but not its mirror image. In keeping with his conviction that "in the fields of observation, chance favors only the mind which is prepared," he followed the implications of this observation on to fundamental studies of the role of microorganisms in fermentation. When Pasteur was appointed Professor of Chemistry and Dean of Sciences at the University of Lille, he was urged to assist local industries. Applying the methodology he had used in his studies of crystals to fermenting vats of beet juice, Pasteur discovered microorganisms and optically active products of fermentation. His stereochemical studies led him to the hypothesis that the fermentation process was dependent on living germs or ferments.

Previous speculations about the role of yeasts in fermentation had been ridiculed by the most illustrious organic chemists of the period, who argued that fermentation was a purely chemical process and that microorganisms were the *product* rather than the *cause* of fermentation. Further experiments on a variety of fermentations led Pasteur to the conclusion that all fermentations are caused by specific, organized ferments. Moreover, Pasteur suggested that living ferments might be the cause of infectious diseases as well as fermentations. As we have seen, Joseph Lister's work on the antiseptic system owed a great deal to Pasteur's fermentation studies, but most physicians rejected the idea that the diseases of beer and wine were related to human disease. Pasteur's fermentation studies had great economic importance by providing improved control over the production of wine, beer, and vinegar. Proper understanding of the conditions for fermentation, partial sterilization (pasteurization), and pure inocula were developments immediately applicable to many industrial problems.

Studies of fermentation led Pasteur into studies of the ancient doctrine of spontaneous generation. Friends warned him against being drawn into a contest that could not be won, for one cannot prove a universal negative; that is, one cannot prove that spontaneous generation never occurred, never occurs, or will never occur. Certainly, Pasteur did not enter the battle with an open mind; he was passionately dedicated to destroying the advocates of spontaneous generation and their allies in the medical profession. Building on an experimental approach that can be traced back to the seventeenth century, Pasteur set out to prove that microbes do not spontaneously arise in sterile medium and that all the so-called evidence in support of the contrary proposition was the result of careless techniques and experimental artifacts.

Philosophical arguments about the origin of life, materialism and atheism, or religion and spiritualism were irrelevant to the daily concerns of wine-makers, hospital administrators, and surgeons. The practical point established in this contest was that fermentation, putrefaction, and infectious diseases were caused by specific microbes found in the air and on surfaces. The germ-carrying capacity of the air accounted for fermentation, putrefaction, and infection. The germ-carrying capacity of air could be measured by sucking air through cotton filters to trap the germ-laden dust particles. The numbers and kinds of germs in the air depended on many environmental factors; for example, the germ content of hospital air was quite high, while that of mountain air was low. While almost all kinds of media could be sterilized by fairly simple means, certain apparent exceptions were eventually traced to the existence of heat-resistant spores. Thus, in jousting with the advocates of spontaneous generation, Pasteur and his followers created the sterile techniques that made modern microbiology and surgery possible.

Pasteur was convinced that a revolution in medicine would only become possible when the defenders of spontaneous generation were totally defeated; the development of rational methods for the prevention and treatment of disease depended on rejecting this erroneous doctrine. Well aware of the skepticism with which the conservative medical profession regarded his theories, Pasteur seems to have been reluctant to begin a direct assault on the diseases of higher animals. However, in 1865 at the request of his friend Jean Baptiste Dumas and the Minister of Agriculture, Pasteur became involved in studies of the silkworm diseases that were devastating French sericulture. By 1870, Pasteur had demonstrated the existence of two microbial diseases in silkworms. The epidemic was the result of complex interactions among environmental factors, nutritional deficiencies, and microbes.

Research on silkworms provided a transition between Pasteur's studies of fermentations and diseases of higher animals and humans, such as chicken cholera, swine erysipelas, anthrax, puerperal fever, cholera, and rabies. Contrary to the Pasteur mythology, not all of these studies were successful. For example, Pasteur's studies of a microbe found in victims of childbed fever led him to warn hospital personnel that they carried the microbe from infected women to healthy women, but like Oliver Wendell Holmes and Ignaz Philipp Semmelweis, he failed to convince the medical community. Indeed, an outraged opponent challenged Pasteur to a duel for this assault on the honor of the medical profession. Such violent and personal animosity was not characteristic of the entire medical and public health community. Among those who enthusiastically accepted Pasteur's work as a spur to their own public health reform campaigns were France's scientific, statistically based hygienists. While many French physicians resisted Pasteur's ideas because they anticipated a new form of preventive medicine that would threaten the profession and practice of medicine, by about 1895 this opposition was essentially disarmed by the dazzling prospects of powerful new therapeutic tools that actually strengthened the medical profession.

Rabies, a rare but fatal human disease, and its invisible microbe provided Pasteur's most famous triumph. In his development of a protective vaccine against rabies Pasteur provided ample proof of his contention that microbiology was a demonstration of how the role of the "infinitely small in nature is infinitely great." The first step in his previous studies had been to find the microbe, but all efforts to identify the causative agent for rabies proved futile. At a time when scientists were just beginning to formulate the technical and theoretical problems of immunization, Pasteur was able to take the great intellectual leap of developing a vaccine against an invisible virus. The term "virus" was traditionally used in a nonspecific sense in referring to an unknown agent, or poison of disease.

Why did Pasteur elect to study a disease as rare as rabies when there were so many common diseases that might have been easier to work with? Several answers have been offered. Perhaps it really was the haunting memory of the howls of the mad wolf that invaded Arbois when Pasteur was a boy and the screams of its victims as their wounds were cauterized. Alternatively, the choice may have reflected Pasteur's ambition and his flair for the dramatic. However, Pasteur had done enough to achieve immortality before embarking on what was obviously a dangerous project, for research on rabies must begin with one of the most feared of all creatures, the mad dog. Another factor influencing Pasteur's choice may have been the tension between his condemnation of experimentation on human beings and his desire to prevent human disease. Pasteur was convinced that human experimentation was not only immoral, but criminal. Moreover, his entry into the study of human diseases was apparently inhibited by a deep antipathy for vivisection and his ambivalence towards physicians. To reconcile these conflicts Pasteur needed a disease shared by humans and animals which was invariably fatal so that an experimental treatment could not make the outcome any worse. Whatever the motive might have been, Pasteur had chosen well; the success of his quest was greeted throughout the world as the greatest achievement of microbiological science, and Pasteur was hailed as genius, hero, and saint. The real Pasteur, who was certainly one of the greatest scientists who ever lived, all but disappeared under the weight of myth, romanticism, and adoration. (Those old enough to remember the fear aroused by polio might reflect upon the similar outbursts of joy, hope, and gratitude that greeted Jonas Salk and the polio vaccine.)

The difficulty of predicting the outcome of dog bites is a complicating factor in assessing Pasteur's rabies vaccine. That is, rabies was invariably fatal if contracted, but not all encounters with mad dogs result in human rabies; and not all mad dogs are actually rabid. Moreover, the incubation period for rabies is so variable that in some cases the association between bite and disease was difficult to assess. For example, John Hunter (1728–1793) noted a report of a dog which supposedly bit 21 people. None of these people received any medical attention, but only one became ill. If all of them had been treated, the attending doctors would have claimed 20 cures.

In order to isolate the rabies virus and prepare a vaccine, Pasteur needed a laboratory culture of the organism. Obviously, it was difficult to find rabid dogs on a routine basis and even harder to secure their cooperation. Not surprisingly, kennels for rabid dogs were as welcome in any neighborhood as an AIDS clinic or a toxic waste dump. A reliable and relatively safe system of transmitting rabies, which involved trephining experimental animals and inoculating infectious material through the dura mater, was used to study the disease in rabbits and other animals. Rabies was transmitted from rabbit to rabbit so that a "fixed virus" with a reproducible degree of virulence and a shortened incubation period was always available. Finally, Pasteur and his colleagues discovered that when the isolated spinal cord of a rabid animal was subjected to increasing periods of air drying, the rabies virus became progressively weaker. To test the use of the air-dried material as a preventive vaccine, dogs were inoculated daily with suspensions of increasingly virulent preparations of spinal cord. At the end of this procedure, dogs were resistant to rabies even if the most virulent preparations were inoculated directly into the brain. By 1885 Pasteur was satisfied that he could reliably induce immunity to rabies in dogs.

The question of the safety and effectiveness of this vaccine in human beings could not be avoided once the results on dogs became known. Protecting people by immunizing all the dogs in France was surely an impossible task; moreover, wild animals served as an infinite reservoir of disease. Obviously, rabies vaccine was not a candidate for mass immunizations because human rabies was too rare a condition to justify a dangerous series of painful injections. But Pasteur's vaccine was the only hope against the pain, suffering, and death that were inevitable for victims of the disease. On July 6, 1885, 9-year-old Joseph Meister was brought to Pasteur's laboratory. He had sustained at least 14 wounds, some very deep, when attacked by a mad dog 2 days before. Physicians who examined the boy did not doubt that he would contract rabies and that death was inevitable. After consultation with colleagues at the Academy of Medicine, Pasteur's immunization procedure was begun. Despite the discomfort entailed by the long course of injections, Joseph made a complete recovery. The second patient was a 15-year-old boy who had been savagely bitten by a rabid dog 6 days before treatment began. News of the apparently successful use of Pasteur's vaccine created both bitter criticism and excessive hope. Pasteur was attacked by physicians, veterinarians, antivivisectionists, and antivaccinators, while terrified victims of the bites of rabid, or presumably rabid, animals besieged his laboratory.

The uncertainties inherent in the course of human rabies and the crudeness of the vaccine led to tragic failures as well as successes. Successful immunization depends on how soon the inoculations are begun and the individual's reaction to the vaccine; a certain number of deaths due to reactions to the vaccine were inevitable. Critics could always charge that success measured only by the failure of patients to die of rabies was meaningless. When some patients developed paralysis, Pasteur's critics called him an assassin and charged him with infecting human beings with "laboratory rabies." However, when victims of dog bites compared the risks of the Pasteur method to rabies, thousands decided that the vaccine was a great victory in the battle between science and disease and chose the Pasteur treatment. Throughout the world people echoed Joseph Lister's tribute to Louis Pasteur: "Truly there does not exist in the whole world a person to whom medical science owes more than to you." Perhaps Pasteur's German counterpart Robert Koch would have quarreled with that assessment. The hostility between Koch and Pasteur was due, at least in part, to nationalistic rivalries inflamed by the Franco-Prussian War, but there were also major differences in their goals, objectives, scientific styles, and personalities.

ROBERT KOCH

In contrast to Louis Pasteur, whose road to microbiology began with chemistry, Robert Koch (1843–1910) came to bacteriology as a physician, and his investigations were primarily motivated by medical questions. Lacking Pasteur's flair for the dramatic, Koch's gift was for attention to detail and simple but ingenious techniques

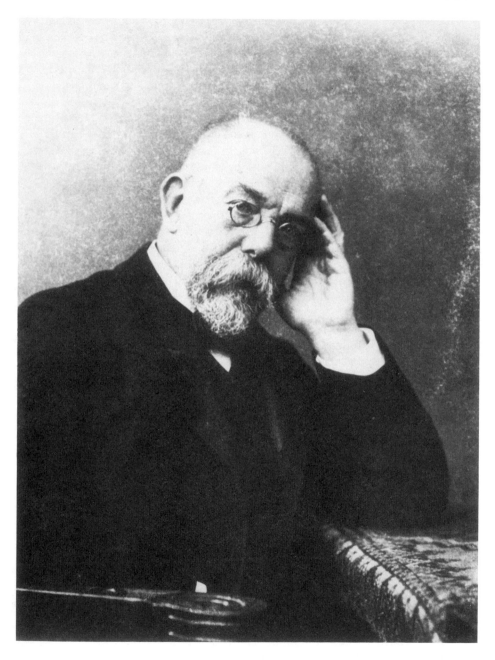

Robert Koch

that made modern microbiology possible. To his contemporaries, Koch was "a man of genius both as technician and as bacteriologist."

Robert Koch was the third of 13 children born to Hermann Koch, a mining administrator, and his wife Mathilde. When Koch began his medical studies at the University of Göttingen, the faculty included many eminent scientists, but in the 1860s not even Jacob Henle seemed to have any interest in the relationship between bacteria and disease. In 1866 Koch received his doctor's degree and passed his state medical examination. He spent several months in Berlin observing medical care at the Charité hospital and attending a course of lectures by Germany's most famous physician, Rudolf Virchow (1821–1902), the founder of cellular pathology. Given to romantic dreams, despite his rather phlegmatic personality, Koch originally hoped for a career as a ship's doctor or military surgeon, but he abandoned this plan in order to become engaged to Emmy Fraatz. His first position as a medical assistant at the Hamburg General Hospital gave him some practical experience in working with cholera, a disease he would return to later. In 1867, after finding another position and establishing a modest private practice, he was able to marry Emmy and appeared to be doomed to spending his life in rural isolation as a general practitioner and district medical officer. A brief interruption occurred during the Franco-Prussian War of 1870, when Koch enlisted in the medical corps. His experience with typhoid fever and battle wounds would later prove valuable in his research. Despite his official duties and private practice, Koch found time for hobbies such as natural history, archaeology, photography, and for research concerning hygiene, public health, and bacteriology. A trip taken in 1875 to attend scientific and medical meetings and visit research centers provided further stimulation for a more serious commitment to scientific research. Thus, when anthrax appeared in his district, Koch was prepared to investigate the relationship between bacteria and disease.

Anthrax is primarily a disease of sheep and cattle, but in humans it can cause severe, localized skin ulcers known as malignant pustules, a dangerous condition known as gastric anthrax, or a virulent pneumonia known as woolsorter's disease. Proponents of the germ theory were particularly interested in anthrax and the relatively large bacilli associated with it. Franz Pollender (1800–1879) had observed bacteria in the blood of anthrax victims as early as 1849, but he did not publish his findings until 1855. Pierre Rayer (1793–1867) claimed to have seen the bacillus in the blood of sheep he had inoculated with blood from animals that had died of anthrax. However, it was Casimir Joseph Davaine (1812–1882) who first presented good, albeit circumstantial evidence of a link between the bacillus and anthrax. Davaine demonstrated that inoculations of blood from anthrax victims transmitted the disease to experimental animals. In 1863 Davaine published important papers on the infectivity of the "filiform bodies" that appeared in the blood of animals dying of anthrax. Identical bacilli could be found in the malignant pustules of human victims. These experiments were suggestive, but not compelling; Davaine had not isolated and purified the anthrax bacillus, nor had he satisfied the criteria of proof suggested by Jacob Henle.

By 1876, Koch had obtained cultures of *Bacillus anthracis* and had worked out the life cycle of the bacillus and the natural history of the disease. Like Davaine, Koch transferred anthrax from infected cattle to rabbits and mice. An important new step was Koch's discovery that bacteria could be cultured outside the whole animal in the fluid taken from the eyeballs of cattle. Bacilli were grown in aqueous humor and injected into experimental animals. Koch's pure laboratory cultures produced anthrax just as if a sample of blood from a naturally infected farm animal had been used. In order to have fresh anthrax material always available and to determine whether the bacilli would change after a certain number of generations, Koch inoculated mice in series (a chain of mouse-to-mouse inoculations). Even after the bacilli had been passed through a series of 20 mice, they remained true to form. These experiments ruled out the possibility that some poison from the original animal caused the disease in experimental animals. Only an agent capable of multiplying within the bodies of infected animals could create these chains of transmission. While observing anthrax bacilli on microscope slides, Koch saw thread-like chains of bacteria become bead-like spores. When fresh medium was added, the spores were transformed into active bacilli which began to multiply again. The extreme hardiness of the spores explained many of the mysteries surrounding the persistence of anthrax in contaminated pastures. Because spores were resistant to harsh conditions, a carcass deposited in a shallow grave could furnish enough spores to infect other animals for many years. Thus, an understanding of the natural history of anthrax immediately suggested measures for controlling the disease through proper disposal of contaminated carcasses.

Convinced that he had solved the riddle of anthrax, Koch sent an account of his work to Ferdinand Cohn (1828–1898), the eminent botanist who was Germany's leading expert on bacteriology. Despite some initial skepticism, Cohn invited Koch to come to the University of Breslau to demonstrate his experiments. Certainly Koch was not the first amateur to invade the academic community claiming to have found a solution to the problem of contagion. In this case, however, Cohn and his associates found the experimental results and demonstrations absolutely convincing. Under Cohn's sponsorship, Koch's paper "The Etiology of Anthrax, Based on the Life Cycle of *Bacillus anthracis*" was published in *Contributions to Plant Biology*.

On the basis of his work with anthrax, Koch confidently predicted that bacteriological science would lead to control over infectious diseases. To overcome the opposition of conservative physicians and scientists, Koch urged advocates of the germ theory of disease to learn to cultivate pure strain of microbes, abandon careless and speculative work, and demonstrate the value of microbiology in the prevention and treatment of disease. In the long run, Koch's predictions were richly validated. However, it was Louis Pasteur who produced an anthrax vaccine to prevent the disease in sheep and cattle and explained how earthworms participated in the chain of transmission by bringing anthrax spores to the surface where they were ingested by grazing animals. While quantity is not necessarily a sign of quality, it is interesting to note that Pasteur published 31 papers on anthrax to Koch's total of two. Such differences in approaching a problem, and achieving practical solutions, aggravated the conflict between Koch and Pasteur. Attacking Pasteur's work openly and directly, Koch called the results of the French microbiologists into question for their alleged failure to produce pure cultures. Koch even stooped to trying to discredit Pasteur by calling attention to the obvious and well-known fact that Pasteur was not a physician. In referring to the praise Pasteur had received as a "second Jenner," Koch contemptuously noted that Jenner's work had involved humans, not sheep.

Having demonstrated the etiology of a specific disease, Koch turned to the general problem of wound infection, which Lister had begun to master through the antiseptic system. Many investigators had observed bacteria in traumatic infective diseases, but they could not determine whether the bacteria were the cause of the disease, the product of pathological processes, or nonspecific entities. In part, the wound infection work was meant to support the concept of the existence of distinct, fixed species of bacteria against an attack by Karl von Nägeli (1817–1891), the Swiss botanist who holds a special place in the history of genetics for his failure to appreciate Gregor Mendel's (1822–1884) theory of inheritance. If bacteria did not exist as separate species, then it made no sense to say that a specific bacterium—such as *Bacillus anthracis*—caused a specific disease. Many critics of the doctrine of specific etiology had indeed "seen" transformation; Koch realized that this was due to sloppy techniques which could only be eliminated by creating simple procedures for obtaining pure cultures and standardized methods of preparing bacteria for microscopic examination.

Studies of experimentally induced traumatic infective diseases led Koch to believe that each septic condition was caused by a different microorganism; he also demonstrated that bacteria were not found in the blood or tissues of healthy animals. Unfortunately, the medical community misinterpreted Koch's general proof of the applicability of germ theory to wound infection as a series of laboratory curiosities involving gangrene and septicemia in mice. Koch excelled in the rigorousness of his techniques, but he was quite lacking in Pasteur's flair for choosing and staging dramatic, attention-getting events. His colleagues would have been more impressed if he could have clearly demonstrated the relationship between his work on sepsis in mice and human disease. In this case the disadvantages of working in rural isolation instead of an urban medical center with access to clinical material were critical. However, Lister was impressed by this work and was instrumental in having Koch's book *The Aetiology of Traumatic Infective Disease* translated into English.

After years of struggling to pursue his research while maintaining a private practice, Koch finally obtained a position as head of a newly established laboratory for bacteriological research with the Imperial Health Office in Berlin. In 1885 he became Professor of Hygiene at the University of Berlin and Director of the

University's Institute of Hygiene, a title he held until 1891 when the Institute for Infectious Diseases was created for him. Despite his professional success, Koch's private life was evidently unhappy until he met 17-year-old Hedwig Freiberg and divorced his first wife. He and Emmy had been estranged for some time, and their daughter Gertude had married Koch's research associate Eduard Pfuhl. Koch was almost 50 and Hedwig was 20 when they married in 1893. The romance between the eminent scientist and the young artist's model raised a "moral storm" among his colleagues. At the 1892 Congress of German Physicians, colleagues admitted that there was more excitement about Koch's love affair than the scientific papers.

Frustrated by the skepticism with which the medical community viewed germ theory, Koch became obsessed with the idea that finding reliable methods of obtaining pure cultures was the key to progress. The animal body might well be the optimum cultivation apparatus for pathogenic bacteria, but microbiologists had to cultivate pure strains outside the animal body in order to establish the role of bacteria in causing disease. Finding it impossible to construct a universal medium suitable for all bacteria, Koch sought a method that would convert the usual nutrient broths into a solid form on which bacterial colonies would stand out like islands, like the colonies one might find on slices of bread or potatoes. Ancient kitchen lore solved his problem when he substituted agar-agar, a polysaccharide derived from seaweed which is used in Oriental cooking, for gelatin. (Gelatin liquifies at normal body temperature, $37°C$, and is digested by many bacteria; gels made with agar-agar are inert to bacterial digestion and remain solid up to $45°C$.) Use of this method was called "Koch's plate technique." A special plate for use with agar cultures was invented by Richard Julius Petri (1852–1921), the curator of Koch's Hygiene Institute. Thanks to the universal adoption of the petri dish, Petri's name is generally more familiar to biology students than that of Robert Koch. Another technical problem addressed by Koch and his associates at the Imperial Health Office was a re-examination of various public health measures, such as disinfection. Microbiology made it possible to understand the difference between disinfection (killing vegetative cells, but not necessarily all spores) and sterilization (completely killing both spores and vegetative cells). In testing the activity of reputed antiseptics, Koch discovered that some old favorites had virtually no disinfecting powers, while others inhibited the growth of bacteria, but did not kill them.

When Lister, Pasteur, and Koch met in London at the Seventh International Medical Congress in 1881, Koch enjoyed the opportunity to demonstrate his plate technique in Lister's laboratory. Shortly after returning from this triumphant visit, Koch began his work on tuberculosis. Committing all his energies to the task of identifying the causal agent of tuberculosis and finding a cure for this ubiquitous malady, Koch worked indefatigably in strict secrecy. The first experiments were performed in August 1881; in March 1882, at a meeting of the Berlin Physiological Society, he announced his discovery of the tubercle bacillus, *Mycobacterium tuberculosis*. News of Koch's discovery caused great excitement throughout the world. The physicist John Tyndall, one of Pasteur's most dedicated supporters, published an English summary of Koch's paper as a letter to the London *Times*. A few weeks later Tyndall's letter was published in the *New York Times*. Reports and editorials immediately took up the theme that Koch's discovery would soon lead to a treatment for tuberculosis, perhaps along the lines of Pasteur's vaccine for anthrax.

During the golden age of bacteriology, Koch recalled, the bacterial agents of many infectious diseases seemed to fall into the hands of microbiologists "like ripe apples from a tree," but the tubercle bacillus did not fall so easily. Of all the microbes studied by Koch, the tubercle bacillus was the most difficult to identify, isolate, and culture. On appropriate nutrient agar, most bacteria produce large colonies within 2 days; the tubercle bacillus took 2 weeks to form visible colonies. In these investigations, superb microbiological technique, special media and staining techniques, and appropriate experimental animals were indispensable. But so too was the conviction that tuberculosis was a contagious bacterial disease, strong faith that the causative agent could be isolated, and almost infinite patience. The discovery of the tubercle bacillus and proof of its existence in diseased tissue swept away the confusion that had so long thwarted efforts to understand tuberculosis in all its many forms. Because *Mycobacterium tuberculosis* can attack virtually every part of the body, it produces a bewildering array of clinical patterns known as phthisis, consumption, scrofula, miliary tuberculosis, meningitis, and so forth. Identification of the tubercle bacillus proved that the various clinical forms were manifestations of the work of a specific pathogen.

To understand the profound effect of Koch's announcement requires an appreciation of the ways in which this disease permeated the fabric of life in the nineteenth century. Tuberculosis was, in terms of the number of victims claimed, more devastating than the most dreaded epidemic diseases, including smallpox and cholera. Even in the seventeenth century, Richard Morton (1637–1698), author of *Phthisiologia: A Treatise of Consumptions* (1694), found it difficult to believe that anyone could reach adulthood without at least a touch of consumption. Already established as the "captain of the men of death" by the seventeenth century, in the nineteenth century tuberculosis was the cause of about one in seven deaths. Its impact on society was greatly amplified by the fact that it was particularly likely to claim victims in their most productive adult years. The tragic deaths of young artists, writers, composers, and musicians supported the myth that tuberculosis was related to artistic genius. Robust artists complained that it was fashionable for poets to suffer from consumption and die before reaching the age of 30. The brief life of John Keats (1795–1821) reflects the romantic view of tuberculosis and the medical mismanagement that often accelerated the inevitable. Although the poet's mother and brother had died of tuberculosis, his illness was misdiagnosed as "gastric fever," and he was subjected to a debilitating regimen of bleeding and starvation diets. At autopsy his lungs were found to have been almost totally destroyed.

Victims of most infectious diseases died or recovered too quickly to indulge in the deep, dark meditations of consumptive artists brooding on the slow, but inexorable progress of their disease. To Franz Kafka, tuberculosis was not an ordinary disease but the "germ of death itself." In Romantic imagery, consumptives were possessed by a nervous force that drove them to artistic accomplishments. But with the disease running rampant in city slums and impoverished villages, the connection was obviously fortuitous, not causal. Perhaps the threat of early death, the chronic mild fever, and the opiates taken to control coughing intensified the creative drive of consumptives who were artists and enhanced the allure of tubercular women. Only an "angel of phthisis" fit the Romantic ideal of femininity: young, pale, thin, with eyes bright from fever, discreetly coughing up blood into her white lace handkerchief, before her inevitable, but redemptive death. As Keats lamented: "Youth grows pale, and spectre thin, and dies."

After Koch's discovery of the tubercle bacillus, the perverted sentimentalism associated with the disease was gradually superseded by acceptance of the fact that it was more intimately linked to poverty and filth than to genius and art. Worse yet, as Koch noted in his early papers on tuberculosis, the tubercle bacillus was very similar in form, size, and staining properties to that which caused leprosy. Medical thinking about the cause and management of tuberculosis reflected peculiar regional differences. Physicians in northern Europe generally believed in a noncontagious, hereditary "tubercular diathesis" (which essentially means that people who are susceptible to tuberculosis are susceptible to tuberculosis). It was common knowledge that the disease "ran in families," sometimes for several generations. Moreover, the fact that only certain individuals developed the disease, although almost everyone was exposed to it, was used to argue against contagion. This is rather like saying that bullets do not kill, because not every soldier on the battlefield was killed by a barrage of bullets.

Koch was not the first scientist to argue for the "unitary theory" of tubercular disease, nor even the first to demonstrate that consumption was contagious. William Budd (1811–1880), an English epidemiologist best known for his classic treatise on typhoid fever, argued that the epidemiology of tuberculosis among blacks in England and Africa indicated that it was a contagious disease. The distinguished French physician Jean Antoine Villemin (1827–1892), attempted to demonstrate the contagiousness of tuberculosis by inoculating rabbits and guinea pigs with sputum and other materials from victims of tuberculosis. The transmission of human tuberculosis to rabbits allowed Villemin to demonstrate the infectiousness of sputum, blood, and bronchial secretions. He even argued that tuberculosis in humans was identical to that occurring in cattle. However, Villemin's work had little immediate impact, and attempts by other physicians to repeat his experiments were inconclusive. Indeed, Rudolf Virchow argued that pulmonary tuberculosis and miliary tuberculosis were different diseases, although René Laënnec (1781–1826) had shown that tuberculosis caused morbid effects throughout the body; in some individuals this resulted in the miliary pattern while others exhibited the symptoms of pulmonary tuberculosis. Despite the brilliance of Virchow's work in cellular pathology, his views on tuberculosis seem to have been limited by his lack of clinical experience and, perhaps, clouded by nationalistic pride and prejudice. Just as Koch belittled French microbiology, Virchow denigrated the combination of clinical observation and autopsy studies that characterized the work of René Laënnec and other members of the "Paris school." Of course, Virchow's resistance was not entirely a matter of nationalism; even after inspecting Koch's demonstrations, Virchow continued to speak of the "so-called tubercle bacillus."

Having cultured a specific microbe apparently associated with tuberculosis in all its manifestations, Koch provided unequivocal evidence that the tubercle bacillus was the specific cause of the disease. In doing so, he formalized the criteria now known as "Koch's postulates" which must be satisfied in order to prove that a particular microbial agent is the cause of a particular disease. To satisfy Koch's postulates, the investigator must prove that a specific microorganism is invariably associated with the disease. Combining such observations with evidence that the microbe was not found in healthy individuals or in those suffering from other diseases was suggestive, but not compelling. Unequivocal proof depended upon culturing the microbe in the laboratory to separate it from contaminating tissue and other organisms. After the alleged pathogen had been serially cultured, it should be inoculated into healthy animals. If pure laboratory cultures induced the disease in experimental animals, the investigator should isolate the microbe from those animals in order to prove that a causal relationship existed between microbe and disease. For human diseases like cholera, typhoid, and leprosy it was impossible to satisfy Koch's Postulates because no suitable experimental animal had been found. To provide unequivocal evidence in such cases would require unethical human experimentation. Koch's postulates were formulated for studies of infectious disease, but his general approach has been extended to guide studies of other disorders, such as the health hazards posed by asbestos and other chemicals.

Even though Koch's discovery of the tubercle bacillus was not immediately followed by a preventive vaccine or specific therapeutic agent, it stimulated hope that conscientious patients might recover their health through appropriate medical guidance. Nevertheless, Koch was under considerable pressure to match the achievements of his great French rival. In 1889, after several years devoted to his official duties and travels, he began to work in the laboratory again, with great intensity and complete secrecy as to the nature of the experiments producing such large numbers of dead guinea pigs. In August 1890, in a speech for the Tenth International Congress of Medicine in Berlin, Koch implied that he had discovered a cure for tuberculosis. A close examination of what Koch actually said should have prevented the excess of hope and the sense of betrayal that followed distorted newspaper accounts of his tentative assessment of the prospects for a cure. Koch announced that he had found a substance that arrested the growth of the tubercle bacillus in the test tube and in living bodies. The living bodies, however, were those of guinea pigs, not human beings. This is an important point, because guinea pigs do not acquire tuberculosis naturally, but become diseased when properly inoculated. Nevertheless, Koch incautiously referred to his agent as a remedy. Press reports immediately labeled the mysterious agent "Koch's lymph," "Kochin," or "Koch's fluid"; Koch called his preparation "tuberculin." Based on the preliminary results obtained with guinea pigs, large-scale human trials were premature, but a world full of consumptives was not willing to wait for controlled clinical tests to validate tuberculin's promise. Some of Koch's colleagues suggested that Koch had been pressured (or perhaps bribed) into revealing his preliminary results by the government. In any case, before the safety and efficacy of tuberculin had been evaluated, the German Emperor personally conferred the medal of the Grand Cross of the Red Eagle upon Koch and the magistrates of Berlin presented him with the freedom of the city.

Despite the fact that Germany had a law prohibiting "secret medicines," Koch refused to reveal the nature of tuberculin. He did provide the name and address of a doctor named Libbertz who was preparing tuberculin under the direction of Dr. Pfuhl (Koch's son-in-law). Dr. Arthur Conan Doyle (creator of Sherlock Holmes), who was sent to Berlin by the *Review of Reviews* to report on the German remedy, visited Dr. Libbertz in November 1890 and found his office literally knee-high in piles of letters begging for Koch's miraculous remedy. Even Joseph Lister, who brought his niece to Berlin for treatment, had to wait a week before Koch had time to see him. Impressed by the work on tuberculin, as well as the discovery of new methods for the prevention and treatment of diphtheria and tetanus, Lister complained that German science was far ahead of British science.

Within a year of Koch's revelation, thousands of people had received tuberculin treatment. Patients were treated without order, system, or controls. Tuberculin seemed to help some patients in the early stages of tuberculosis of the skin, bone, or joints. Unfortunately, further experience showed that tuberculin was useless, or even dangerous for patients with pulmonary tuberculosis. Disappointment was quickly followed by violent condemnation of Koch and his secret remedy. A study prepared for the German government, flawed as it was by the way in which treatments had been carried out, found remarkably little evidence to justify the claims made for tuberculin. Nevertheless, anecdotal reports of cures and improvements led government officials to continue support for tuberculin and to allow its use in prisons and in the army.

In a paper published in January 1891, Koch finally described the nature and preparation of his remedy. Tuberculin was simply a glycerine extract of tubercle bacilli. Critics cynically noted that he revealed the great secret because it had become obvious that tuberculin was worthless. In his own defense Koch later explained that preparing tuberculin was very difficult, and he was afraid that doctors and quacks all around the world would attempt to prepare and inoculate harmful imitations, causing great damage to patients and to the reputation of German science. As the storm gathered in 1891, Koch arranged a long vacation in Egypt, leaving his son-in-law in charge of tuberculin and the Institute for Infectious Diseases.

To the end of his life, Koch continued to hope that an improved form of tuberculin would serve as an immunizing agent or cure. This dream was never realized, but tuberculin was recognized as a valuable diagnostic aid in the detection of early, asymptomatic tuberculosis. In the heroic tradition of the time, Koch had tested tuberculin on himself. His strong reaction indicated that like most of his contemporaries he had not escaped a "touch of tuberculosis." What he had actually stumbled upon was the complex immunological phenomenon now called delayed-type hypersensitivity. Tuberculin was not a cure, but the discovery of the tubercle bacillus and tuberculin provided the weaponry for a crusade against tuberculosis. The tuberculin test could detect asymptomatic cases, and microbiology laboratories could help the physician monitor the patient's status by analyzing throat cultures or sputum samples. The need for caution and for critical clinical trials should have been the lesson of the tuberculin fiasco. The demands that the whole apparatus of clinical trials be abandoned in the search for AIDS remedies 100 years later suggests that the lesson has been completely forgotten. AIDS in the 1980s, like tuberculosis in the 1880s, was perceived as a mysterious, dreaded, and fatal illness. Withholding a drug that might cure, or at least slow the progress of a fatal illness is, doubtless, a cruel and unethical act. It is more difficult to come to grips with the more subtle, but still cruel process of dispensing ineffectual drugs and unjustified hope for a disease with so complex and uncertain a natural history as AIDS or tuberculosis.

Expressing the despair caused by tuberculosis, Charles Dickens characterized this inexorable enemy as the disease that medicine never cured and wealth never warded off. Nevertheless, rates of tuberculosis morbidity and mortality declined significantly well before the advent of specific antibiotic therapy. Progress in controlling tuberculosis was gradually achieved as public health workers assimilated the idea that tuberculosis was a preventable disease and taught physicians and patients to think in terms of a complex web of causation. Detecting early cases and accurately measuring the incidence of infection was made possible by the development of sensitive tuberculin tests and X-ray examinations. Even though the bacillus remained ubiquitous, the incidence of sickness declined with changes in living standards that allowed more people access to fresh air, light, and improved nutrition. Scientists suggested that with biological wisdom directing social and individual behavior, the disease could be eradicated without vaccines. However, medical and public health authorities have rarely reached a workable consensus as to the nature of "biological wisdom."

When marked variations in the virulence of different varieties of tubercle bacilli were discovered, scientists hoped that a particular strain could play the role cowpox served in preventing smallpox. But evaluating tuberculosis vaccines is very difficult; in some areas almost everyone has been exposed to the bacillus and many have had a primary infection. The most widely used vaccine against tuberculosis is derived from the live, attenuated strain produced by Albert Léon Charles Calmette

(1863–1933) and coworkers. Since the 1920s BCG (Bacille Calmette-Guérin) has been used as a vaccine against childhood tuberculosis. Despite recurring questions about the safety and efficacy of BCG, preventive vaccination remains the basis of anti-tuberculosis efforts in many developing nations.

An important step towards controlling tuberculosis was recognition of the danger posed by contaminated milk. In July 1901 at the First British Congress of Tuberculosis in London, Koch announced that bovine and human tuberculosis were two distinct diseases. Counter to prevailing opinion at the time, he declared that humans could not be infected with the bovine organism. This announcement was stunning, not just because it was absolutely wrong, but because in his early work on tuberculosis Koch had said that bovine and human tuberculosis were caused by the same microbe. Bacteriologists rushed to confirm or disprove this proclamation. A British commission reached the conclusion that bovine tuberculosis was a public health menace; a German commission agreed with Koch. Emil von Behring (1854–1917), who won the first Nobel Prize in Physiology or Medicine for discovering diphtheria antitoxin, argued that contaminated milk was the major source of infection for children. This view was confirmed by the American bacteriologist Theobald Smith (1859–1934). Children between the ages of 1 and 5 were particularly susceptible to infection from the ''pale cultures of tuberculosis'' sold as milk.

While pursuing his early work under primitive and difficult conditions, Koch had been a patient and conscientious worker. After achieving his greatest victories, he seems to have become increasingly opinionated, arrogant, and dogmatic. Many critics pointed to the militaristic approach and authoritarian environment of German science as a factor. Perhaps even Koch fell victim to the Koch mythology and was swept up by official pressure and public adulation. When a scientist of Koch's standing was wrong, his oracular pronouncements could endanger the public health. In 1908 the major issue of contention at the International Tuberculosis Congress in the United States was the problem of bovine tuberculosis. To the delight of America's ''anti-pasteurizers,'' Koch focused on pulmonary tuberculosis, which he said accounted for 11 out of every 12 deaths from tuberculosis, and he declared that the issue of intestinal infection of children was irrelevant. This seems to be a very strange way to look at childhood illness. Critics contended that Koch had taken this position to shield the German government and the German meat industry. When Koch returned to Berlin after the bitter 1908 meeting, he attempted to resume his research on tuberculosis, but his health deteriorated rapidly and he died at Baden-Baden, May 27, 1910, of a heart attack. Two years later, the Institute for Infectious Diseases was renamed the Robert Koch Institute.

Since the time of Hippocrates, consumptives have been subjected to bizarre diets, noxious remedies, and a soothing elixir of ''opium and lies.'' Probably the most colorful cure was the ritual of the Royal Touch, performed by kings of England and France from the Middle Ages to the eighteenth century. Because the scrofulous wretches selected for the ceremony received a coin as a souvenir, records of the alms disbursed during such rituals provide estimates of the number of touches. Perhaps a few skeptics like Michael Servetus (1511–1553) could see that many were touched and few were cured, but because of the unpredictable nature of the disease, the Royal Touch might have worked as well as any other remedy. Depending on the shifting tides of medical fashion, physicians have prescribed rest, exercise, starvation diets, rich foods, fresh air, sunshine, tonics, and tranquilizers for their consumptive patients. Folk remedies for phthisis included wolf's liver boiled in wine, weasel blood, pigeon dung, and essence of skunk; eating live snails was said to prevent the disease. Twentieth-century physicians prescribed creosote, digitalis, opium, cod-liver oil, heavy metals, gold salts, and Fowler's solution (a tonic rich in arsenic). Public and private agencies established tuberculosis dispensaries and sanatoriums. Some physicians prescribed mountain air, hiking and horseback riding, and carefully graduated work programs, while others warned that exercise placed too much stress on the lungs. Complete rest for the afflicted lung was produced by artificial pneumothorax (collapsing the lung with injections of air between the pleural membranes). Many standard remedies for tuberculosis were useless, and some, like gold salts, were found to exacerbate the illness when therapeutic trials were conducted under controlled conditions.

During the early decades of the twentieth century, tuberculosis remained the "captain of the men of death." The work of Koch and the scientific hygiene movement made it possible to believe that tuberculosis could be controlled, perhaps ultimately eradicated, by new medical techniques, institutions, administrative structures, and the authority of the state. But twentieth-century campaigns against tuberculosis emphasized individual responsibility, while neglecting the deep-seated social and economic problems that established close links between poverty and tuberculosis. Many physicians ignored the implications of Koch's work and minimized the role of the microbe and the contagiousness of the disease. Old ideas about the hereditary nature of the disease, or an innate predisposition, were not abandoned. The social and environmental factors responsible for the association between poverty and tuberculosis, such as malnutrition, crowding, lack of fresh air and sunlight, were neglected. Victims of the disease were isolated, shunned, and confined in sanatoriums in a manner reminiscent of the medieval leper.

The romantic notion of the tuberculosis sanatorium as a place located on a "Magic Mountain" offering rest, sunshine, nourishing food, and a healing atmosphere has been largely dispelled by further studies of the suffering endured by patients who experienced the isolation, rigidity, and degradation characteristic of many of these proprietary institutions. In the nineteenth and twentieth centuries, the sanatorium regime evolved from a benign program of fresh air and rest to more rigid and medicalized programs involving strict prescriptions of graduated work, drug trials, and surgery. Criteria of success were remarkably low, as indicated by claims of success for injections of gold salts in which nine out of 42 patients died. Many patients were subjected to artificial pneumothorax, although, in some institutions, the mortality rate for this operation was about 50%. The analysis of such disappointing results convinced many investigators that it was impossible to find a specific chemotherapeutic agent for a disease as intractable and complex as tuberculosis.

For complex reasons that are still the subject of heated debate, by the time effective antibiotics were available, the great "white plague" was already subsiding. As in the case of leprosy, the history of tuberculosis, when considered in a broad social and global context, reminds us that the pattern of human suffering and death associated with a specific disease cannot be reduced to a description of its microbial agent. All detailed studies of tuberculosis reveal that a large decline in mortality occurred before the introduction of specific and effective treatment in 1947. Efforts to evaluate the contribution antibiotics made to the subsequent fall in mortality rates from tuberculosis are complicated by the fact that the BCG vaccination was adopted only shortly before streptomycin. Drugs that were effective against experimental tuberculosis in laboratory animals were not necessarily useful in the treatment of the disease in humans. However, reports that streptomycin, an antibiotic discovered by Selman A. Waksman (1888–1973) in 1943, was effective against tuberculosis in guinea pigs were soon followed by evidence of efficacy in humans. The early, impure preparations of streptomycin caused serious side effects, including deafness; moreover, in some trials only 51% of the treated patients improved after 6 months of therapy (8% of the controls also improved). Nevertheless, the appearance of streptomycin and other chemotherapeutic agents transformed the management and treatment of tuberculosis patients and virtually emptied the sanatoriums.

From the public health standpoint, even a partial course of treatment is useful in arresting an active infection and breaking the chain of transmission. A complete cure may take many months. As in the case of leprosy, the long course of treatment is costly and creates ideal conditions for the proliferation of drug-resistant bacteria. While tubercle bacilli grow slowly, they are remarkably persistent; bacteria have been cultured from surgical and autopsy specimens immersed in formalin solutions for many years. However, the disease is virtually 100% curable, and by the 1960s global eradication was regarded as well within the technical possibilities of medical science. Nevertheless, in the 1980s for complex socioeconomic and political reasons, eradication remained a remote possibility; each year the "germ of death" claims 2 to 3 million lives and infects about an equal number of new victims. Even in the United States, 100 years after Koch discovered the tubercle bacillus, public health authorities detected localized increases in the incidence of tuberculosis in areas where poverty and the spread of AIDS provided a zone of vulnerability. Tuberculosis, especially in its association with AIDS, highlights the vast chasm between what medical science and public health measures could accomplish and the dreadful toll preventable diseases continue to take.

By the end of the nineteenth century, microbiology was a well-established discipline which had sprouted several specialized branches. Textbooks, journals, institutes, and courses in microbiology multiplied almost as rapidly as bacteria. In 1879 Pasteur's associate Émile Duclaux established a course in microbiology at the Sorbonne. Koch introduced a comprehensive course in medical microbiology at the University of Berlin in 1884. American science and medicine still lagged far behind its European models, but by the 1890s, even American medical schools and agricultural colleges were beginning to include bacteriology in their curricula. Medical microbiology was an important stimulus for the emerging acceptance of laboratory-based medical education, which the 1910 Flexner Report on medical education in the United States and Canada presented as an absolute necessity.

While most physicians and surgeons learned to reconcile professional practice with the germ theory of disease, some physicians and scientists continued to battle against the germ theory well into the twentieth century. Many of those who rejected germ theory were actively involved in sanitary or hygienic reform movements which had significant successes in improving the health of cities. In practice, an all-out attack on filth and pollution may be even more effective in the long-range control of epidemic and endemic diseases than an attack on specific pathogens, because of the general improvements in hygienic conditions. The first Institute of Hygiene in the world was founded by the indomitable Max von Pettenkofer (1818–1901), a man who had little sympathy for the germ theory of disease. After pursuing interests that ranged from acting to physiology and chemistry, Pettenkofer settled into the study of medicine and was awarded his medical degree at Munich in 1843. In 1847 he was appointed professor of medicinal chemistry at Munich; he became Munich's first professor of hygiene in 1878 in recognition of his pioneering work on hygiene and epidemiology.

Pettenkofer believed that the science of hygiene would reveal the origin of infectious diseases and the most effective means of preventing them. His approach to medicine was sanitarian, or what would now be called environmental medicine. While the germ theory of disease was winning its place as one of the most powerful branches of experimental medicine, Pettenkofer continued to argue that poisonous miasmata, soil conditions, and climatological disturbances were primarily responsible for the generation and spread of disease. For example, while minimizing the discovery of the microbe that causes cholera, he developed his own "ground-water theory" of the generation of cholera-producing miasmata and followed this with a successful campaign for the improvement of the city's sewage systems. As a consequence of these sanitary reforms, Munich enjoyed a significant reduction in the burden of intestinal diseases. Pettenkofer's attitude towards germ theory is exemplified in his challenge to Koch's claim that the causal agent of cholera was the so-called comma bacillus or cholera vibrio. In 1892, in the presence of unimpeachable witnesses, the 74-year-old founder of modern hygiene swallowed a broth culture of cholera vibrios. Pettenkofer later admitted to some slight intestinal discomfort, but refused to diagnose this as cholera. If Pettenkofer could have investigated the cholera epidemic centered in Peru in 1991 which threatened much of South and Central America, as well as the more chronic cholera outbreaks in Africa, he would claim vindication for the sanitarian doctrine that poverty and the lack of hygienic conditions were the most significant factors in generating and disseminating epidemic cholera. Despite the apparent conflict between Pettenkofer's miasmatic theory and Koch's germ theory, both physicians were dedicated to the idea that the scientific study of the discipline of hygiene would have a great and beneficial impact on the burden of infectious diseases. Nevertheless, in the long run it was Koch's discoveries that focused attention on how best to integrate hygiene into medical research and the medical curriculum.

INVISIBLE MICROBES AND VIROLOGY

Long before scientists could define the nature of specific viruses, viral diseases—smallpox and rabies—had provided the most significant and dramatic examples of the potential of preventive inoculations. Because the meaning of the Latin word *virus* has undergone many changes in two millennia of usage, the modern reader is likely to be confused upon finding the term in ancient texts. The first and most general meaning of "virus" was "slime," presumably unpleasant, but not necessarily dangerous. However, Latin authors increasingly used the term with the implication of poison or venom, something menacing to health, or a mysterious, unknown infectious agent. Thus, both the Roman writer Celsus and Louis Pasteur could speak of the virus of rabies.

Medieval scholars generally used "virus" as a synonym for "poison." In medical treatises of the sixteenth and seventeenth centuries, translators usually replaced the Latin "virus" with the English "venom." Seventeenth-century writers referred to a "virus pestiferum" or "virus pestilens" in discussing infectious diseases. Eighteenth-century medical writers applied the term "virus" to the contagion that transmitted an infectious disease, as in Edward Jenner's discussion of the "cow-pox virus" in the pustular lymph that transmitted the disease. For medical writers in the early nineteenth century, "virus" stood for the obscure causative principles of infectious diseases; the vagueness of the term made it particularly attractive.

After the establishment of germ theory in the late nineteenth century, "virus" was used in the general sense of "an agent with infectious properties," and when submicroscopic filterable infectious agents were discovered, the term virus was applied to them. Even if the causative agent for an infectious disease had not been identified, Pasteur's message was that "Every virus is a microbe." In 1891, Koch made a speech in which he implied that bacteriology was not the answer to all questions concerning infectious disease and that other kinds of organisms might be involved in various diseases. The exceptional agents that he knew of were larger than bacteria, most notably the protozoan that caused malaria, but there was no theoretical reason to rule out the existence of peculiar forms of smaller parasites. Nevertheless, the reverence for Koch's postulates may have inhibited virology, as well as protozoology, because it was virtually impossible to culture such entities in artificial media. Koch himself did not let bacteriological dogma inhibit his work on tropical medicine even where the microbes could not be cultured in the laboratory.

By the end of the nineteenth century, the techniques of microbiology were sufficiently advanced for scientists to name, with a high degree of confidence, many diseases caused by specific bacteria or protozoa. But the infectious agents of some diseases refused to be isolated by conventional techniques. Eventually, exotic but visible pathogens (rickettsias, chlamydias, mycoplasmas, and brucellas) joined the classical fungi, bacteria, and protozoa. Because some of the exotic pathogens had complicated life cycles and were difficult to culture in vitro, it seemed possible that members of these groups might be the undiscovered agents of various infectious diseases. Therefore, in the early twentieth century the term virus was generally restricted to the class of filterable-invisible microbes; such microbes were defined operationally in terms of their ability to pass through filters that trapped bacteria and their ability to remain invisible to the light microscope. But technique-based criteria provided little insight into the genetic and biochemical nature of viruses. As scientists closed in on the invisible-filterable viruses, they discovered that their operational criteria were not necessarily linked. The failure of infectious agents to grow in vitro was not a satisfactory criterion either, because scientists could not exclude the possibility that exotic microbes might need special media and growth conditions. A more radical explanation for this phenomenon was that some microbes might be obligate parasites of living organisms that could not be cultured in vitro on any cell-free culture medium.

Although for the sake of human health, it would have been better if viruses had totally destroyed all tobacco plants, progress in virology owes a great deal to this pernicious product of the New World, because it was the tobacco mosaic virus that established Adolf Eduard Mayer, Martinus Beijerinck, and Dimitri Ivanovski as the founders of virology. The study of plant virology can be traced to 1886 when Adolf Eduard Mayer (1843–1942) discovered that tobacco mosaic disease could be transmitted to healthy plants by inoculating them with extracts of sap from the leaves of diseased plants. Unable to culture a tobacco mosaic disease microbe on artificial media, Mayer filtered the sap and demonstrated that the filtrate was still infectious. Mayer was certain that his microbe must be a very unusual bacterium. In 1892, Dimitri Iosifovitch Ivanovski (1864–1920) demonstrated that the infectious agent for tobacco mosaic disease could pass through the finest filters available. All attempts to isolate or culture the "tobacco microbe" were failures. Frustrated by this apparent dead end, Ivanovski turned to research on alcoholic fermentations.

Martinus Willem Beijerinck (1851–1931) was introduced to tobacco mosaic disease by Adolf Mayer while he was pursuing his doctoral degree at the University of Leiden. However, their early attempts to isolate the virus were unsuccessful. In 1895 Beijerinck became professor of microbiology at the Polytechnical School in Delft, where he devoted himself to research in botany, microbiology, chemistry, and genetics. Eventually, he returned to the problem of tobacco mosaic disease. Like

Ivanovski, Beijerinck found that the sap of plants with tobacco mosaic disease remained infectious after passage through a porcelain filter. Because filtered sap could transmit the disease to a large number of plants in series, he concluded that tobacco mosaic disease must be caused by an agent which had to incorporate itself into the living protoplasm of a cell in order to reproduce. Beijerinck's theory of the *contagium vivum fluidum* (contagious living fluid) was a first step towards a new theory in which the fundamental difference between bacteria and virus was not a matter of size or filterability, but in the virus's lifestyle as an obligate intracellular parasite, an agent that can only reproduce within living cells.

Friedrich Loeffler (1852–1915) and Paul Frosch (1860–1928), disciples of Robert Koch, are remembered primarily for their work on foot-and-mouth disease, the first example of a filterable virus disease of animals. Although Loeffler and Frosch were well qualified to isolate pathological bacteria, the microbial agent of this important cattle disease eluded them. Nevertheless, they could transmit the disease to cattle and pigs with minute amounts of bacteria-free filtrates from the vesicles of infected animals. After proving that cattle could be immunized against foot-and-mouth disease with mixtures of blood and lymph from the vesicles, Loeffler and Frosch suggested that the disease might be caused by a soluble poison or an agent small enough to pass through the pores of their filters. Their experiments and calculations suggested that only a living agent capable of reproducing itself could continue to cause the disease after passage through a series of animals. Loeffler and Frosch did not think of their virus in modern terms; they believed that the infectious agent was a special small microbe, rather than a fundamentally different entity.

In 1915, Frederick William Twort (1877–1950) discovered that even bacteria can suffer from viral diseases. "Twort particles" were filterable, like the infectious agents of many mysterious plant and animal diseases. Twort's work on this problem was interrupted by World War I and his paper had little immediate impact on microbiology. However, while working on the dysentery bacillus at the Pasteur Institute, Félix d'Hérelle (1873–1949) discovered what he called an invisible microbe that was capable of destroying the dysentery bacillus. D'Hérelle concluded that the invisible microbe, which he named "bacteriophage" (bacteria-eater), must be an obligate parasite of the dysentery bacillus. D'Hérelle's particles sparked the hope that bacteriophages might be turned into weapons against pathogenic bacteria. Unfortunately, the bacteriophage refused to become the "microbe of immunity." Until pressed into service as the "experimental animal" of molecular biology, bacterial viruses remained a laboratory curiosity.

In a practical rather than philosophical sense, many arguments about the nature of viruses faded from the picture as researchers in the 1930s and 1940s examined them with new biochemical techniques. By the 1940s biochemical techniques were revealing just how complicated biological macromolecules could be. Advances in biochemistry supported the concept of the virus as a complex entity on the borderline between cells, genes, and molecules. In 1939, scientists obtained the first portrait of the tobacco mosaic virus by electron microscopy. Today viruses are generally described as particles composed of a protein overcoat and an inner core of nucleic acid which is capable of entering a host cell and taking over its metabolic apparatus. As to just what the viruses are and where they fit into the scheme of things among plants and animals, microbes and macromolecules, living and nonliving, André Lwoff's paraphrase of a famous line by Gertrude Stein seems the most appropriate answer: "Viruses should be considered viruses because viruses are viruses." However, research on diseases caused by entities called slow viruses, viroids, and prions indicates that there are still many fascinating, and perhaps menacing, creatures in the submicroscopic world.

SUGGESTED READINGS

Ackerknecht, E. H. (953). *Rudolf Virchow: Doctor, Statesman, Anthropologist.* Madison, WI: University of Wisconsin Press.

Bradbury, S. (1967). *The Evolution of the Microscope.* Oxford, England: Pergamon.

Bloch, Marc (1973). *The Royal Touch: Sacred Monarchy and Scrofula in England and France.* Trans. J.E. Anderson. London: Routledge & Kegan Paul.

Brock, Thomas D. (1988). *Robert Koch. A Life in Medicine and Bacteriology.* Scientific Revolutionaries. Madison, WI: Science Tech.

Brock, Thomas D., ed. (1961). *Milestones in Microbiology.* Englewood Cliffs, NJ: Prentice-Hall.

Bryder, Linda (1988). *Below the Magic Mountain: A Social History of Tuberculosis in Twentieth-Century Britain.* Oxford, England: Clarendon Press.

Budd, William (1984). *On the Causes of Fever (1839).* Ed. Dale C. Smith. Baltimore, MD: Johns Hopkins University Press.

Cairns, John, Stent, G. S., and Watson, J. D., eds. (1966). *Phage and the Origins of Molecular Biology.* Cold Spring Harbor, NY: Cold Spring Harbor Laboratory of Quantitative Biology.

Caldwell, Mark (1988). *The Last Crusade: The War on Consumption, 1862-1954.* New York: Atheneum.

Casida, L. E., Jr. (1976). Leeuwenhoek's Observations of Bacteria. *Science* 192: 1348-1349.

Chanock, Robert M., and Lerner, Richard A. eds. (1984). *Modern Approaches to Vaccines: Molecular and Chemical Basis of Virus Virulence and Immunogenicity.* Cold Spring Harbor, NY: Cold Spring Harbor Laboratory.

Corbin, Alain (1986). *The Foul and the Fragrant. Odor and the French Social Imagination.* Cambridge, MA: Harvard University Press.

Diener, Theodor O., ed. (1987). *The Viroids.* New York: Plenum.

Dobell, C. (1960). *Antony van Leeuwenhoek and His 'Little Animals.'* New York: Dover.

Doetsch, R. N., ed. (1960). *Microbiology: Historical Contributions from 1776-1908.* New Brunswick, NJ: Rutgers University Press.

Dowling, Harry F. (1977). *Fighting Infection: Conquests of the Twentieth Century.* Cambridge, MA: Harvard University Press.

Dubos, René (1986). *Louis Pasteur: Free Lance of Science.* New York: Da Capo Series in Science.

Dubos, René, and Dubos, Jean (1952). *The White Plague: Tuberculosis, Man and Society*. Boston, MA: Boston-Little, Brown, & Co.

Duclaux, Emile (1920). *Pasteur, The History of a Mind*. Trans. E. F. Smith and F. Nedges. Philadelphia: W. B. Saunders.

Farley, John (1977). *The Spontaneous Generation Controversy from Descartes to Oparin*. Baltimore, MD: Johns Hopkins University Press.

Fenner, F., and Gibbs, A., eds. (1988). *A History of Virology*. Basel: Karger.

Flexner, Abraham (1910). *Medical Education in the United States and Canada*. New York: Carnegie Foundation.

Forster, Robert, and Ranum, Orest, eds. (1980). *Medicine and Society in France*. Baltimore, MD: Johns Hopkins Press.

Foster, W. D. (1970). *A History of Medical Bacteriology and Immunology*. London: William Heinemann Medical Books.

Gallo, Robert (1990). *Virus Hunting. Cancer, AIDS, and the Human Retrovirus: A Story of Scientific Discovery*. New York: Basic Books.

Henle, Jacob (1938). *Jacob Henle: On Miasmata and Contagia*. Trans. by George Rosen. Baltimore, MD: Johns Hopkins University Press.

Hirsch, A. (1883-6). *Handbook of Geographical and Historical Pathology*. 3 vols. London: New Sydenham Society.

Hudson, Robert P. (1983). *Disease and Its Control: The Shaping of Modern Thought*. Westport, CT: Greenwood Press.

Hughs, Sally Smith (1977). *The Virus: A History of the Concept*. New York: Science History Publications.

Hume, Edgar Ersking (1927). *Max von Pettenkofer. His Theory of the Etiology of Cholera, Typhoid Fever and Other Intestinal Diseases. A Review of His Arguments and Evidence*. New York: Paul B. Hoeber.

James, Walene (1988). *Immunization. The Reality Behind the Myth*. Granby, MA: Bergin & Garvey.

Johnson, Joseph E., ed. (1970). *Rational Therapy and Control of Tuberculosis, A Symposium*. Gainesville, FL: University of Florida Press.

Koch, Robert (1932). *The Aetiology of Tuberculosis*. Trans. of the 1882 paper by Dr. and Mrs. Max Pinner. New York: National Tuberculosis Association.

Koch, Robert (1880). *Investigations into the Etiology of Traumatic Infective Diseases*. Trans. W. Watson Cheyne. London: The New Sydenham Society.

Koch, Robert et al. (1886). *Microparasites in Disease*. London: New Sydenham Society.

Koprowski, Hilary, and Plotkin, S.A., eds. (1985). *World's Debt to Pasteur. Proceedings Centennial Symposium Commemorating the First Rabies Vaccination*. New York: Alan R. Liss.

Latour, Bruno (1988). *The Pasteurization of France*. Trans. by Alan Sheridan and John Law. Cambridge, MA: Harvard University Press.

Lechevalier, H.A. and Solotorovsky, M. (1965). *Three Centuries of Microbiology*. New York: McGraw-Hill. (Repr., New York: Dover, 1974.)

Marton, L. (1941). The Electron Microscope. A New Tool for Bacteriological Research. *J. Bacteriology* 41:397-413.

McKeown, Thomas (1979). *The Role of Medicine. Dream, Mirage, or Nemesis?* Princeton, NJ: Princeton University Press.

Metchnikoff, Élie (1939). *The Founders of Modern Medicine. Pasteur. Koch. Lister.* New York: Walden Publications.

Nutton, Vivian (1990). The Reception of Fractoro's Theory of Contagion. *Osiris.* 2nd series. 6: 196-234.

Nutton, Vivian (1983). The Seeds of Disease: An Explanation of Contagion and Infection from the Greeks to the Renaissance. *Medical History* 27: 1-34.

Oxford, John S., and Oberg, Bo (1985). *Conquest of Viral Diseases: A Topical Review of Drugs and Vaccines.* New York: Elsevier.

Parish, H. J. (1965). *A History of Immunization.* Edinburgh, Scotland: Livingstone.

Pasteur, Louis (1968). *Correspondence of Pasteur and Thuillier Concerning Anthrax and Swine Fever Vaccinations.* Trans. and ed. by R. M. Frank and Denise Wrolnowska. Tuscaloosa, AL: University of Alabama Press.

Porter, J. R. (1972). Louis Pasteur Sesquicentennial (1822-1972). *Science* 178:1249-1254.

Sargent, Frederick II (1982). *Hippocratic Heritage: A History of Ideas about Weather and Human Health.* New York: Pergamon Press.

Silverstein, Arthur M. (1989). *A History of Immunology.* New York: Academic Press.

Smith, F. B. (1988). *The Retreat of Tuberculosis, 1850-1950.* New York: Croom Helm.

Smith, F. B. (1979). *The People's Health 1830-1910.* New York: Holmes & Meier.

Smith, Theobold (1934). *Parasitism and Disease.* Princeton, NJ: Princeton University Press.

Stevenson, L. G. (1955). Science down the Drain. *BHM* 29:1-16.

Swazey, Judith P., and Reeds, Karen (1978). *Today's Medicine, Tomorrow's Science: Essays on Paths of Discovery in the Biomedical Sciences.* Washington, DC: U.S. Dept. of HEW, PHS, NIH.

Turner, Gerard L'E. (1980). *Essays on the History of the Microscope.* Oxford, England: Senecio.

Vallery-Radot, R. (1923). *The Life of Pasteur.* Trans. by R.L. Devonshire. New York: Doubleday, Page.

Vandervliet, Glenn (1971). *Microbiology and the Spontaneous Generation Debate During the 1870s.* Lawrence, KS: Coronado University Press.

Virchow, Rudolf (1971). *Cellular Pathology.* New York: Dover.

Waksman, Selman A. (1964). *The Conquest of Tuberculosis.* Berkeley, CA: University of California Press.

Waterson, A. P., and Wilkinson, Lise (1978). *An Introduction to the History of Virology.* New York: Cambridge University Press.

Winslow, Charles-Edward Amory (1980). *The Conquest of Epidemic Disease. A Chapter in the History of Ideas.* Madison, WI: University of Wisconsin Press.

DIAGNOSTICS AND THERAPEUTICS

For many hundreds of years, medical theory and practice changed so little that Hippocrates and Galen might easily have rejoined the community of learned physicians. But the most knowledgeable physician of the 1880s would be completely mystified by the diagnostic and therapeutic techniques of medicine in the 1980s, as well as its scientific, institutional, educational, and economic components. Nevertheless, it could be argued that the conceptual framework within which physicians are educated and within which they practice today belongs to the era of Pasteur and Koch at the very beginning of a century of profound change, that is, the idea that medicine is a biological construct and that health and disease are strictly biological parameters. Moreover, if we look at the history of medicine from the point of view of the diseased and distressed person, it seems likely that in terms of dealing with the patient's experience, suffering, hope, despair, expectations of help from the physician, and tendency to disobey medical orders and resort to self-medication, Hippocrates and Galen might well have valuable advice for the modern physician. Indeed, their emphasis on the prevention of disease, the individuality of the patient, the interplay between patients and their environment, the notion of treating the patient as a whole, and the role of the physician in prescribing a life-long, health-promoting regimen would enjoy a powerful resonance with public hopes and expectations.

By the beginning of the twentieth century, medical microbiology made it possible to identify the cause and means of transmission of many infectious diseases, but it had little impact on therapeutics, and in surgery, if asepsis failed, the surgeon was as helpless against infection as his medieval counterpart. The golden age of microbiology was a time of great excitement with respect to the science of medicine, but from the point of view of the sick, knowing the cause of their disease was not as important as having a remedy. The major public health benefit of germ theory was the guidance provided in stopping the spread of waterborne diseases like typhoid fever and cholera through improved sanitation and rational public health measures, such as the purification of drinking water, proper sewer systems, food inspection, and pasteurization. While public health authorities could rationalize the need for compulsory measures, such as vaccination, isolation of the sick, and the identification of healthy carriers (as exemplified by the semi-legendary Typhoid Mary and Patient Zero of the AIDS epidemic), such measures conflicted with cherished concepts of individual liberties and the right to privacy.

THE ART AND SCIENCE OF DIAGNOSIS

The triumphs of medical microbiology discussed previously tend to overshadow another important aspect of nineteenth-century medicine which grew out of what we might think of as the unhappy junction of clinical medicine practiced at the patient's bedside, with pathological investigations conducted in the autopsy room. Achieving a more precise understanding of the nature and seats of disease within the dead body was eventually coupled with more precise diagnosis of disease in living patients. Symptoms were correlated with localized internal lesions, but, until the development of instruments such as the stethoscope, the lesions could only be detected at the postmortem. The gradual development and recent enthusiastic reception of the technological aids used in the diagnosis of disease represent remarkable aspects of the evolution of medical practice over the course of the last 200 years. Beyond their obvious role in transforming the art of diagnosis, medical instruments have profoundly affected the relationship between patient and physician, the education and practical training of physicians, the demarcation between areas of medical specialization, the locus of medical practice, and even the financial base of medical care and treatment. From the time of Hippocrates until well into the nineteenth century, the average physician relied on essentially subjective information, such as the patient's own account of the course of illness and the physician's observations of notable signs and symptoms. Which signs and symptoms were considered notable was determined by prevailing medical philosophy, tempered by the experience of the individual physician. Physical examination involving touching the patient was extremely limited, except for some attention to the quality of the pulse. Under these conditions, the physician could diagnose and prescribe by letter without even seeing the patient. Indeed, the fee for advising the patient by letter was higher than that for an office visit.

During the nineteenth century, even the average physician was being encouraged to follow the path marked out by the great clinicians and morbid anatomists of the previous century towards a more active role in obtaining objective information concerning signs and symptoms of illness by direct physical examination. In 1761, the year in which Morgagni published his monumental five-volume examination of *The Seats and Causes of Diseases*, Leopold Auenbrugger (1722-1809) of Vienna published another landmark in the history of medicine entitled *Inventum Novum*. In little more than 20 pages, Auenbrugger set forth an account of a new diagnostic method called "chest percussion" by means of which the physician could gain insight into the internal state of the chest cavity by carefully evaluating the sounds produced by chest percussion, less elegantly known as "chest thumping." Of course a great deal of experience was needed before a doctor learned to distinguish between the sounds of a healthy chest and those which betrayed the earliest signs of tuberculosis or pneumonia made by a "morbid chest." Auenbrugger, who was considered a gifted amateur musician and composer, presumably had a better trained ear than most physicians. Chest percussion, which depends on the differences in sound transmitted through air and fluid, is rather like tapping a wine cask or beer barrel to determine whether it is empty or partially full. Presumably Auenbrugger was familiar with this phenomenon because his father was a tavern keeper. Although Auenbrugger considered his method revolutionary, some physicians saw little difference between percussion and other methods of diagnosis by auscultation (listening) dating back to the time of Hippocrates, such as shaking the patient and listening for the sound of fluid sloshing about in the chest. Indeed, Auenbrugger's teacher had employed percussion of the abdomen in cases of ascites (fluid accumulation in the peritoneal cavity).

Few physicians expressed any interest in Auenbrugger's work until Jean Nicolas Corvisart (1755-1821) published a translation and commentary in 1808. By this time, thanks to the work of the so-called Paris school of morbid anatomy, humoralism had been essentially eclipsed by the concept of localized pathological anatomy. Corvisart's disciples, especially René Théophile Hyacinthe Laënnec (1781-1826), established the value of direct (immediate) and indirect (mediate) auscultation and transformed the art and science of physical examination. Working at the Necker Hospital and the Charité, Laënnec adopted the goals and methods of the Paris school of hospital medicine. Eventually, his invention of the stethoscope would make him one of the most famous exemplars of this school, and a symbol of French science, but during his life he was generally treated with indifference and hostility by his peers.

Proponents of early nineteenth-century "hospital medicine" tended to see themselves as disciples of Hippocrates for their emphasis on clinical observation, but the context in which they worked was quite different from that of the ancients. Leaders of the French Revolution had imagined a new era in which hospitals, medical schools, and doctors would disappear. Instead, in the aftermath of the Revolution, new hospitals, medical schools, doctrines, and professional standards emerged. In the major hospitals of Paris, clinicians could see thousands of cases and carry out many

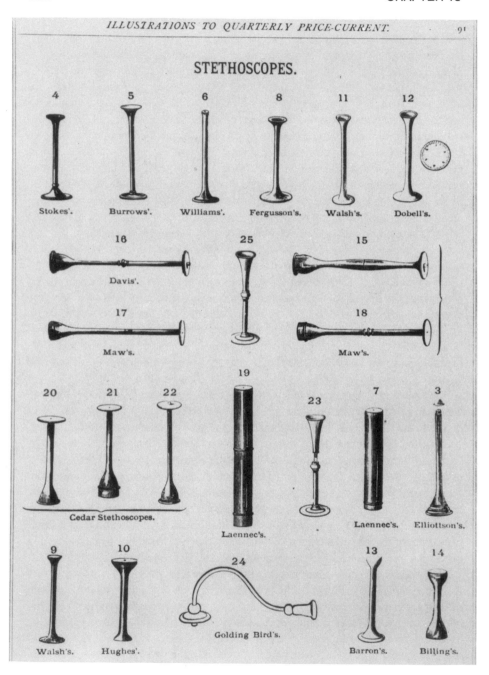

ILLUSTRATIONS TO QUARTERLY PRICE-CURRENT.   91

STETHOSCOPES.

Stethoscopes for sale in 1869

hundreds of autopsies. American students flocked to the great hospitals to supplement their limited education and lack of clinical experience.

The large scale of nineteenth-century hospital medicine provided the "clinical material" for more active and intrusive methods of physical examination and diagnosis, statistical evaluation of various therapeutic interventions, and confirmation of correlations among symptoms, lesions, and remedies by investigations performed in the autopsy room. Although immediate auscultation and chest percussion were becoming valuable aids to diagnosis and research into what Corvisart called "internal medicine," many physicians were reluctant to practice these methods. Given the great abundance of fleas and lice on many patients and the general neglect of bathing, this was understandable. The stethoscope not only provided some distance between physician and patient, it improved the quality of the sounds that could be heard within the chest. The name stethoscope was coined from the Greek for "chest" (*stethos*) and "to view" (*skopein*).

In *On Mediate Auscultation* (1819), Laënnec described the difficulties he encountered when examining a young woman with signs of heart disease. Discreet percussion with a gloved hand did not reveal anything about the state of the inside of her chest, because of the rather stout state of the outside of her chest. Considerations of propriety precluded immediate auscultation, but with a flash of inspiration Laënnec took a sheaf of paper and rolled it into a cylinder. When he applied one end of the cylinder to the chest and the other to his ear, he could hear the heart beat with remarkably clarity. Improvements in his cylinder made it possible to listen to all kinds of sounds and movements within the chest.

Laënnec warned physicians not to neglect Auenbrugger's methods when using the stethoscope, because the physician should use as many aids to diagnosis as possible. More important, it was essential to realize that a great deal of practice was required before the instrument could be used effectively. To learn the technique, the young physician should work in a hospital where he had access to many kinds of patients and expert guidance. Large numbers of post-mortems were needed to confirm diagnostic accuracy. Like many of his colleagues, Laënnec succumbed to tuberculosis, the disease that was often the subject of his research. France, which had contributed so much to the study of tuberculosis, had the highest mortality rate from consumption in western Europe well into the twentieth century, perhaps largely due to lingering beliefs that heredity was more significant than contagion and indifference to available public health measures.

Dr. John Forbes, who translated excerpts from Laënnec's 900-page treatise on auscultation into English in 1821, noted that the stethoscope was extremely valuable, but he doubted that mediate auscultation would ever come into general use among English doctors, because its use required too much time and trouble. His most serious objection was that it was so totally foreign in character and incompatible with British traditions. Its use could be imposed on patients in the army and navy and in hospitals, but not on private patients. Like many of his colleagues, Dr. Forbes saw something ludicrous about a dignified physician listening to the patient's chest through a long tube. Such a practice was foreign to the calm, cautious, and philosophical habits of the English physician. In other words, instruments were associated with surgeons and manual labor, not with learned physicians.

It is interesting that the thermometer was not accepted into diagnostics as quickly as the stethoscope, although Santorio had praised the value of his clinical thermometer in the seventeenth century. The concept of localized pathology is generally given credit for the acceptance of physical aids to diagnosis, as well as advances in surgery, but the thermometer, which reflected a general condition of bodily heat, did not fit the pattern of a pathology of solids. The advantages of objective aids to diagnosis also seemed small and uncertain compared to the dangers such instruments were thought to pose to the bond that was supposed to exist between physician and patient.

Dr. Forbes proved to be a very poor prophet; the stethoscope soon became the very symbol of medicine and a necessary part of the doctor's apparel. Few doctors were able to match Laënnec's extraordinary skill at auscultation, but many learned that it was possible to gain objective information about the nature of a patient's condition and to distinguish between diseases such as tuberculosis and pleurisy. The stethoscope made it possible for physicians to "anatomize" the living body, but it was only on the autopsy table that the diagnosis could be confirmed. Even the most selfless patient was unlikely to sympathize with a physician who referred to the post-mortem as one of the best ways to diagnose disease because several autopsies shed more light on pathology than 20 years spent observing symptoms.

The stethoscope was, of course, only the first of the many new "scopes" that allowed physicians to view every nook and cranny of the interior of the body. It is obviously a long way from Laënnec's cylinder to nuclear magnetic resonance imaging, but it is a brief interval compared to the many centuries that separated Hippocrates from Laënnec. From the patient's point of view, progress in diagnostics which was not coupled with progress in therapeutics was of dubious value. Although increasingly sophisticated and expensive new instruments have contributed to the power and prestige of medicine, and may have relieved the patient of the burden of uncertainty, they do not necessarily improve the treatment of disease or the healing of wounds. An accurate diagnosis at an early stage of a disease like tuberculosis, which was made possible by tuberculin and chest X-rays, or AIDS could be interpreted as simply increasing the length of time in which the patient brooded on the inevitability of death. In less that 200 years, diagnostic and therapeutic technologies have become a central and enormously expensive aspect of medicine. Technological success has created an avalanche of expectations and questions about the actual risks and benefits associated with this transformation of medical practice. Faith in the diagnostic power of medical instruments led to decreased interest in the step that the pioneers in this field thought so fundamental: confirmation at the post-mortem. In an attempt to shed light on this problem, a team of researchers analyzed 100 randomly selected autopsies performed in 1960, 1970, and 1980 at one university teaching hospital. In each year studied, about 10% of the autopsies revealed major diagnoses that might have led to changes in therapy if known before death. The number of systemic bacterial, viral, and fungal infections had significantly increased in the 1980s; diagnosis of these infections had been clinically missed 24% of the time. Ironically, the researchers found that over-reliance on new procedures such as radionuclide scans, ultrasound, and computerized tomography sometimes contributed directly to major diagnostic errors.

One of the persistent complaints issued against the medicine practiced in the great hospitals of Paris and Vienna was that physicians were too interested in diagnosis and pathology, but too little interested in therapy. A nineteenth-century cynic assessing the battle between practitioners who favored active interventions and heroic bleeding and researchers who relied on a passive or expectative approach could conclude that Viennese hospital doctors no longer killed their patients, they just let them die. In the Parisian hospitals, a variety of approaches to therapy competed for attention. Some physicians favored bleeding, others relied on antimony or other chemical remedies, while some remained loyal to complex ancient remedies derived from plants, animals, and minerals. Even the standard definition of therapeutics as the art of curing diseases was called into question by those who claimed that the term referred to the most convenient means of treating disease. Oliver Wendell Holmes suggested that patients might be better off if the entire materia medica, except for quinine and opium, was thrown into the sea, but most doctors agreed that it was better to try something doubtful than to do nothing. Moreover, advances in chemistry were providing new drugs—such as morphine, emetine, strychnine, codeine, and iodine—which were unquestionably powerful, as demonstrated by experimental pharmacologists using animal models, even if questions of safety and efficacy remained in doubt.

SERUM THERAPY

As a new generation of scientists looked back on the golden age of bacteriology, their enthusiasm was tempered by the realization that microbe hunting did not in itself lead to the cure of disease. A reevaluation of the factors that determined the balance between health and disease involved rejecting too narrow a bacteriological focus and working towards an understanding of the physiological responses of the host. Certainly the observation that surviving one attack of a particular disease provided protection from subsequent attacks was not new; this was the basis of the immunity earned in exchange for submitting to the risks of smallpox inoculation or vaccination. The Latin term ''immunity'' originally referred to an ''exemption'' in the legal sense. Since the introduction of Jennerian vaccination, it was clear that protective vaccines took advantage of the body's own defense mechanisms, but the modern era of immunization began in the 1880s when Louis Pasteur proved that it was possible to attenuate pathogenic microbes and create specific vaccines. Building on the work of Louis Pasteur and Robert Koch, Shibasaburo Kitasato, Emil von Behring, and Paul

Ehrlich developed new forms of treatment known as serum therapy and chemotherapy. Behring's work also provides a paradigm for an era in which the search for profits, glory, and patents is sometimes pursued more energetically than the search for knowledge.

Emil Adolf von Behring (1854–1917) was one of 13 children fathered by a schoolmaster in Hansdorf, West Prussia. The family could not afford to send Behring to a university, but he was able to obtain a free medical education at the Army Medical College in Berlin in exchange for 10 years of service in the Prussian Army. Military medicine provided an important route into the profession for many men of modest means. Behring obtained his medical degree in 1878 and passed his State Examination in 1880. Ten years later he joined Robert Koch's staff at the Institute of Hygiene in Berlin; their association continued when Koch moved to the Institute for Infectious Diseases. Behring was appointed Professor of Hygiene at Halle in 1894, but one year later he took a professorship at Marburg. After 1901 Behring gave up lecturing because of the state of his health and devoted himself to the study of tuberculosis and an entrepreneurial approach to serum therapy. In 1914 he founded the Behringwerke for the production of sera and vaccines.

Trained as a military doctor in the Listerian era, Behring was intrigued by the possibility of using "internal disinfectants" against infectious diseases. Experiments with iodoform initiated a life-long preoccupation with antitoxic substances and an appreciation for the fact that chemical disinfectants were often more damaging to the tissues of the host than to the invading bacteria. Some preliminary experiments indicated that while iodoform did not kill microbes, it seemed to neutralize bacterial toxins. Eventually, Behring focused his attention on the fact that guinea pigs which survived the effects of both the infection and the antitoxin were resistant to reinfection. By 1890, researchers at the Pasteur Institute in Paris had demonstrated that bacteria-free filtrates of diphtheria cultures contained a toxin that produced the symptoms of diphtheria when injected into experimental animals. Koch's associate Shibasaburo Kitasato (1852–1931) isolated the tetanus bacillus and proved that it also produced a specific toxin. Working together on the toxins of diphtheria and tetanus bacilli, Behring and Kitasato developed a new form of therapy. When animals were given a series of increasing doses of sterilized cultures of diphtheria or tetanus bacilli, they produced "antitoxins," substances in their blood which neutralized the bacterial toxins. Antitoxins produced by experimental animals could be used to immunize other animals, and could even cure infected animals.

Encouraged by these early results, Behring predicted that his toxin-antitoxin mixtures would lead to the eradication of diphtheria. A first step in the transformation of serum therapy from a laboratory curiosity into a therapeutic tool was accomplished by turning sheep and horses into antitoxin factories. Prof. August Laubenheimer, who had arranged for the German chemical company Hoechst to produce Koch's tuberculin, encouraged Behring to enter into a similar commercial relationship. However, Behring's preparations were too variable, unreliable, and weak for commercial distribution. Fearing that French scientists would overtake them, Koch urged Behring to ask Paul Ehrlich for help. Having systematically worked out methods of immunization with the plant toxins ricin and abrin, Ehrlich knew how to increase the production of antitoxins and measure the activity of antisera with precision. Ehrlich's quantitative methods for producing very active, standardized sera made serum therapy practical. According to an agreement with Hoechst, Behring and Ehrlich were to share in the profits from diphtheria antitoxin, but Behring persuaded Ehrlich to give up his share of the profits by promising to help him get his own research institute. For reasons that remain obscure, Behring did not carry out his part of the deal. He did, however, keep his enlarged share of the profits and became a very wealthy man. Relations between Ehrlich and Behring rapidly deteriorated as Behring became richer and more arrogant. Perhaps Ehrlich could take some comfort in the fact that after their collaboration ended all of Behring's scientific projects were failures.

Diphtheria might have been a minor disease when compared to tuberculosis, but while tuberculin was causing bitter disappointment, serum therapy was being hailed as a major contribution to medicine. In 1901, Behring was awarded the first Nobel Prize in Physiology or Medicine for his pioneering work in serum therapy and the establishment of a science that would surely provide the physician with victorious weapons against death and disease. Behring's Nobel lecture was addressed to the topic "Serum Therapy in Therapeutics and Medical Science." The Nobel Prize of 1901 acknowledged a century of remarkable progress since Edward Jenner's vaccine had been accepted by the medical community. Louis Pasteur had demonstrated that it was possible to create vaccines in the laboratory, Robert Koch had shown that it was possible to isolate pure cultures of microbes, tuberculin had failed as a remedy but provided a diagnostic tool and a clue to a complex immunological puzzle, and Behring and Kitasato had demonstrated that active and passive immunity could be induced. Serum therapy seemed to be the final blow to all infectious diseases. Yet within 10 years euphoria was replaced by profound frustration and the dawn of a period that has been called the "Dark Ages of Immunology."

Since the discovery of serum therapy, diphtheria has been the most successfully studied of the once common childhood diseases. Diphtheria is an acute infection caused by toxin-producing *Corynebacterium diphtheriae*. Case fatality rates for diphtheria rarely exceeded 10%, but sometimes exceptional epidemics took such a heavy toll that the disease was still greatly feared at the beginning of the twentieth century. In 1883 the bacillus was discovered by Edwin Klebs (1834–1913) and Friedrich Loeffler (1852–1915). Autopsies of victims revealed that the disease caused considerable damage to the internal organs, but the bacteria usually remained localized in the throat. Pasteur's associates Émile Roux (1853–1933) and Alexandre Yersin (1863–1943) proved that the bacteria release toxins that enter the bloodstream and attack various tissues. The disease is acquired by inhaling bacteria released when a patient or carrier coughs and sneezes. Within a week after infection, the victim experiences generalized illness and the characteristic "false membrane" in the throat that can cause death by suffocation.

Because immunity can be brought about by antibodies directed against the toxin itself, researchers could focus on the toxin rather than the bacillus. In 1928, Gaston Léon Ramon (1886–1963) discovered that diphtheria toxin treated with formaldehyde retained serological specificity and immunogenicity, while losing its toxicity. Modified toxins were called "toxoids." Evidence for the proposition that there is nothing new under the sun can be found in nineteenth-century reports about certain "wizards" in central Africa who told visiting Europeans that they could protect people against snake bites with a potion containing snake heads and ant eggs. Similar methods have been employed by native healers in other parts of the world. By exploiting the fact that ants contain formol, such so-called primitive healers had accomplished the chemical detoxification of toxins and venoms. Massive immunization campaigns have almost eradicated the threat of diphtheria in the wealthy industrialized nations. It should be noted that diphtheria remains the only major human infectious disease of bacterial origin to be so successfully managed by preventive immunizations. Unfortunately, a generation unfamiliar with the threat once posed by diphtheria is unable to understand the dangers posed by the breakdown of "herd immunity."

Diphtheria toxin is only one of several bacterial toxins to have found a valuable place in therapeutic medicine and biomedical research. Just as alchemists once began their quest for powerful elixirs with powerful poisons, genetic engineers have turned to bacterial toxins, proteins which are the product of "natural engineering" to find natural products suitable for appropriate modification. Knowledge of pathogens and their products thus provides materials with valuable properties; the diphtheria toxin, for example, was naturally engineered as a protein which could penetrate cell membranes. Linking a polypeptide toxin to an antibody would produce a hybrid immunotoxin; the antibody part of the molecule would be selected to guide the molecule to the surface of the target cells; the toxin part could then enter the cell and perform its killer role. The idea seems simple in theory, but it is difficult to apply in practice. A genetically engineered drug combining the diphtheria toxin with a protein that binds to certain white blood cells may serve as the prototype for a new approach to the treatment of rheumatoid arthritis in the 1990s. (Technically, the drug is known as an interleukin-2 fusion toxin. Rheumatoid arthritis appears to be an autoimmune disease in which certain white blood cells known as activated T cells mistakenly attack the lining of the joints.)

CHEMOTHERAPY, ANTIBIOTICS, AND IMMUNOLOGY

Throughout his career, Paul Ehrlich (1854–1915) struggled to understand the body's immunological defenses and to develop ways of augmenting them by means of an approach to therapeutics that has been called experimental therapy. Like Pasteur, his

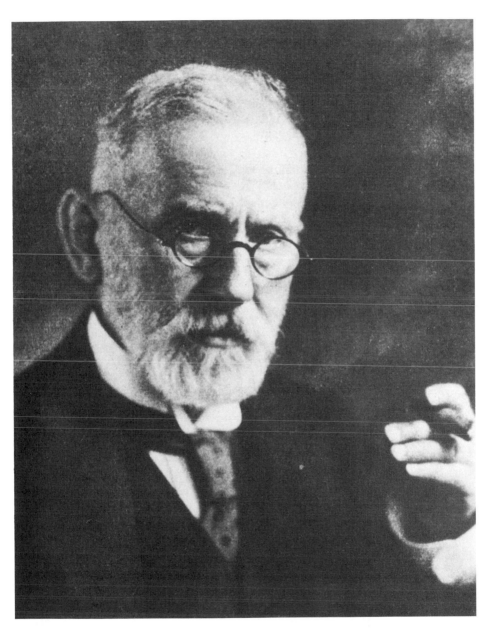

Paul Ehrlich

theoretical interests were closely linked to practical issues; this interplay resulted in major contributions to immunology, toxicology, pharmacology, and therapeutics. Ehrlich's achievements include the development of salvarsan, clarification of the distinction between active and passive immunity, recognition of the latent period in the development of active immunity, and an ingenious conceptual model for antibody production and antigen-antibody recognition. Salvarsan, the first chemotherapeutic agent specifically aimed at the microbe that causes syphilis, provided an effective demonstration for Paul Ehrlich's belief that it was possible to fight infectious diseases through a systematic search for drugs that would kill invading microorganisms without damaging the host; such drugs have been called "magic bullets."

Ehrlich's doctoral thesis, "A Contribution Towards the Theory and Practice of Histological Staining," contains the germ of his life's work: the concept that specific chemicals can interact with particular tissues, cells, subcellular components, or microbial agents. In 1878, after studying at the Universities of Breslau, Strasbourg, and Leipzig, Ehrlich graduated and qualified as a doctor of medicine. A position as assistant to Professor Friedrich Theodor Frerichs at the Berlin Medical Clinic allowed Ehrlich to continue his research. But Frerichs committed suicide in 1885, and Ehrlich's new supervisor expected his senior physicians to devote more time to the clinic than to research. Depressed and somewhat ill, Ehrlich seized the opportunity provided by a positive tuberculin test to leave the hospital and embark on a consumptive's pilgrimage to Egypt. Returning to Berlin with his health restored, Ehrlich was distressed to find himself almost totally excluded from the academic community; he was not nominated for a professorship or offered a position in a scientific institute for 15 years. During this period he conducted studies of the nervous system that involved testing the effect of methylene blue on neuralgia and malaria. Selective staining also allowed Ehrlich to distinguish different types of white blood cells and leukemias. Somewhat later, using bacteriological techniques and transplantable tumors, Ehrlich initiated a new approach to cancer research in which cancer cells were treated like microbes and the host organism served as the nutrient medium. The success of the diphtheria program led to the establishment of a new Institute for Serology and Serum Testing in 1896 with Ehrlich as Director. Facilities at the Institute were rather limited, but Ehrlich told friends he could work in a barn, as long as he had test tubes, a Bunsen burner, and blotting paper. Three years later the Institute was transferred from Berlin to Frankfurt and renamed the Royal Institute for Experimental Therapy. Next door to the Royal Institute, thanks to a large bequest from Franziska Speyer, Ehrlich established the Georg Speyer Institute for Chemotherapy.

In 1908 Ehrlich shared the Nobel Prize in Physiology or Medicine with Élie Metchnikoff (1845–1916) for their work on immunity. Ehrlich's Nobel Prize lecture, entitled "Partial Cell Functions," began with a tribute to the concept of the cell as "the axis around which the whole of the modern science of life revolves." However, he thought that the problem of cell life had reached a stage of investigation in which it was necessary to "break down the concept of the cell as a unit into that of a great number of individual specific partial functions." Such a research program required focusing on the chemical nature of the many processes occurring within the cell. He anticipated that this chemical approach would provide a real understanding of the life processes and "the basis for a truly rational use of medicinal substances." Progress in this direction had come about as a result of attempts to find the key to the mysterious processes underlying Behring's discovery of the antitoxins. "Key" was the operative word, because as the great chemist Emil Fischer (1852–1919) had said of enzymes and their substrates, antibodies and antigens entered into a chemical bond of such strict specificity that they interacted like lock and key.

Ehrlich used the term "immunotherapy" as early as 1906 in a period of great hope that many diseases would be prevented or cured by serum therapy. His shift from immunology to chemotherapy was stimulated in part by recognition of the limitations of serum therapy, especially in the case of cancer. Ehrlich came to believe that further progress would have to come from synthetic drugs rather than antibodies. In the mid-nineteenth century many researchers had questioned the value of all remedies, but Ehrlich's era was a time in which experimental pharmacology flourished along with experimental medicine. In studying the marvelous specificity of the antibodies generated in response to the challenge of poisons, toxins, and other foreign invaders, Ehrlich became convinced that it should be possible to design chemotherapeutic substances by exploiting the specific interactions between synthetic chemicals and biological materials. Because the body did not produce effective antibodies for every challenge, Ehrlich considered it the task of medical science to provide chemical agents that would substitute for or augment the natural defenses. Antibodies were nature's own "magic bullets"; chemotherapy was an attempt to imitate nature by creating drugs lethal to pathogenic microbes, but harmless to the patient.

Using the "disinfection" produced by quinine for malaria as a model, Ehrlich planned an extensive series of tests of potential drugs and their derivatives. Despite the ambitious scope of his research program, he encouraged his associates to take time for reflection. Ehrlich believed that the keys to success in research were "Geld, Geduld, and Gluck" (money, patience, and luck), and that spending too much time in the laboratory meant wasteful use of supplies and experimental animals. The first targets for the new chemotherapy were the trypanosomes, the causative agents of African sleeping sickness, Gambia fever, and nagana. Following his "chemical intuition," along a path that had begun with his early studies of dye substances, Ehrlich began an investigation of a drug called atoxyl and related arsenic compounds. Atoxyl was quite effective in the test tube, but was not a suitable therapeutic agent because it caused neurological damage and blindness. The distinction between killing microbes in the test tube and killing them in a living being without causing damage to the patient is often forgotten, especially today in the midst of the AIDS crisis. Ehrlich's experiments proved that the accepted chemical formula for atoxyl was incorrect and that it was possible to create myriads of derivatives, many of which proved to be safer and more effective than atoxyl.

Because spirochetes were thought to be similar to trypanosomes, Ehrlich's group also conducted tests on spirochetal diseases. Fritz Schaudinn (1871–1906) and Erich Hoffmann (1868–1959) had discovered the causative agent for syphilis in 1905. Within a year, scientists succeeded in establishing syphilitic infections in rabbits. An expert in the use of this model system, Sahachiro Hata (1872–1938), conducted systematic tests of Ehrlich's arsenical compounds on the microbes that cause syphilis, chicken spirillosis, and relapsing fever. Some of the atoxyl derivatives were quite toxic, but birds infected with chicken spirillosis were cured by one injection of Preparation 606. This chemical also cured relapsing fever in rats and syphilis in rabbits. After two physicians offered to be guinea pigs, Ehrlich's collaborators began intramuscular injections of 606 on some of their most hopeless patients, mental patients with progressive paralysis, an invariably fatal condition thought to be of syphilitic origin. Expecting at most a slight increase in survival, they were surprised at the improvements caused by a single injection of the drug. The possibility that toxic effects might be delayed remained unresolved; moreover, the remissions, relapses, and complications that were part of the natural history of syphilis made evaluating remedies extremely difficult.

By September 1910 about 10,000 syphilitics had been treated with Preparation 606, which had been named salvarsan. The testing undergone by salvarsan was quite extensive compared to the usual practice at the time. The drug had been tested in nearly 30,000 cases before Hoechst and Ehrlich announced that salvarsan would be made available to the medical community at large. When congratulated on this remarkable achievement, Ehrlich often replied that salvarsan accounted for one moment of good luck after 7 years of misfortune. With tens of thousands successfully treated for syphilis he could not anticipate the years of misfortune still to come.

Alchemists often began the search for their elixirs of life with poisons, because the fact that a substance was a known poison proved that it was powerful. It is unreasonable to expect any drug to be both effective and completely harmless, but some of Ehrlich's supporters argued that salvarsan was totally nontoxic, while his critics accused the drug of causing a wide range of adverse reactions. One of the first attacks on salvarsan was made by a dermatologist named Richard Dreuw. Although most doctors were complaining that Ehrlich had been too cautious, Dreuw accused Ehrlich of releasing salvarsan without sufficient testing. When medical journals rejected his papers, Dreuw became obsessed with the idea that a "salvarsan syndicate" was controlling the Germany medical community and suppressing all criticism. Joined by some members of the Reichstag and anti-Semitic newspapers, Dreuw attacked Ehrlich personally and demanded that the Imperial Health Office establish a national ban on salvarsan. The anti-salvarsan crusaders claimed that salvarsan caused deafness, blindness, nerve damage, and hundreds of fatalities, but ignored the fact that over one million people had been successfully treated. Compared to the deaths caused by syphilis, and the suffering of its victims, salvarsan was relatively benign, although prolonged treatment involved real dangers of side effects in some patients. Another problem was that patients who had been cured often returned to the behavior that allowed them to contract syphilis in the first place; they blamed the "relapse" not on themselves, but on salvarsan.

The most bizarre member of the anti-salvarsan crusade was Karl Wassmann, a writer who habitually dressed as a monk. Hearing prostitutes complain that salvarsan was being forced on them at the Frankfurt Hospital, Wassmann concluded that Prof. Herxheimer, director of the Dermatology Department, was an agent of the salvarsan syndicate. From 1913 on, Wassmann made the battle between prostitutes and the medical authorities a major theme of his magazine, *The Freethinker*. According to Wassmann, salvarsan caused permanent damage to patients who had been forced to receive injections. Wassmann also charged that the government was suppressing the truth about the salvarsan syndicate. Proclaiming himself champion of the abused underclass, Wassmann courted controversy to call attention to himself and his writings. Ehrlich and Hoechst wanted to ignore him, but Herxheimer brought suit for slander. Salvarsan was so completely vindicated by the evidence brought out at the trial that when the prosecution requested a 6 month prison term for Wassmann, the court doubled the sentence. Nevertheless, Ehrlich was extremely distressed by the trial and the futility of trying to present complex scientific and medical issues in the hostile, adversarial environment of the courtroom. Ehrlich died of a heart attack in August 1915. Salvarsan, with the addition of mercury and bismuth, remained the standard remedy for syphilis until it was replaced by penicillin after World War II.

As in the case of salvarsan, evaluating the safety and efficacy of any drug or medical innovation is always difficult. Indeed, rigorous statistical analyses are likely to demonstrate that various "miracle drugs" are ineffective, or are no more effective than the previously used remedies. Worse yet, some drugs pose dangers not only to the patients for whom they were prescribed, but also for their future children, as demonstrated by the tragic cases of thalidomide and diethylstilbesterol (DES). Thalidomide, which was prescribed as a sleeping aid and tranquilizer for pregnant women, caused profound malformations and deaths in their children. DES, a synthetic estrogen, was widely prescribed from the 1940s to the 1970s, in the mistaken belief that it would prevent miscarriages. Not only did DES increase the risk of complications during pregnancy, it caused a rare form of cancer in DES daughters, reproductive disorders in both DES sons and daughters, and increased the risk of various cancers in the women who had taken the drug.

Attempts to create an arsenal of magic bullets were thwarted until the 1930s when Gerhard Domagk (1895–1964) found that a sulfur-containing red dye called prontosil protected mice from streptococcal infections. This led to the synthesis of a series of related drugs called the sulfonamides or "sulfa drugs" which were highly effective against certain bacteria. Domagk was the director of research in experimental pathology and bacteriology at the German chemical firm I. G. Farben. Like Ehrlich,

Domagk turned to the study of dyes as a means of understanding the vital functions of pathogenic microorganisms. Preliminary studies of bacterial staining led to a systematic survey of the aniline dyes in hopes of finding chemicals that would kill bacteria. In a typical experiment, the quantity of a particular strain of bacteria needed to kill inoculated mice (the lethal dose) was determined. Then a number of mice were infected with 10 times the lethal dose and half of the animals were given a test substance, such as the aniline dye prontosil. By 1932 Domagk had shown that prontosil protected mice against staphylococci and streptococci. As early as 1933 the drug had been in secret use in humans with life-threatening staphylococcal and streptococcal infections. However, Domagk's report, "A Contribution to the Chemotherapy of Bacterial Infections," was not published until 1935. Domagk may have delayed publication because of Farben's interest in patent protection, but the delay might also have been caused by some difficulty in reproducing the initial results. Domagk was awarded the 1939 Nobel Prize in Physiology or Medicine "for the discovery of the antibacterial effects of prontosil," but Nazi officials would not allow him to accept it. German leadership in the development of chemotheraputic agents was essentially lost during the period from 1933 to 1945 because of National Socialistic politics, which isolated Germany from the international research community, and forced many Jewish scientists to seek refuge in England and America. Domagk finally received the Nobel medal in 1947 and delivered a very emotional lecture on progress in chemotherapy.

As soon as Domagk's results were published, prontosil was tested in laboratories in France, America, and Britain. Researchers at the Pasteur Institute proved that prontosil was inactive until it was split in the animal body and that the antibacterial activity was due to the sulfonamide portion of the molecule. Not only was sulfanilimide more active than prontosil, it did not have the disadvantage of being a messy red dye. Prontosil was synthesized and patented by I. G. Farben in 1932, but an account of the synthesis of sulfanilamide had been published in 1908. Thus, Farben did not have patent protection for derivatives of sulfanilamide. With open season on the sulfa drugs, over 5000 derivatives were synthesized in the decade after Domagk's report. In the entire series of sulfonamides, so laboriously synthesized and tested, fewer than 20 clinically useful compounds were identified. Chemists began to realize that the odds of finding a safe and effective drug were rather like those of winning the lottery. Nevertheless, studies of the sulfa drugs flooded the literature. Laboratory tests showed that these drugs were effective against many bacteria in vitro. Clinical trials in hospitals throughout the world provided promising results in the treatment of pneumonia, scarlet fever, gonococcal infections, and so forth. Unfortunately, drug-resistant strains of bacteria appeared almost as rapidly as new drugs. The sulfa drugs were indiscriminately prescribed for infections of unknown origin, casually given for suspected gonorrheal infections, and liberally sprinkled into wounds.

Hailed as "miracle drugs" in the 1930s, by the end of World War II the sulfa drugs were considered largely obsolete. Domagk suggested that part of the problem might have been caused by a decrease in natural resistance due to wartime stress and malnutrition, the spread of resistant strains through natural selection abetted by "the general upheaval during and after the war," and the development of resistant strains during the course of treatment. He warned that the same disappointments would follow the use of penicillin unless physicians learned to appreciate the factors that led to the development and spread of resistant strains.

The next generation of "wonder drugs" for infectious disease were derived from a previously obscure corner of nature's storehouse. By the 1870s, several scientists had called attention to the implications of "antibiosis" (the struggle for existence between different microorganisms), but according to popular mythology, the antibiotic era began in 1928 when Alexander Fleming (1881–1955) discovered penicillin. Of course, the real story is much more complicated. Indeed, in his Nobel lecture Fleming suggested that the discovery of "natural antiseptics" had taken so long because bacteriologists of his generation had taken the fact of microbial antagonisms for granted rather than as a phenomenon to be explored. Fleming discovered the effect of the mold *Penicillium notatum* on bacteria in 1928; within a year he demonstrated that crude preparations of penicillin killed certain bacteria, but were apparently harmless to higher animals. Penicillin was not the first anti-bacterial agent Fleming discovered. In 1922 he found a "powerful antibacterial ferment" in nasal secretions, tears, and saliva. Although this enzyme, which was named "lysozyme," plays a role in the body's natural defense system, it was not a practical "magic bullet." As Fleming often said, he was no chemist; Howard Florey and Ernst Boris Chain who later tested and purified penicillin worked out the chemical nature and mode of action of lysozyme.

Alexander Fleming was only 7 when his elderly father, a Scottish farmer, died. Because his family's resources were limited, he worked as a clerk for several years before a small legacy made it possible for him to enter St. Mary's Medical School in London. More mature than the other students, Fleming excelled at competitive examinations, swimming, and shooting. After graduating in 1908, he became assistant to the eminent and eccentric bacteriologist, Sir Almroth Wright (1861–1947). Fleming's interest in agents that kill bacteria was stimulated by his experience in the Royal Army Medical Corps during World War I. Attending to the infected wounds that were the common aftermath of battle, Fleming was convinced that chemical antiseptics were generally more lethal to human tissues than to the invading bacteria. After the war, Fleming returned to St. Mary's to continue his research on antibacterial substances. According to what we might call the penicillin myth, a spore supposedly drifted through an open window into Fleming's laboratory and settled on a petri dish on which he was growing staphylococci. Contamination of bacteriological materials with molds is a common laboratory accident, generally considered a sign of poor technique. Fleming often said that he would have made no discoveries if his laboratory bench had been neat and tidy. Thus, his contaminated plate was left among stacks of dirty petri dishes when Fleming went off on vacation. On his return, Fleming

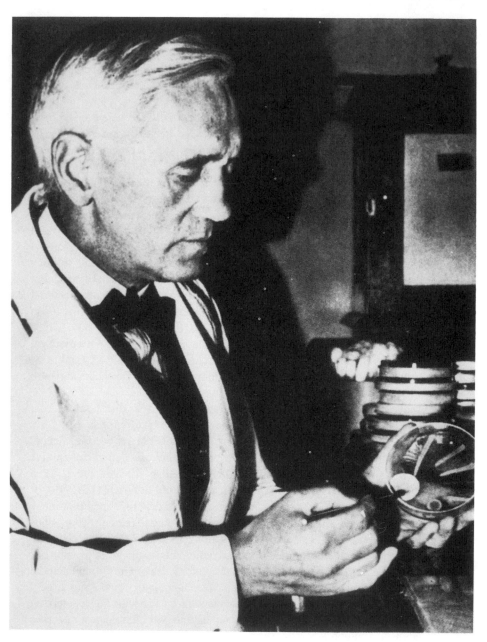

Alexander Fleming in 1944

noticed that staphylococci had been destroyed in the vicinity of a certain mold colony and decided that this case of antibiosis was worth pursuing.

Scientists who tried to recreate this great moment in medical history suggest an alternative scenario: staphylococci were sown on the plate but did not grow because of an unusual cold spell. A spore of the relatively rare mold *Penicillium notatum* that had previously fallen on the plate grew during this period; then the warming trend triggered the growth of the staphylococci, and the penicillin that had been released into the medium around the mold killed the growing bacteria. It was necessary to imagine such a sequence of events in order to explain Fleming's observation, because penicillin cannot dissolve fully grown colonies of staphylococci. Fleming discovered that even in very crude, dilute preparations, penicillin stopped the growth of bacteria and caused them to die, but it was essentially harmless to white blood cells in the test tube. It was also unstable and extremely difficult to purify. Not being an active clinician or a chemist, Fleming and his students rarely managed to have a supply of penicillin and a suitable patient available at the same time. Nor did Fleming perform the animal experiments that would have demonstrated penicillin's effectiveness in fighting bacteria in infected animals. Fleming later recalled that neither bacteriologists nor physicians paid any attention to penicillin until the introduction of sulphonamide changed attitudes towards the possibilities for the chemotherapy of bacterial infections. However, in 1930 one of Fleming's former students had successfully used crude penicillin by means of local applications for the treatment of eye infections.

The story of Fleming's "accidental discovery" is well known, but often forgotten is the fact that penicillin remained a laboratory curiosity until World War II. In 1945, the Nobel Prize for Physiology and Medicine was awarded to Alexander Fleming, Howard Walter Florey (1898–1968), and Ernst Boris Chain (1906–1979) "for the discovery of penicillin and its curative effect in various infectious diseases." In 1938, Florey, Director of the Sir William Dunn School of Pathology at Oxford University, and Chain, who had recently fled from Nazi Germany, began a systematic study of naturally occurring antibacterial agents, including lysozyme and substances produced by various microbes. Within 2 years, partially purified penicillin was tested in mice infected with virulent streptococci. Further experiments proved that penicillin was active against streptococci, staphylococci, and several other pathogens. The Oxford group quickly moved on to human tests; the first patient was a 43-year-old man who had contracted a mixed infection of staphylococci and streptococci. Although the patient was close to death when treatment began, penicillin produced a remarkable improvement. Unfortunately, even though the drug was recovered from the patient's urine, the supply was soon exhausted and the patient died. An account of the first successful clinical trial was published, but further studies became part of the secret war effort.

With Britain's resources strained by the war, it was obvious that British pharmaceutical companies could not develop a new drug. Florey was forced to seek American support. The path from laboratory curiosity to the industrial production of penicillin was full of obstacles, not all of them technical and scientific. Research on penicillin was closely associated with military needs and goals. Within 2 years of Florey's visit to the United States about 16 companies were producing penicillin and major clinical trials were under way. As hundreds of patients were treated with penicillin, researchers became more optimistic about its therapeutic potential. Penicillin proved to be effective against syphilis, gonorrhea, and infections caused by staphylococci, streptococci, and pneumococci. Penicillin was hailed as a panacea that would deliver armies from both venereal diseases and battle injuries. Where supplies were limited, military authorities had to decide whether to use it on those wounded in battle, or those wounded in the brothels. In his delayed Nobel Prize lecture of 1947, Domagk attributed differences in mortality rates for American soldiers in the two world wars to the new chemotherapy. Of course many other aspects of battlefield conditions, weaponry, military medicine, surgery, and hygiene had changed during the years between the wars, but differences between the nations that had access to penicillin and those that did not reflected, at least in part, the role played by antibiotic treatment. Florey was more cautious in evaluating the impact of penicillin on battle casualties than Domagk. When the war ended, although American and British firms were selling millions of units of penicillin, there was still a flourishing black market where penicillin bottles were refilled with worthless chemicals and sold for hundreds of dollars. By 1948 pharmaceutical plants all over the world were producing penicillin. When penicillin became readily available, many physicians adopted treatment regimens reminiscent of the era of "heroic medicine." Penicillin was combined with bismuth, arsenicals, sulfonamides and other drugs, and injected at frequent intervals over a lengthy course of treatments. Further work proved that a single dose of penicillin was effective in treating certain diseases. The promise of a simple cure for venereal infections drove moralists to denounce penicillin as a stimulus to promiscuity.

During the war, some scientists insisted that chemical synthesis of the penicillin molecule would be more productive than further modifications of fermentation methods. By the late 1940s chemists had decided that the synthesis of penicillin was impractical, if not impossible. In commercial terms, this remains essentially true, however, the total synthesis of penicillin was achieved by the organic chemist John C. Sheehan. Sheehan also discovered that in the new antibiotic era patent battles and commercial considerations could overwhelm scientific aspects of drug development. Sheehan synthesized penicillin in 1957, but it took 23 years to clear up patent disputes.

Inspired by lessons learned and profits earned with penicillin, researchers sifted through samples of dirt from every corner of the world in search of new "miracle molds." As Selman A. Waksman (1888–1973) reminded his audience when he delivered his 1952 Nobel Prize lecture: "The Lord hath created medicines out of the earth; and he that is wise will not abhor them" (Ecclesiastes 38:4). During his search for such medicines, Waksman, a biochemist and pioneer in soil microbiology,

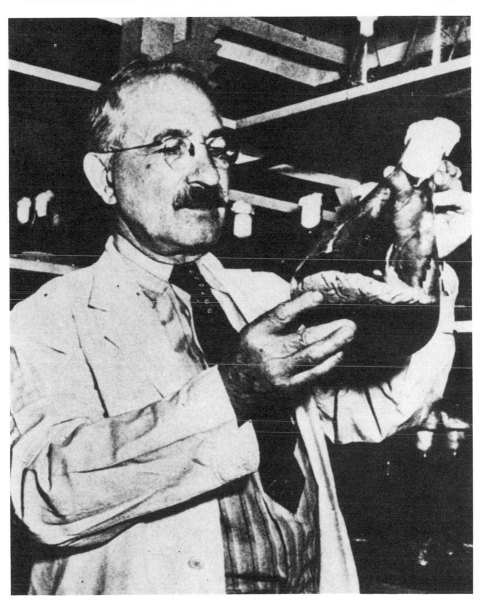

Selman A. Waksman

discovered streptomycin, neomycin, and many other antibiotics, most of which were too weak to serve as therapeutic agents, or too toxic for human use. Waksman coined the term "antibiotics" to refer to a group of compounds produced by microorganisms which can inhibit the growth of other microorganisms, or even destroy them.

According to bacteriological folklore, the normally persistent tubercle bacillus could be destroyed in soil. Therefore, Waksman turned his systematic studies of soil microbes into a search for agents antagonistic to the tubercle bacillus. More than 10,000 different soil microbes were investigated before Waksman, Elizabeth Bugie, and Albert Schatz reported the discovery of streptomycin in 1944. One year later William H. Feldman and H. Corwin Hinshaw of the Mayo Clinic announced that streptomycin was effective against tuberculosis in humans. Evaluating remedies for tuberculosis is very difficult because the disease is unpredictable, develops slowly, and is affected by nonspecific factors, such as improved diet, fresh air, and rest. By 1948 eight companies were producing the drug. Unlike the long barren years between Fleming's discovery of penicillin and the exploitation of its therapeutic potential, streptomycin went from laboratory curiosity to major pharmaceutical product within a few brief years. Indeed, the success of penicillin and streptomycin proved to be a tremendous stimulus to the growth of the pharmaceutical industry and the expansion of research.

During the 1940s and 1950s, the golden age of antibiotics, chloramphenicol, neomycin, aureomycin, erythromycin, nystatin, and many other valuable antibiotics were discovered. Waksman optimistically predicted that future research would lead to the discovery of more active and less toxic agents and to powerful combinations of antibiotics and synthetic compounds. However, the golden age of discovery of novel antibiotics seemed to have ended by about 1960; most of the antibiotics introduced since then have been slight modifications of previously known drugs. Moreover, the warnings issued earlier were found to be true; overuse and misuse of antibiotics revealed adverse side effects and promoted the development of drug-resistant strains of bacteria.

By the 1880s it was recognized that the virulence of infectious diseases varied with many factors, including the means and duration of exposure, the way in which the germ entered the body, and the physiological status of the host. By the end of the century, the fundamental question concerning scientists investigating the immune response was: is the mechanism of innate and acquired immunity humoral or cellular? When Behring was awarded the first Nobel Prize in Medicine for his work on serum therapy, he made a special point of reviewing the history of the dispute between cellular and humoral pathology. He considered antitoxic serum therapy "humoral therapy in the strictest sense of the word." Humoral therapy, Behring predicted, would put medicine on the road to a strictly scientific etiological therapy in contrast to traditional, nonspecific, symptomatic remedies. The scientific debate often degenerated into vicious personal attacks, but Joseph Lister, ever the gentleman, delicately referred to this controversial era as the "romantic chapter in pathology."

As serology was transformed into immunology, researchers saw their new discipline rapidly outgrowing its parent disciplines of microbiology and toxicology. Studies of cellular mechanisms of defense seemed to be a relic of a less sophisticated era of biology closely associated with old-fashioned ideas such as those of Élie Metchnikoff. Metchnikoff, discoverer of phagocytes (the "eating cells" that devour invading microorganisms) and the process of phagocytosis, was more interested in the defenses of the host than the depredations of the pathogen. While most scientists argued that specific chemical entities in the blood defended the body from bacteria and toxins, Metchnikoff followed his own idiosyncratic hypotheses concerning evolution, inflammation, immunity, senility, and phagocytosis. He shared the 1908 Nobel Prize with Paul Ehrlich.

Born in Russia in 1845, Metchnikoff died in Paris in 1916 after a life devoted to researches that were creative and original to the point of eccentricity. Through personal experience he knew how little physicians could do for victims of infectious diseases. His first wife had been so weakened by tuberculosis that she had to be carried to their wedding. When she died 5 years later, Metchnikoff tried to end his own life by swallowing a large dose of opium. With his second wife close to death from typhoid fever, Metchnikoff inoculated himself with relapsing fever so that his death would be of service to science. The discovery of phagocytosis seems to have rescued Metchnikoff from the depression that had driven him to attempt bacteriological suicide. From 1888 on, the Pasteur Institute provided a refuge in which Metchnikoff could pursue his researches and dreams. Primarily a zoologist, influenced as much by Charles Darwin as by Pasteur or Koch, Metchnikoff's theories of inflammation and immunity grew out of his evolutionary vision of comparative pathology.

Studies of inflammation that began with starfish larvae led Metchnikoff to the conclusion that phagocytosis was a biological phenomenon of fundamental importance. While observing the interaction between phagocytes and bacteria, Metchnikoff discovered that phagocytosis was greatly enhanced in animals previously exposed to the same bacteria. He, therefore, concluded that phagocytes were the primary agents of inflammation and immunity. In his Nobel Prize lecture, the impractical dreamer expressed his hope that people would see his work as an example of the "practical value of pure research." Inspired by Metchnikoff's "phagocyte theory," some surgeons attempted to rush white blood cells to the rescue by introducing various substances into the abdominal cavity or under the skin. Another follower of Metchnikoff's theories systematically applied cupping-glasses and rubber ligatures around the site of abscesses and similar infections; the localized edema produced by these procedures was supposed to attract an army of protective phagocytes.

Confident that science would eventually free human beings from the threat of disease, Metchnikoff applied his theory of the phagocyte to the specter of senility. Reflecting upon the principles of comparative pathology, he concluded that senility was primarily brought about by phagocytes. From gray hair and baldness to weakness of bone, muscle, and brain, Metchnikoff saw the telltale footprints of myriads of motile cells "adrift in the tissues of the aged." Noxious influences, such as bacterial toxins and the products of intestinal putrefaction, allegedly triggered the transformation of friendly phagocytes into fearsome foes. Even though senility was caused by phagocytes, life could not be extended by destroying these misguided cells, because the body would then be left defenseless in the struggle against pathogenic microbes. After comparing the life spans of various animals, Metchnikoff concluded that duration of life was determined by the organs of digestion. Specifically, the problem resided in the large intestine where microbial mischief produced "fermentations and putrefactions harmful to the organism." Stopping just short of a call for prophylactic removal of this "useless organ," Metchnikoff suggested that life might be lengthened by disinfecting the digestive tract. Unfortunately, traditional purges and enemas seemed to harm the intestines more than the microbes. Since acids could preserve animal and vegetable food, Metchnikoff concluded that lactic fermentation might prevent putrefaction within the intestines. In practical terms his advice could be summarized by the motto: "Eat yogurt and live longer."

Although Metchnikoff's concept of the treacherous phagocytes won few defenders, other surprising findings about the immune system proved that it was not wholly beneficent. Of course the body's failure to mount an effective defense to some pathogens was well known, but the discovery by Charles Robert Richet (1850–1935) and Paul Jules Portier (1866–1962) that the immune system could react to certain antigens with life-threatening hypersensitivity was unexpected. Richet, who won the Nobel Prize in 1913, coined the term "anaphylaxis" to describe this dangerous response. Based in the Greek word "phylaxis" meaning protection, he formed "anaphylaxis" to refer to a state of hypersensitivity characterized by violent itching, vomiting, bloody diarrhea, fainting, choking, and convulsions. In its most severe form, anaphylactic shock could cause death within a few minutes of exposure to the offending antigen. Further investigations proved that just as it was possible to transfer passive immunity, it was also possible to transfer the anaphylactic condition via serum.

Anaphylaxis seemed to be a peculiar exception to the generally beneficial working of the immune system. Thus, studies of immunology seemed to be the key to providing powerful new approaches to therapeutics. A good example of the optimism characteristic of this early phase of immunology is provided by Almroth Wright (1861–1947), a man who was expected to take the torch from Pasteur and Koch and illuminate new aspects of experimental immunization and medical bacteriology. Wright expected his work in the Inoculation Department at St. Mary's Hospital to bring about a revolution in medicine, but he is generally remembered only as mentor to Alexander Fleming. A man of broad interests, Wright published about 150 books and papers on science, intellectual morality, and ethics. While Professor of Pathology at the Army Medical School at the Royal Victoria Hospital, Wright developed sensitive laboratory methods of diagnosing the "army fevers" that killed more soldiers than bullets. His diagnostic test was based on the "agglutination effect," that is, the clumping of microbes by serum from patients recovering from a disease. These studies led to the development of a vaccine that protected monkeys from Malta fever. In the great tradition of scientists who served as their own guinea pigs, Wright injected himself with his vaccine, but he was not as lucky as his monkeys.

While recovering from Malta fever, Wright began planning a major study of typhoid fever. During the 1890s this dreaded disease claimed tens of thousands of lives in the United States and Great Britain. The case fatality rate varied from 10 to 30%, but recovery was a slow and unpredictable process. Using himself and his students as guinea pigs, Wright found that heat-killed cultures of typhoid bacilli could be used as vaccines. Sir William Boog Leishman's (1865-1926) study of typhoid cases in the British Army between 1905 and 1909 provided the first significant documentation of the value of anti-typhoid inoculations. According to Leishman, the death rate of the unvaccinated men was 10 times that of the inoculated group.

Openly contemptuous of the "military mentality," Wright was happy to resign from the Army Medical Service when he was offered the position of pathologist at St. Mary's Hospital in 1902. Although he received only a small salary, meager facilities, and was responsible for many tedious and time-consuming duties, he attracted eager disciples and hordes of desperate patients. With the fees charged for vaccine therapy, Wright's Inoculation Department became a flourishing and financially rewarding enterprise. According to Wright, ingestion of microbes by white blood cells required the action of certain substances in the liquid part of the blood which he called "opsonins," from the Greek *opsono* meaning "I prepare victuals for." His vaccines were designed to increase the "opsonic index" of the blood. Patients suffering from acne, bronchitis, carbuncles, erysipelas, and even leprosy submitted to Wright's experimental inoculations and blood tests. Doubtless many patients recovered despite the therapy rather than because of it, but Wright had no interest in statistical evaluation of medical trials. Wright exhibited great confidence in his methods and warned reactionary physicians that they would be "degraded to the position of a head nurse" as the art of medicine was transformed into a new form of applied bacteriology. By the end of World War II it was obvious that Wright's opsonically calibrated vaccines were no more successful than Metchnikoff's yogurt. Even Wright's admirers were forced to conclude that the vaccines dispensed by his Inoculation Department were generally "valueless to the point of fraudulence." George Bernard Shaw immortalized Almroth Wright's eccentricities in *The Doctor's Dilemma*, but scientists remembered him as "Sir Almost Wright."

Reviewing what was known about immunology in the 1920s, the eminent physiologist Ernest H. Starling concluded that the only thing perfectly clear about the immune system was that "immunity, whether innate or acquired, is extremely complex in character." Further studies of the system have added more degrees of complexity and controversies at least as vigorous as those that characterized the conflict between humoral and cellular theory. Immunology is a relatively young field, but its twentieth-century evolution has been so dynamic that it has become one of the fundamental disciplines of modern medicine and biology. Discussions of AIDS, cancer, rheumatoid arthritis, metabolic disorders, and other modern plagues are increasingly conducted in the complex vocabulary of immunobiology and molecular biology.

Modern explanations for the induction of antibodies and their remarkable diversity and specificity can be divided into information, or instructive theories and genetic, or selective theories. According to the information theory of antibody synthesis, the antigen dictates the specific structure of the antibody by direct or indirect means. Direct instruction implies that the antigen can enter a randomly chosen antibody-producing cell where it acts as a template for the production of antibodies with a configuration complementary to the antigen. An indirect template theory suggests that the antigen modifies the transcription of immunoglobulin genes in such a manner as to affect the sequence of the amino acids incorporated into antibody in the affected cell and its daughter cells. The genetic theory of antibody production assumes that information for the synthesis of all possible configurations of antibodies is contained in the genome and that specific receptors are normally present on immunocompetent cells, as suggested by Paul Ehrlich. Selective theories presuppose sufficient natural diversity to provide ample opportunities for accidental affinity between antigen and immunoglobulin producing cells; the antigen acts as a kind of trigger for antibody synthesis.

One of the first modern theories of antibody formation, Paul Ehrlich's side-chain theory, was an attempt to provide a chemical explanation for the specificity of the antibody response and the nature of toxins, toxoids, and antibodies. According to this theory, antibody-producing cells were studded with "side-chains," that is, groups capable of specific combination with antigens such as tetanus toxin and diphtheria toxin. When a particular antigen entered the body, it reacted with its special side-chain. In response, the affected cell committed itself to full-scale production of the appropriate side-chain. Excess side-chains became detached and circulated in the body fluids where they neutralized circulating toxins. Like a key in a lock, the fit between antigen and antibody was remarkably specific, although it was presumably due to accident rather than design.

Karl Landsteiner (1868–1943) argued that Ehrlich's theory was untenable primarily because it presupposed an "unlimited number of physiological substances." However, it was Landsteiner's demonstration that the body is capable of making antibodies against "haptens" (small molecules, or synthetic chemical radicals) when they were linked to a large carrier protein that transformed the supposed number of antibodies from "unlimited" in the sense of very large to "unlimited" in the sense of almost infinite. The implications of this line of research were so startling that Landsteiner, who won the Nobel Prize in Medicine in 1930 for his discovery of the human blood groups, considered his development of the concept of haptens and the chemical approach to immunology a much greater scientific contribution.

It had always been difficult to imagine an antibody-producing cell carrying a large enough array of potentially useful side-chains to cope with the entire range of naturally occurring antibodies; it was essentially impossible to believe that evolution had equipped cells with side-chains for the synthetic antigens produced by ingenious chemists. However, no significant alternative to the genetic theory emerged until 1930 when Friedrich Breinl (1888–1936) and Felix Haurowitz (1896–1988) proposed the first instructionist theory, which they called the template theory. According to this theory, the antigen enters the lymphocyte and act as a template for the specific folding of the antibody. Many kinds of objections were offered in response to this hypothesis, but proof that antibodies differ in their amino acid sequence made early versions of this theory untenable. A long line of complex clinical puzzles and methodological challenges culminated in the complete determination of the amino acid sequence of an entire immunoglobulin molecule in 1969 by Gerald M. Edelman (b.1929) and his associates. Rodney R. Porter (1917–1985) and Edelman were awarded the Nobel Prize in 1972 in recognition of their work on the chemical structure of antibodies.

The instructionist theory was challenged in 1955 by Niels Kaj Jerne's (b.1911) "natural selection theory." According to this theory, the antigen seeks out a globulin with the appropriate configuration, combines with it, and carries it to the antibody-producing apparatus. Modified versions of Jerne's theory solved the primary difficulty of Jerne's original concept by substituting randomly diversified cells for randomly diversified antibody molecules, that is, it is the cells that are selected, not the antibodies. The cell, or clonal selection theory, independently proposed by Sir Frank Macfarlane Burnet (1899–1985) and David Talmage (b.1919), revolutionized ideas about the nature of the immune system, the mechanism of the immune response, and the genesis of immunologic tolerance. Burnet's clonal selection theory encompasses both the defense mechanism aspect of the immune system and the prohibition against reaction to "self." During development, "forbidden clones" (cells that could react against "self") are presumably eliminated or destroyed. Macfarlane Burnet and Sir Peter Medawar (1915–1987) were awarded the Nobel Prize in 1960 for their work on immunological tolerance.

When Macfarlane Burnet reviewed the state of immunology in 1967, 10 years after he had proposed the clonal selection theory, the field seemed to have "come of age." Unlike Ehrlich and Landsteiner, who had emphasized the importance of a chemical approach to immunology, Burnet's emphasis was on biological concepts: reproduction, mutation, and selection. By the 1980s, the cell selection theory had gone beyond general acceptance to the status of "immunological dogma." This transformation was stimulated by the explosive development of experimental cellular immunology. Immunology laboratories were awash with T cells and B cells, helper cells, suppressor cells, killer cells, and fused cells producing monoclonal antibodies. Throughout the 1970s and 1980s immunologists were awarded Nobel Prizes for remarkable theoretical and practical contributions to our understanding of organ transplant rejection, cancer, and autoimmune diseases, and new diagnostic and therapeutic tools of great power and precision. A century of progress in immunology since the time of Louis Pasteur had created as many questions as it had answered, but it clearly established the fact that much of the future of medical theory and practice would be outgrowths of immunobiology.

As cardiovascular disease and cancer replaced the infectious diseases as the leading causes of morbidity and mortality in the wealthy, industrialized nations, immunology seemed to offer the answer to the riddle of health and disease just as microbiology had provided answers to the diseases that had posed the greatest threats in the nineteenth century. In the 1950s, Macfarlane Burnet expressed the belief that immunology was ready for a new phase of activity which would reach far beyond the previous phase that had been inspired by Ehrlich at the beginning of the century. Microbiology and chemotherapy had provided a powerful arsenal of magic bullets directed against the infectious diseases; the new combination of immunology and molecular biology promised to create a new generation of genetically engineer drugs that some have called "poisoned arrows" or "smart-bombs." These new weapons would be designed to target not only old microbial enemies, but also the modern epidemic conditions and chronic diseases, such as cardiovascular disease, cancer, autoimmune disorders, allergies, and organ rejection.

In 1984, Niels Kaj Jerne, who had been called immunology's greatest theoretician, shared the Nobel Prize in Medicine with Cesar Milstein (b.1927) and Georges Köhler (b.1946) who were honored for the development of the hybridoma technique for the production of monoclonal antibodies, one of the most significant technological breakthroughs in the biomedical sciences in the 1970s. Jerne had predicted in 1969 that all the interesting problems of immunology would soon be solved and that nothing would remain except the tedious details involved in the management of disease. Such drudgery, he suggested, was not of interest to scientists, but would provide plenty of work for physicians. The technique developed by Milstein and Köhler in 1975 has made it possible to explore many details of the workings of the immune system and has provided a new approach to diagnostics and therapeutics. Contrary to Jerne's prediction, researchers have not run out of questions to ask about the immune system, nor have there been any complaints that the field has become less exciting.

The characteristic of the immune system that is so important in guarding the body against foreign invaders, i.e., the ability to produce an almost unlimited number of different antibodies, represents a problem for the immunologist trying to understand the system. Immunologists who have struggled with the phenomenon of antibody diversity estimate that a mouse can make millions of different antibodies. The technique developed by Milstein and Köhler has transformed the study of antibody diversity and made it essentially possible to order what Milstein calls "antibodies à la carte." Thus, just as Ehrlich was able to make hundreds of derivatives from atoxyl, and hundreds of sulfa drugs were created as derivatives of dyestuffs, hybridomas can be manipulated to create a new generation of magic bullets. Hybridomas are made by fusing mouse myeloma tumor cells with spleen cells derived from a mouse that has been previously immunized with the antigen of interest. The hybrid cells produce large quantities of specific antibodies, called monoclonal antibodies (Mabs). In the not too distant future, by combining the techniques of immunology and molecular biology, scientists will be able to design hybrid molecules that will function as poisoned arrows or smart bombs. And, as Sir Almroth Wright predicted, the healer of the future will be an immunologist.

By 1980, only 5 years after Köhler and Milstein first published an account of their technique, Mabs were well-established tools in many areas of biological research; by 1990, thousands of Mabs had been produced and described in the literature. In 1990 researchers were predicting that "second-generation Mabs" and "human Mabs" would replace the conventional antisera introduced by Behring 100 years ago. Mabs might also serve as novel vaccines and as diagnostic and therapeutic molecules for use against various cancers. In cancer threapy, Mabs might function as smart bombs, targeted against cancer cells to provide site-specific delivery of chemotherapeutic drugs. The concept is simple in theory, but difficult to achieve in practice. In part this is due to the fact that, although advances in molecular biology have led to profound changes in our understanding of cancer, we are still at a stage rather like that of medical microbiology 100 years ago. When we speak of "cancer" it is like speaking of fevers, plagues, pestilences, and infectious diseases. The complex constellation of disorders subsumed by the category of cancer looks quite different to the physician, patient, pathologist, and molecular biologist. There is a great gap between understanding the nature of oncogenes (genes which appear to induce malignant changes in normal cells when they are affected by carcinogenic agents), transforming retroviruses (RNA viruses that can transform normal cells into malignant cells), proto-oncogenes, and so forth, and cure and prevention.

With so many dazzling therapeutic possibilites in view since 1980, some observers have asked why the revolution in therapeutics had not been accomplished by 1990. Many difficulties exist, but prominent among them is the problem that thwarted seventeenth-century blood transfusions and twentieth-century heart transplants. The experimental work on Mabs has generally involved mouse antibodies; the human immune system fails to realize that they are magic bullets and attacks the mouse Mabs as foreign invaders. Although the use of Mabs in humans will doubtlessly involve some risks, the potential benefits of the new biopharmaceuticals are so important that great efforts will be expended to develop appropriate modifications.

Mabs are only one example of the potential therapeutic products that are theoretically possible through the union of molecular biology and immunology. Recombinant DNA technology makes it possible to modify the animo acid sequence of a protein, to fuse proteins to form hybrid proteins, or to synthesize genes for entirely new proteins. Such techniques will make it possible to design proteins with specific desirable functions: drugs, antibodies, hormones, growth factors, antibiotics, pesticides, vaccines, and so forth. For example, in 1991, a field trial of a genetically engineered rabies vaccine was initiated on an isolated island off the shores of Virginia.

Scientists had been ready to test the vaccine several years before, but were unable to get permission to conduct the experiment at a suitable site. It should not be surprising that the reaction to requests for releasing a genetically engineered vaccine consisting of a combination of the rabies virus and the vaccinia virus into the environment was not greeted with enthusiasm. (The vaccine consists of a glycoprotein from the rabies virus inserted into an attentuated strain of the vaccinia virus.) The goal of the trial was to immunize racoons, a major natural reservoir of the rabies virus, by introducing the vaccine into their food supply.

Although the excitement generated by the techniques of immunology and molecular biology are justified by the promise of future contributions to the control of disease, expectations tend to affect the balance between preventive and therapeutic medicine before promises have been tested against reality. The situation is rather like that in 1882 when Koch isolated the tuberculosis bacillus; the discovery led to the expectation of cure and control that were not immediately justified. The analysis of specific examples and general trends in mortality and morbidity have led some historians, epidemiologists, demographers, and critics of medicine to question the role of medical practice, medical education, and medical research throughout history. When epidemiologists look at the rise and fall of diseases in a global setting over long periods of time, they provide a perspective quite different from that available to the patient and the physician confronted by immediate problems. Such a perspective suggests a cautious response to the hyperbole surrounding the latest medical miracles and suggests that high technology applied to the major modern killers, cardiovascular disease and cancer, will not have a great impact on mortality and morbidity in the foreseeable future. On the other hand, preventive measures—even changes as obvious and simple as eradicating cigarette smoking and lowering fat intake—would have a more immediate and certainly more cost-effective impact. Indeed, in looking closely at the three leading causes of death in the United States today—cardiovascular disease, cancer, and trauma—epidemiologists and policy advisors generally suggest that the most important focus of attention is no longer the conquest of disease, but the containment of medical costs.

One issue raised by the widespread misconception that the infectious diseases have been conquered is whether interest in public health and preventive immunizations can be sustained without the threat of epidemics. In wealthy, industrialized nations few individuals recall the heavy toll once taken by tuberculosis, diphtheria, smallpox, or even polio. Moreover, many people believe that antibiotics can cure all infectious diseases and that there is a miracle drug for every conceivable condition. Some observers warn that the declining status of state and city public health departments indicates that in the absence of fear, the essential, but generally routine work of such institutions is neither understood nor appreciated. As Rudolf Virchow warned his bacteria-hunting colleagues, simplistically attributing contagious diseases to bacteria "hinders further research and lulls the conscience to sleep." Understanding the tensions that derive from changing patterns of health, disease, and demography, and the differences in patterns found in the wealthy nations and the developing nations requires familiarity with history, geography, ecology, and economics, as well as knowledge of medicine and science. The global spread of AIDS, which is devastating villages and cities in central Africa where the disease perhaps originated, is one proof of the need for a global and historic perspective. AIDS first appeared as a diagnostic entity in 1981 when the Centers for Disease Control began to report strange clusters of illnesses that were usually associated with a severely compromised condition of the immune system in previously healthy gay men in New York and Los Angeles. In 1984, the causative agent, a retrovirus which was named the human immunodeficiency virus (HIV), was identified. Within 5 years of the first reports, the United States Public Health Service estimated that perhaps as many as 1 1/2 million Americans were infected with HIV. Further studies of HIV suggested that the virus had not simply appeared in the 1980s, but had been incubating as a silent epidemic in areas of the world where the deaths of children and young adults from fevers and diarrheal diseases were not at all uncommon. Perhaps the fears generated by AIDS will fully reverse the tendency in the wealthy nations to assume that the infectious diseases have been conquered and that the archaic contagious diseases of third world countries are inconsequential. AIDS has made it clear that the most powerful chemotherapeutic agents are ultimately powerless against the onslaught of germs if the natural immunological defenses cannot participate in the battle. Of course, in much of the world old specters, such as cholera, typhoid fever, leprosy, tuberculosis, malaria, measles, and, above all, poverty and malnutrition, have not given up their role as "million-murdering death." Presumably, other still unrecognized diseases remain submerged among the common killers.

Both the idea of progress and the role of medicine become problematical when morbidity and mortality are analyzed in terms of a transition from the infectious diseases to diseases of affluence and diseases of medical progress, and when patients find their rising expectations for cure and comfort increasingly frustrated. Such controversial issues have been addressed judiciously in professional journals and the scholarly literature, and passionately in popular books, magazines, and TV talk shows. Another 500 pages would hardly begin to address these problems, but perhaps even a bare survey of the history of medicine will provide some of the facts and concepts that every person needs to know in order to appreciate the complex relationships among disease, health, medicine, and society. A century after Pasteur extended his methods of protective immunization from animals to humans, biomedical science is certainly entering a new era in the development of vaccines and therapeutic agents. But as always, there are no remedies without risk; therefore, the words of the wise doctors of Salerno still provide an appropriate conclusion to any considerations of the history of medicine:

And here I cease to write, but will not cease
To wish you live in health, and die in peace;
And ye our Physicke rules that friendly read,
God grant that Physicke you may never need.

SUGGESTED READINGS

Ackerknecht, E. H. (1973). *Therapeutics from the Primitives to the Twentieth Century*. New York: Hafner Press.

Altschule, Mark D. (1989). *Essays on the Rise and Decline of Bedside Medicine*. Philadelphia: Totts Gap Medical Research Laboratories Inc.

Amler, R. W., and Dull, H. B., eds. (1987). *Closing the Gap: The Burden of Unnecessary Illness*. New York: Oxford University Press.

Apfel, Roberta J., and Fisher, Susan M. (1984). *To Do No Harm: DES and the Dilemmas of Modern Medicine*. New Haven, CT: Yale University Press.

Auenbrugger, Leopold (1936). On Percussion of the Chest. Trans. by John Forbes from the 1761 Latin edition. *Bulletin of the History of Medicine* 4: 373-403.

Bäumler, Ernest (1984). *Paul Ehrlich. Scientist for Life*. Trans. by Grant Edwards. New York: Holmes and Meier.

Bayer, Ronald (1989). *Private Acts, Social Consequences. AIDS and the Politics of Public Health*. New York: Free Press.

Borrebaeck, Carl A. K., and Larrick, James W., eds. (11990). *Therapeutic Monoclonal Antibodies*. New York: Stockton Press.

Burnet, F. M. (1959). *The Clonal Selection Theory of Acquired Immunity*. Nashville, TN: Vanderbilt University Press.

Burnet, Sir Frank Macfarlane (1969). *Cellular Immunology*. Cambridge, England: Melbourne University Press.

CDC (1982). Historical Perspective. Centennial: Koch's Discovery of the Tubercle Bacillus. *MMWR* 31(10): 121-123.

CDC (1985). A Centennial Celebration: Pasteur and the Modern Era of Immunization. *MMWR* 34(26): 189-390.

Chain, E. B. (1954). The development of bacterial chemotherapy. *Antibiotics and Chemotherapy* 4:215-241.

Clark, Ronald W. (1985). *The Life of Ernst Chain. Penicillin and Beyond*. New York: St. Martin's Press.

Cold Spring Harbor Symposia on Quantitative Biology (1977). Vol. 41: *Origins of Lymphocyte Diversity*. Introduction by N. K. Jerne and Summary by G. M. Edelman. New York: Cold Spring Harbor Laboratory.

Colebrook, Leonard (1954). *Almroth Wright: Provocative Doctor and Thinker*. London: William Heinemann Medical Books, Ltd.

Crellin, John K. (1981). Internal Antisepsis or the Dawn of Chemotherapy? *JHMAS* 36:9-18.

Davies, Audry B. (1981). *Medicine and Its Technology: An Introduction to the History of Medical Instrumentation*. Westport, CT: Greenwood Press.

Dowling, Harry F. (1977). *Fighting Infection: Conquests of the Twentieth Century*. Cambridge, MA: Harvard University Press.

Duke, Martin (1991). *The Development of Medical Techniques and Treatments. From Leeches to Heart Surgery*. Madison, CT: International Universities Press., Inc.

Dutton, Diana B. (1988). *Worse than the Disease. Pitfalls of Medical Progress*. New York: Cambridge University Press.

Ehrlich, Paul (1960). *The Collected Papers of Paul Ehrlich*. F. Himmelweit, ed. New York: Pergamon.

Fleming, Sir Alexander, ed. (1946). *History and Development of Penicillin*. London: Butterworth.

Florey, H.W., Chain, E., Heatley, N. G., Jennings, M. A., Sanders, A. G., Abraham, E. P., and Florey, M.E. (1949). *Antiobiotics. A Survey of Penicillin, Streptomycin, and Other Antimicrobial Substances from Fungi, Actinomycetes, Bacteria and Plants*. Oxford, England: Oxford University Press.

Gelfand, Toby (1980). *Professionalizing Modern Medicine: Paris Surgeons and Medical Science and Institutions in the 18th Century*. Westport, CT: Greenwood Press.

Grabar, Pierre (1984). The historical background of immunology. In Stites, Daniel P., Stobo, J. D., Fundenberg, H. H., and Wells, J. V., eds. *Basic and Clinical Immunology*. 5th ed. Los Altos, CA: Lange Medical Publications.

Grmek, Mirko D. (1990). *History of AIDS. Emergence and Origins of a Modern Pandemic*. Trans. by R.C. Maulitz and J. Duffin. Princeton, NJ: Princeton University Press.

Hare, Ronald (1970). *The Birth of Penicillin*. London: George Allen and Unwin.

Hobby, Gladys L. (1984). *Penicillin: Meeting the Challenge*. New Haven, CT: Yale University Press.

Illich, Ivan (1975). *Medical Nemesis: The Expropriation of Health*. London: Calder and Boyars Ltd.

Inlander, Charles B., Levin, L. S. and Weiner, E. (1988). *Medicine on Trial*. New York: Prentice Hall.

Inouye, Msayori and Sarma, Raghupathy, eds. (1986). *Protein Engineering: Applications in Science, Medicine, and Industry*. Orlando, FL: Academic Press.

Insight Team of the Sunday Times of London (1979). *Suffer the Children: the Story of Thalidomide*. New York: Viking Press.

Kawakita, Yosio, Sakai, Shizu, and Otsuka, Yasuo, eds. (1990). *History of Therapy*. Proceedings of the 10th International Symposium on the Comparative History of Medicine—East and West. Tokyo: Ishiyaku EuroAmerica, Inc.

Kennett, Roger H., McKearn, Thomas J. and Bechtol, Kathleen B. (1980). *Monoclonal Antibodies. Hybridomas: A New Dimension in Biological Analyses*. New York: Plenum Press.

Köhler, G. and Milstein, C. (1975). Continuous Cultures of Fused Cells Secreting Antibody of Predefined Specificity. *Nature* 256: 495-497.

Landsteiner, Karl (1962). *The Specificity of Serological Reactions*. New York: Dover.

Lappé, Marc (1982). *Germs That Won't Die. Medical Consequences of the Misuse of Antibiotics*. New York: Anchor/Doubleday.

Lasagna, Louis (1969). The Pharmaceutical Revolution: Its Impact on Science and Society. *Science* 166:1227-1238.

Macfarlane, Gwyn (1985). *Alexander Fleming. The Man and the Myth*. New York: Oxford University Press.

Maulitz, Russell C., ed. (1988). *Unnatural Causes: The Three Leading Killer Diseases in America*. New Brunswick, NJ: Rutgers University Press.

Mazumdar, Pauline M. H., ed. (1989). *Immunology, 1930-1980: Essays on the History of Immunology*. Toronto: Wall & Thompson.

McKeown, Thomas (1979). *The Role of Medicine. Dream, Mirage, or Nemesis?* Princeton, NJ: Princeton University Press.

McLachlan, Gordon, and McKeown, Thomas, eds. (1971). *Medical History and Medical Care. A Symposium of Perspectives.* Arranged by the Nuffield Provincial Hospitals Trust and the Josiah Macy Jr. Foundation. London: Oxford University Press.

Metchnikoff, Élie (1968). *Lectures on the Comparative Pathology of Inflammation.* Trans. by F. A. Starling and E. H. Starling. New York: Dover.

Metchnikoff, Élie, (1908). *The Prolongation of Life. Optimistic Studies.* New York: G. P. Putnam's Sons, 1908.

Mez-Mangold, Lydia (1986). *A History of Drugs.* New York: Barnes & Noble.

Miller, Norman, and Rockwell, Richard C., eds. (1988). *AIDS in Africa. The Social and Policy Impact.* Studies in African Health and Medicine. Volume 10. Lewiston, New York: The Edwin Mellen Press.

Milstein, Cesar (1981). Monoclonal Antibodies from Hybrid Myelomas. The Wellcome Foundation Lecture, 1980. *Proc. Royal Soc. London B* 211:393-412.

Mitchell, Allan (1988). Obsessive Questions and Faint Answers: The French Response to Tuberculosis in the Belle Epoque. *Bulletin of the History of Medicine* 62: 215-235.

Old, R. W., and Primrose, S. B. (1989). *Principles of Gene Manipulation. An Introduction to Genetic Engineering.* Oxford, England: Blackwell Scientific Publications.

Parascandola, John, ed. (1980). *The History of Antibiotics; A Symposium.* Madison, WI: Amer. Inst. Hist. Pharmacy.

Parascandola, John (1990). The Introduction of Antibiotics into Therapeutics. In Kawakita, Yosio, Sakai, Shizu, and Otsuka, Yasuo, eds. (1990). *History of Therapy.* Proceedings of the 10th International Symposium on the Comparative History of Medicine—East and West. Tokyo: Ishiyaku EuroAmerica, Inc.

Raffel, Marshall W., ed. (1984). *Comparative Health Systems. Descriptive Analyses of Fourteen National Health Systems.* University Park, PA: Pennsylvania State University Press.

Reiser, S. J., and Anbar, M., eds. (1984). *The Machine at the Bedside. Strategies for using Technology in Patient Care.* New York: Cambridge University Press.

Rothman, David J. (1990). *Strangers at the Bedside. A History of How Law and Bioethics Transformed Medical Decision Making.* New York: Basic Books.

Sheehan, J. C. (1982). *The Enchanted Ring: The Untold Story of Penicillin.* Cambridge, MA: MIT Press.

Silverstein, Arthur M. (1989). *A History of Immunology.* New York: Academic Press.

Starling, Ernest H. (1926). *Principles of Human Physiology.* 4th ed. Philadelphia: Lea & Febiger.

Swann, John Patrick (1983). The Search for Synthetic Penicillin During World War II. *Brit. J. Hist. Sci.* 16: 154-190.

Talmage, David W. (1986). The Acceptance and Rejection of Immunological Concepts. *Annual Review of Immunology* 4: 1-12.

Wainright, Milton (1987). The History of the Therapeutic Use of Crude Penicillin. *Med. Hist.* 31: 41-50.

Waksman, Selman A. (1954). *My Life with the Microbes.* New York: Simon & Schuster.

Weisz, George (1987). The Posthumous Laennec: Creating a Modern Medical Hero, 1822-1870. *Bulletin of the History of Medicine* 61: 541-562.

Williams, T. I. (1984). *Howard Florey: Penicillin and After*. New York: Oxford University Press.

Woodruff, H. B., ed. (1968). *Scientific Contributions of Selman A. Waksman*. Selected Articles Published in Honor of His 80th Birthday, July 22, 1968. New Brunswick, NJ: Rutgers University Press.

Yelton, Dale E., and Scharff, Matthew D. (1980). Monoclonal Antibodies. *Amer. Sci.* 68:510-516.

Young, James Harvey (1967). *The Medical Messiahs; A Social History of Health Quackery in Twentieth-Century America*. Princeton, NJ: Princeton University Press.

INDEX